Care Management of Skin Diseases

LIFE QUALITY AND ECONOMIC IMPACT

Care Management of Skin Diseases

LIFE QUALITY AND ECONOMIC IMPACT

edited by

Rukmini Rajagopalan
Glaxo Wellcome, Inc.
Research Triangle Park, North Carolina

Elizabeth F. Sherertz
Roger T. Anderson
Bowman Gray School of Medicine of Wake Forest University
Winston-Salem, North Carolina

MARCEL DEKKER, INC. NEW YORK • BASEL • HONG KONG

ISBN: 0-8247-0128-3

The publisher offers discounts on this book when ordered in bulk quantities. For more information, write to Special Sales/Professional Marketing at the address below.

This book is printed on acid-free paper.

Marcel Dekker, Inc.
270 Madison Avenue, New York, New York 10016
http://www.dekker.com

Current printing (last digit):
10 9 8 7 6 5 4 3 2 1

PRINTED IN THE UNITED STATES OF AMERICA

Foreword

This book covers the right subject matter for the health care debate of the '90s and beyond. It addresses what skin diseases do to real people in the real world, and how much impact physicians' efforts on their patients' behalf really have. Since most skin diseases are not fatal, there has been a tendency to trivialize the impact of skin disease as something merely cosmetic or of little consequence. This was not always so. In biblical times, skin disease was equated with uncleanness, and this was a cause for separation from society. In those days, chest pain did not lead to exile, but white spots on your skin would.

In today's health care debate, facts rather than opinions are expected, and these facts can result in the flow of (or paucity of) dollars for research. Malcolm Greaves encountered this problem in the United Kingdom and addressed it by studying the quality of life of patients with chronic urticaria, a disease he has researched for years. He found that the impact of chronic urticaria on the quality of life was equivalent to that of coronary artery disease. These data were of assistance in getting continued funding for further research. I was taught by the late Orville Stone at the University of Texas Medical Branch that acne could cause a young person to marry into a lower level of society due to poor self-esteem. The need for sensitivity to the quality of life of patients with skin disease is not lost on dermatologists, but it may be on other health professionals without quantitative data to support these opinions.

Advances in outcomes research and a need to address quality-of-care issues have fostered a debate over how much care should be delivered to various populations of patients, and who should deliver it. Dermatologists have been slow to assemble data that support the role of one treatment vis-à-vis another; such data will be necessary to convince third parties of the merits of our efforts on patients' behalf. This book brings together this type of information for the first time and will likely usher in a new era in which we measure the benefit of our treatments by the real impact on our patients' lives.

Robert L. Rietschel, M.D.
Chairman
Department of Dermatology
Ochsner Clinic and Alton Ochsner Medical Foundation
New Orleans, Louisiana

Foreword

This is a superb collection of chapters on quality of life and the economics of skin diseases, representing the first time that these important issues have been combined into one text. With the concerns about the rising costs of health care, we can no longer provide the best care to patients unless we understand the quality of life and economic aspects of an illness as well as the clinical aspects. The introductory section of the book includes an overview of skin diseases including epidemiology, health-related quality of life, and the patient's perspective. The quality of life section reviews the methods of developing instruments and contains specific chapters on measuring QOL in psoriasis, contact dermatitis, skin cancer, pigment disorders, viral infections, and many other disorders. The economics section includes several important chapters that cover topics such as measuring the cost-effectiveness of treatments for contact dermatitis, eczema, fungal infections, and carcinoma.

The case management section covers treatment strategies for managed care programs and primary care providers. This section also discusses the legal implications for managed care; another chapter elucidates the providers' perspective for managing dermatological patients. There are useful chapters that discuss the prevention of skin diseases and insight into future directions for these important issues. The appendix includes valuable examples of validated QOL instruments.

Health economics and quality of life are rapidly evolving research areas, and an understanding of the concepts in these chapters is critical for dealing with dermatological diseases in the dynamic health care marketplace. This book will be a valuable resource for students, practitioners, and researchers. This is a significant collection of information, and anyone interested in skin disease, economics, or quality of life should find this book useful and informative.

William F. McGhan, Pharm.D, Ph.D.
Professor and Chairman
Department of Pharmacy Practice and Administration
Philadelphia College of Pharmacy and Science
Philadelphia, Pennsylvania

Preface

The first clinical focus on quality of life developed nearly 40 years ago, with the assessment of functional status in patients being treated for cancer. Since then, the concept of health-related quality of life (HRQL) has expanded in both scope and importance in medical care. HRQL is now used to refer specifically to influences on quality of life by illnesses and their treatment rather than by nonmedical conditions. Basically, HRQL comprises an array of information about an individual's physical, social, and psychological well-being. This matrix forms a broader definition of treatment effectiveness by focusing on the ability of an individual to lead a productive and enjoyable life. HRQL also describes the burden of disease in terms of impairment of the patient's day-to-day life as well as the burden to society.

In many fields of medicine, survival and physiological parameters prognostic of survival were long the primary outcomes of interest. The advent of several effective treatment options has now shifted the focus to life quality. In dermatology, HRQL is a natural primary goal of treatment; the patient's perspective is necessary (and should be sought) because of the complexity of the effects of skin diseases on people's lives, such as psychological stress, embarrassment, feelings of stigma, and physical discomfort. These are not measurable by any known objective clinical indicator. Since for many conditions successful treatment in terms of total alleviation of all or even some of the disease's effects on life quality is difficult, a key advance in developing a matrix for quality of life is that information can be integrated across domains of functioning and used to understand how manipulation through treatment of one aspect of life quality would affect other aspects. Also, this matrix would reveal which aspects of life quality a disease has affected. For instance, a disease that produces intense itching and skin pain may initially disrupt sleep quality and cause mental stress from the irritation. Over time, other domains of functioning become affected as the person grows fatigued and despondent. Failing a cure from a first-line therapy, a disease-management plan might be developed with the goal of episodic control of bothersome symptoms during flare-ups as well as teaching coping skills that encourage resumption of daily activities. Here, the HRQL matrix can be used to systematically identify the areas of concern and to formulate a problem list. If the application of more intensive medical interventions might produce unwanted side effects, this probability must be weighed against the known probability of any gains in life quality from clinical trials. Obviously, the more information there is about the magnitude of improvement in life quality and which patient groups respond most favorably, the more precision there will be in selecting an effective therapy that can deliver the treatment goals valued by the patient.

It has been only in the last decade or so that HRQL has been used as a major outcome in clinical trials of therapeutic interventions to differentiate among medications, dosages, or regimens in terms of costs and benefits to the patient, and the value added to society. In dermatology, owing to the lack of development of HRQL assessment tools, more is currently known anecdotally about life quality with skin diseases than through the use of standard comprehensive instruments. We note that the first formal HRQL assessment tool in dermatology was developed by Finlay and colleagues about a decade ago, and was intended for clinical care. Recently, several new HRQL measures for skin disease have been developed by other investigators expressly for use in clinical trials in dermatology. This book, the first dedicated solely to issues of quality of life in dermatology, is intended to document and discuss the considerable growth evident in HRQL assessments in skin disease, and its importance.

We have organized information ranging from the selection of HRQL instruments to the development of models to test treatment effects and describe the impact of dermatological diseases on life quality. An essential point in HRQL assessment is that appropriate use of an HRQL instrument is conditional upon such issues as the purpose for which the instrument was originally developed, the range of severity of illness or nature of the patient population to be studied, the conceptualization and operationalization of HRQL, and whether transitory or chronic diseases or symptoms are to be measured. Since dermatological diseases present a myriad of conditions and limitations not represented in generic health-status measures, the trend has been to develop instruments specific to skin disease. In some cases, these disease-specific measures can be used in conjunction with generic measures to describe a broader range of HRQL assessment. For example, disease manifestations from psoriatic arthritis or vulvar dermatoses may include considerable impact on physical and social functioning, through physical discomfort, sleep disturbance, and negative self-appraisals. In addition to disruption in gross physical and emotional functioning assessed by a generic HRQL instrument, such as the SF-36, additional items would be needed to capture these skin-disease-specific effects. At the other end of the continuum, conditions such as acne vulgaris may impose relatively little physical disability but have considerable impact on self-perception and social life. In this case, generic measures of life quality would tend to undervalue or miss much of the impact of skin disease.

The next area of interest is the responsiveness of the instrument to clinically significant changes. In dermatology, such measures can include the physician's ratings of improvement, lessening disease severity, and reductions in signs and symptoms associated with skin disease. It should be realized, however, that there is no "gold standard" by which to evaluate HRQL changes. At some point, we need to rely on validated HRQL instruments to tell us what changes in HRQL are important, perhaps by asking patients to weigh the magnitude of improvement obtained from the treatment.

The book also addresses the economic impact of disease and therapy. As we approach the turn of the century, the use of every resource must be examined in terms of the benefit it will produce. For example, when financial resources are to be allocated to treat a disease, the comparative benefits of the available alternative measures should be reviewed before the decision is made. From a societal perspective, on the other hand, the choices will be twofold: 1) the most cost-effective treatment alternative and 2) based on the amount of resource outlay, the alternative issue to solve that would benefit a large proportion of the population. As people's awareness of the economic aspects of diseases and treatments grows, it is hoped that they will make sound decisions not only for their own benefit but also in the context of society.

Chapters 21–25 provide economic evaluations of treatments for major diseases such as psoriasis, eczema, atopic dermatitis, onychomycosis, and cutaneous T-cell lymphoma. All the assessments are not strictly cost-effectiveness analyses. Unlike quality-of-life research, this is almost a maiden attempt at economic evaluation of skin diseases and their treatments. The scope of the subject is far and wide, and we have a long way to go. However, the first step is in the right direction: evaluation of the burden of disease and cost of treatment.

For psoriasis, the cost of each treatment modality is estimated based on the expense of medication, frequency of use and dosage prescribed, maintenance requirements, extent of body surface area involved (for topical therapies), and frequency and type of appropriate laboratory evaluation. Physicians' fees are not included in the calculations because they depend on such factors as the health care system and geographical area. The cost of anticipated treatments over one year are extrapolated and compared. Analyzing the differential costs of available therapies with their benefit–risk ratios allows practitioners to choose cost-effective treatments.

In 1994, the National Center for Health Statistics recorded that, of all visits to physicians, approximately 25% were for contact dermatitis, atopic dermatitis, or eczema. This study evaluates the benefits of the diagnostic method: patch testing to help in early diagnosis of allergic contact dermatitis. The proportion of subjects with a confirmed diagnosis and average time to obtain a confirmed diagnosis are calculated for a patch-tested group and their complement, the non-patch-tested group. The impact on quality of life of the decision to patch-test or otherwise is evaluated using a validated dermatology-specific quality of life instrument. The findings in Chapter 22, even though they are results of an interim analysis of an observational study, are important for providers and decision-makers in understanding the patient's perspective.

With regard to eczema and atopic dermatitis, there have been assessments of national expenditure and resource utilization by economists, providers, and third-party payors. However, there is no detailed literature assessing comparative treatments to provide recommendations as to the most cost-effective course of treatment. The authors of Chapter 23 explain the existing information and the respective sources; further, they provide a plan for performing a methodological evaluation of various available treatments for cost-effectiveness. These plans can be utilized for future research.

Onychomycosis, the subject of Chapter 24, is more than a cosmetic issue for many patients. It is important to realize that pharmacoeconomic studies merely provide general guidelines. The choice of drug is more than likely to be individualized depending on several factors, for example, status of regulatory approval of various drug substances, physician's preference and past experience, etiological agent, concomitant medications, previous treatment for onychomycosis, and patient's preference (e.g., whether to take an antifungal agent in continuous dosing or an intermittent-pulse format). With the help of an experienced physician, patients may be able to make informed decisions regarding their treatment.

Chapter 25, on cutaneous T-cell lymphoma, provides important information regarding the variety of tests and procedures utilized in diagnosing and staging patients with mycosis fungoides. Many effective treatment modalities are described, particularly for early disease. Diagnostic and therapeutic modalities are increasing in number and sophistication every day. Under the circumstances, it is all the more important for the physician to provide the most appropriate and effective treatment while keeping a control on the costs.

Care management is another important topic covered in the book. As we make progress in cost-containment, cost-effectiveness, better resource allocation, and better HRQL from the societal perspective, it seems very logical that health care management should be brought into line with all these objectives in mind. As new managed care systems are emerging, we are bound to find differences among them. Although established systems might provide better service owing to their experience, new organizations may bring in innovative ideas. Ideally, as ideas are shared, all organizations will proceed with better themes and goals.

The managed care industry is still going through its development stages, implementing programs to manage care by disease condition. There is a serious need for information systems that can capture, analyze, and report information related to patients' medical condition. Establishment of national standards of care, identification of specialist providers, information, and education programs, along with nurse intervention services, are all important components in building a condition-management program. Components of such programs are the same for the management of any condition, including skin diseases. Managed care administrators will very quickly realize that the same kind of efforts applied to other disease entities are also essential for skin diseases, to keep up the balance in the health care industry.

In Chapter 27, we have a physician's perspective of how a good working relationship between a primary care physician and a consultant dermatologist may expedite diagnostic work-up and treatment of patients with contact dermatitis. The chapter reviews the scope of the problem, the disease mechanism, primary care management, and appropriate referral patterns and strategies.

Chapter 28 outlines the legal aspects of the relationship between the physician and the managed care system. Options for the physician may be limited, depending on the stage of development of the managed care organization in the city or the locality in question. Suggestions from the legal point of view are provided for the dermatologist to make any situation successful for everybody involved. Working closely with primary care physicians (PCPs) and educating them will minimize overutilization of resources and improve the PCP–dermatologist relationship, and their confidence in each other, which will result in more cost-effective care management.

As people's awareness increases of the economic value of health care, so do their simultaneous and conflicting desires both to preserve their freedom to select providers and to contain costs. Managed care organizations (MCOs) and pharmacy benefit managements (PBMs) need to work collaboratively to analyze a combination of available patient and pharmacy data and garner the benefits of outcomes research so they can make informed decisions to obtain cost-effective interventions to provide best possible health care.

With MCOs increasingly penetrating into the health care arena, specialty independent practice associations (IPAs) may offer unique advantages. Chapter 29 provides information regarding the special advantages of dermatology IPAs as well as legal guidelines for forming a dermatology IPA. The benefits of a dermatology IPA to the dermatologist, the MCO, and the public are illustrated.

An important perspective provided in this volume is that of the patient. Although HRQL instruments focus on the patient's perception of how treatment has impacted his quality of life, we need to know more about what it is like to be a person with skin disease, beyond the aspect of general well-being. Two chapters deal with the issues of being a patient—coming to terms with the diagnoses and prognoses of chronic, recurrent, and bothersome skin diseases, and the social stigma. More emphasis is needed on how to link the treatment of skin disease to the psychological and social needs of the patient at various stages of the process (e.g., from diagnosis to developing patient education and self-management skills). Just as we have begun to focus on the matrix of HRQL as an important outcome of treatment, we likewise need to develop effective combination therapies to address the complex of patient needs. For example, as described in Chapter 6, which offers a patient's perspective on herpes simplex, persons with HSV are prone to become isolated and despondent, and may be considerably handicapped socially. In this regard, patient support groups and psychoeducational interventions may add considerable value to traditional therapies and the recovery process. Persons with scarring or disfigurement from skin disease may likewise benefit from interventions designed to enhance coping strategies and bolster positive self-appraisals. We strongly encourage researchers to conduct the qualitative work in this important area to develop better treatment models for patient care.

Rukmini Rajagopalan
Roger T. Anderson

Contents

COUNSELING FOR LIFE QUALITY

STUDIES ON QUALITY OF LIFE

Contributors

Roger T. Anderson, Ph.D. Department of Public Health Sciences, Bowman Gray School of Medicine of Wake Forest University, Winston-Salem, North Carolina

Steven R. Arikian, M.D.* Faculty of Epidemiology, Columbia University, New York, New York

Betty Bellman M.D. Clinical Instructor, Department of Dermatology and Cutaneous Surgery, University of Miami School of Medicine, Miami, Florida

Debra L. Breneman, M.D. Department of Dermatology, University of Cincinnati, Cincinnati, Ohio

John C. Breneman, M.D. Division of Radiation Oncology, Department of Radiology, University of Cincinnati, Cincinnati, Ohio

Mary-Margaret Chren, M.D.* Dermatology Service and Program in Health Care Research, Cleveland Veterans Affairs Medical Center, and Department of Dermatology, University Hospitals of Cleveland and Case Western Reserve University, Cleveland, Ohio

Peggy Clarke, M.P.H. American Social Health Association, Research Triangle Park, North Carolina

---

***Current affiliation**: Department of Dermatology, University of California at San Francisco, and San Francisco Veterans Affairs Medical Center, San Franciso, California.

Lynda C. Doward Galen Research, Manchester, United Kingdom

John J. Doyle* Columbia University, New York, New York

Thomas R. Einarson, Ph.D. Division of Health Administration, Faculty of Medicine, University of Toronto, and Division of Clinical Pharmacology, Hospital for Sick Children, Toronto, Ontario, Canada

M. Lyn Exum, M.A. Department of Psychiatry and Behavioral Medicine, Bowman Gray School of Medicine of Wake Forest University, Winston-Salem, North Carolina

Steven R. Feldman, M.D., Ph.D. Department of Dermatology, Bowman Gray School of Medicine of Wake Forest University, Winston-Salem, North Carolina

Andrew Y. Finlay, M.B. B.S., F.R.C.P. (London and Glasgow) Department of Dermatology, University of Wales College of Medicine, Cardiff, United Kingdom

Alan B. Fleischer, Jr., M.D. Department of Dermatology, Bowman Gray School of Medicine of Wake Forest University, Winston-Salem, North Carolina

Joseph F. Fowler, Jr., M.D. Division of Dermatology, Department of Medicine, University of Louisville School of Medicine, Louisville, Kentucky

Aditya K. Gupta, M.D., F.R.C.P.(C) Division of Dermatology, Department of Medicine, Sunnybrook Health Science Center, and University of Toronto, Toronto, Ontario, Canada

Madhulika A. Gupta, M.D., F.R.C.P. (C) Department of Psychiatry, University of Western Ontario, London, Ontario, Canada

Christine J. Hashem, M.D. Department of Dermatology, Wake Forest University Medical Center, Winston-Salem, North Carolina

Ron D. Hays, Ph.D. Department of Medicine, University of California, Los Angeles, and RAND Health Program, Los Angeles, California

John T. Jones, M.A., M.S. PharmaResearch Corporation, Wilmington, North Carolina

* *Current affiliation*: The Analytica Group, Scarsdale, New York.

John Kallal, Ph.D. Glaxo Dermatology, a Division of Glaxo Wellcome Inc., Research Triangle Park, North Carolina

Lisa J. Kaplan, J.D. American Academy of Dermatology, Schaumburg, Illinois

John Koo, M.D. Psoriasis Treatment Center and Department of Dermatology, University of California, San Francisco Medical Center, San Francisco, California

Daniel P. Krowchuk, M.D. Departments of Pediatrics and Dermatology, Bowman Gray School of Medicine of Wake Forest University, Winston-Salem, North Carolina

Rebecca J. Lasek, Ph.D. Program in Health Care Research, Cleveland Veterans Affairs Medical Center, and Department of Dermatology, University Hospitals of Cleveland and Case Western Reserve University, Cleveland, Ohio

Gary C. Lee, Ph.D., M.D. Department of Dermatology, University of California, Irvine, Irvine, California

Richard D. Lennox, Ph.D. Outcomes Research Associates, Hillsborough, North Carolina

Barry Leshin, M.D. Department of Dermatology, Wake Forest University Medical Center, Winston-Salem, North Carolina

Stephen P. McKenna, Ph.D. Galen Research, Manchester, United Kingdom

David J. McLean, Ph.D. United Resource Networks, United HealthCare Corporation, Golden Valley, Minnesota

Amy J. McMichael, M.D. Department of Dermatology, Bowman Gray School of Medicine of Wake Forest University, Winston-Salem, North Carolina

Melissa McPheeters, M.P.H. American Social Health Association, Research Triangle Park, North Carolina

Paul I. Oh, M.D., F.R.C.P.(C) Divisions of Clinical Pharmacology and Internal Medicine, Department of Medicine, Sunnybrook Health Science Center, and University of Toronto, Toronto, Ontario, Canada

Patricia O'Hare, M.D. Department of Dermatology, Bowman Gray School of Medicine of Wake Forest University, Winston-Salem, North Carolina

David M. Pariser, M.D., F.A.C.P. Division of Dermatology, Eastern Virgina Medical School, Norfolk, Virginia

Curtis S. Phinney, M.S. Herndon, Virginia

Rukmini Rajagopalan, Dr.P.H., M.B.A., R.N. Biostatistics and Health Economics, Glaxo Dermatology, a Division of Glaxo Wellcome Inc., Research Triangle Park, North Carolina

Stephen R. Rapp, Ph.D. Department of Psychiatry and Behavioral Medicine and Department of Public Health Sciences, Bowman Gray School of Medicine of Wake Forest University, Winston-Salem, North Carolina

David M. Reboussin, Ph.D. Department of Public Health Sciences, Bowman Gray School of Medicine of Wake Forest University, Winston-Salem, North Carolina

Carol M. Retchin, M.P.H. PharmaResearch Corporation, Wilmington, North Carolina

Dennis Revicki, Ph.D. MEDTAP International, Bethesda, Maryland, and School of Public Health, University of North Carolina, Chapel Hill, North Carolina

Syam Sarma, Ph.D. PharmaResearch Corporation, Wilmington, North Carolina

Neil H. Shear, M.D., F.R.C.P.(C) Divisions of Dermatology and Clinical Pharmacology, Departments of Medicine and Pharmacology, Sunnybrook Health Science Center, and University of Toronto, Toronto, Ontario, Canada

Elizabeth F. Sherertz, M.D. Department of Dermatology, Bowman Gray School of Medicine of Wake Forest University, Winston-Salem, North Carolina

John Siebenlist, M.D. Department of Dermatology, University of Texas Health Science Center, San Antonio, Texas

Jeffrey A. Smith, Ph.D. Department of Psychiatry and Behavioral Medicine, Bowman Gray School of Medicine of Wake Forest University, Winston-Salem, North Carolina

Kent H. Summers, R.Ph., Ph.D. Health Outcomes Resarch Consultant, Eli Lilly and Company, Indianapolis, Indiana

Judi A. VanHorn, R.N. Department of Dermatology, University of Cincinnati, Cincinnati, Ohio

Gerald D. Weinstein, M.D. Department of Dermatology, University of California, Irvine, Irvine, California

Martin A. Weinstock, M.D., Ph.D. Dermatology Section, VA Medical Center, and Department of Dermatology, Brown University, Providence, Rhode Island

How to Use this Book

INTRODUCTION

Advances in health care over the last century have conquered life vs. death dilemmas for a broad scope of infectious, neoplastic, and inflammatory diseases. Bacterial pneumonia, early stages of carcinoma, and even life-threatening skin diseases such as pemphigus vulgaris are now manageable or even curable with diagnostic methodologies and therapeutic intervention. As longevity from these devastating diseases has been secured, health care has gradually refocused on primary prevention of disease, and secondary control of disease symptoms and their functional impact. Dermatological diseases have sometimes been discounted in their severity as being "only skin conditions," but as health care management and patient expectation shift toward efficacy, comparisons of specific specialty and treatment approaches and efficiency measurements of health outcome, it is timely to review the groundwork, key concepts, and state of the art with regard to life quality and economic impact of skin diseases. This text is intended to provide the foundation of the current knowledge on quality of life (QOL) and health economics knowledge in the dermatology area.

The information contained herein will be useful to readers with varied backgrounds and goals in utilizing the content.

USE BY CLINICIANS

Dermatologists—Since the skin is visible to others, skin diseases almost by definition have social impact. In explaining a diagnosis, choosing treatment, and assessing improvement, the doctor–patient interaction must take this into account. Even the unique dermatological symptom of itch is often clinically measured by QOL impact, i.e., whether the itching interferes with sleep or with concentration at school or work. Considering QOL can validate the time spent with patients in a single or multiple visits, can aid in patient education and expectation, and can solidify the doctor–patient relationship. QOL and economic evaluation of therapeutic interventions can be utilized in developing algorithms or stepladder approaches as starting points for individual patients. This information can also be used to support direct access of patients to dermatologists.

Nondermatologists—A large percentage of dermatological patients are cared for by physicians and health care providers other than dermatologists. Increasing their understanding of disease impact and cost of care will augment the effectiveness of their management plans as well. The better the understanding of specialists and primary care physicians of the depth of the issues associated with specific diagnoses, the more respect they can gain for each other and the more effective they can function in partnership within the health care system. This may become increasingly important in group health care organizations in which cost-effectiveness and patient wellness are measured concomitantly.

USE BY PATIENTS

Our patients know how their skin disease can impact every aspect of their life, livelihood, and pocketbooks. Some patients are embarrassed or reluctant to verbalize their concerns beyond the obvious symptoms, and may assume that the physician is tacitly aware or simply uninterested in issues peripheral to the medical diagnosis. The studies and topics dealt with in this book should help individual patients validate their own concerns, and lead to recognition that the physicians, pharmaceutical companies, researchers, medical educators, and other health providers are truly involved in the whole disease process.

Patient advocacy groups can use this information, not only to educate those afflicted by a given disease and their caregivers, but also to strengthen their political arguments, for example, to access specialist care and orphan drugs. Patients can also further educate us about the life quality issues not currently being addressed or the specific diseases that are being underestimated so that we can partner in future studies.

USE BY INDUSTRY

The pharmaceutical/medical device industry—As technological and biochemical advances combine with improved understanding of disease pathophysiology, the efficacy of therapeutic intervention has been refined substantially. With the examples of topical corticosteroids or acne medications, many are similar in their benefit by traditional measures such as time and duration of symptom relief, erythema, or lesion count. To aid in differentiation of products for selected patient populations, it is helpful to have documentation of the impact of the treatments on such issues as compliance of dosage vs. lifestyle, duration of treatment, and number and costs of follow-up visits and laboratory monitoring, comparison of generic vs. brand name products, and even aesthetic factors of the disease or treatment that affect the patient's compliance.

Adding this type of HRQL and economic evaluation to pre- and post-marketing clinical studies increases the credibility and practical usefulness to the many "consumers" of the results, including regulatory agencies, restricted pharmaceutical plans, physicians, insurance companies, patients, and manufacturing competitors.

The cosmetic/consumer product industry—By being aware of the QOL and economics of skin diseases and their care, manufacturers of over-the-counter products may gain insight into the advantages of helping to prevent skin diseases, for instance, by reformulating products so that they contain sunscreen, or are less likely to irritate eczema-prone skin, or can supplement prescribed treatment for a given problem. The extensive awareness of these concerns within the cosmetic industry has already set the stage for sophisticated basic dermatology research and product development under industry and academic collaboration. In the long run, this approach will globally improve skin health and knowledge of disease mechanisms.

It is not naive to think that industry "buy-in" to the QOL and health economics trend cannot also have other benefits as well, such as enhancing market share through responsiveness to demands that these trends indicate.

USE BY HEALTH CARE MANAGERS AND MANAGED CARE ORGANIZATIONS

Times are changing for health care in this country. Patients become end-consumers, and the doctor–patient link is affected by issues of availability of services, limited formularies, cost containment, and disease-severity indices. Sometimes these parameters are set anecdotally and without benefit of detailed information, particularly on disease-specific or organ-specified HRQL and health economics. By bringing together the roots of this knowledge for skin diseases, this book can expand the database from which such decisions are made for health maintenance organizations and payors for health care services. The types of measures outlined within can also be invaluable in the ongoing assessment of care effectiveness, which will continue to be important in developing and marketing health plans and services.

USE BY CLINICAL RESEARCHERS

Dermatology research—We should embrace the value of HRQL research for our patients and for our specialty. It provides opportunity to help patients, to expand knowledge that we can share with the next generation of dermatologists and other skin care providers, and to open new horizons for basic and clinical research in dermatology. The topics discussed in this text merely skim the surface of the many "orphan" dermatological diseases that significantly affect relatively few individuals compared to psoriasis or atopic dermatitis but that represent increasingly more of our practices. The approaches to assessment of QOL and pharmacoeconomic and socioeconomic impact can be expanded to investigate other diseases or additional factors that have not been addressed in some of the diseases already studied. For example, occupational skin diseases could be looked at with regard to impact of medical leave, job modification, and early intervention by an occupational dermatologist vs. chronic maintenance management by a company physician.

Further, including this type of research in a protocol facilitates recruitment of subjects, as they sense a commitment to personal well-being as well as a particular measurement of disease activity. This may increase subjects' confidence in choosing to participate in clinical medical research of other types as well.

NONDERMATOLOGY RESEARCH

Those who primarily study other diseases can use this book both for techniques to adapt to their own research and to potentially expand their current investigation to consider dermatological factors. For example, a large study of estrogen replacement could have a side arm assessing skin or hair changes noted by subjects receiving active or placebo therapy. As another example, the manufacturer of an immunosuppressive medication noted to have excessive hair growth as a common side effect could design a study assessing how that side effect affects compliance in the long term.

USE BY OTHERS

Those who deal with individuals with skin disease—teachers, employers, friends, worker's compensation or disability boards, lawyers, pharmacists, social workers—would enrich their understanding of such individuals with insight into the functional life quality and economic impact that the skin disease can have. It is encouraged that this book be shared as a resource.

The introductory section of the book serves to familiarize the reader with the broad scope of dermatological diseases and the genetic, environmental, and epidemiological factors important to consider in approaching prevention, management, and outcome expectations. The progressive development of QOL assessment and the nuances of assessing QOL in patients with skin disease in general are given as background to the later section that deals with QOL studies of specific diagnoses. A philosophical perspective from a dermatologist/psychiatrist provides unique insights into why it is important for all of us who deal with skin disease to go beyond the surface and consider the "ripple effect" that a dermatological diagnosis has on the patient's self-image as well as his or her work and social life. Medical care is clearly enhanced by considering the "total" patient.

Elizabeth F. Sherertz

1

Epidemiology and Scope of Skin Disease

Martin A. Weinstock *VA Medical Center and Brown University, Providence, Rhode Island*

LIFE QUALITY, COST, AND EPIDEMIOLOGY

Epidemiology is the basic science of public health and is basic to the assessment of public health burden of disease. Efforts to systematically assess the health of the public can be traced back more than 300 years to John Graunt, who used tallies of the weekly Bills of Mortality in London (and local church records) for this purpose. While mortality remains the most important parameter in the assessment of the public health burden of disease, it is only one part of the overall picture. Incidence has assumed greater prominence in recent decades as our ability to monitor it has improved, particularly for invasive malignant neoplasms. The limitation of incidence measures, however, is that they do not reveal the degree of impairment, disability, and handicap associated with the incident cases. In an effort to more completely describe the burden of disease, emphasis in recent years has therefore been given to descriptions of morbidity that reflect the impact upon quality of life of the illness being measured. These epidemiological tools are inherently an order of magnitude more difficult to construct than simple counts of the occurrence of the disorder, but their development is nevertheless critical to further refinement of our assessment of morbidity.

As the provision of health care has come to account for a larger portion of our economy, cost has become an increasingly important measure of disease burden. This parameter has various uses other than a straightforward budgetary one. Some policy makers aim to maximize quality of life, provided the associated costs are acceptable; others seek to minimize costs, provided an adverse effect on quality of life (and mortality) has not been demonstrated or is acceptable given the cost savings.

Both quality of life and cost are used as outcome measures for clinical trials and individual therapeutic interventions as well as for measurement of overall public health burden of disease. The latter requires an epidemiological framework.

CONCEPT OF SKIN DISEASE

Definition of the life quality and economic impact of skin disease requires that skin disease itself be precisely defined. Regrettably, diseases do not necessarily fit into the neat categories we set forth.

One natural approach is to define skin disease as those disorders that are treated by dermatologists. This has the advantage that it relates directly to the organization of medical care by physician specialty. The public health burden of skin disease can therefore be used to allocate resources to dermatologists and their activities. Furthermore, the content of dermatological training programs is relatively well defined in the United States. There are major difficulties with this approach, however. Many disorders are treated by both dermatologists and other specialists, depending on the skills and interests of the practitioners and the stage or manifestations of the disease. Second, the scope of a dermatologist's activities in other countries differs substantially from the pattern found in United States. Finally, some disorders, such as thermal burns and other injuries to the skin, primarily affect the skin but are not typically treated by dermatologists.

A second approach is to define skin disease simply as disease that affects the skin. This approach also is fraught with difficulties. First of all, disorders do not restrict themselves to single organ systems. Hence, while some disorders can clearly be categorized as primarily affecting the skin (e.g., basal cell carcinoma), others arise in the skin but primarily affect other organ systems (e.g., metastatic melanoma) or have major effects on both the skin and other organ systems (e.g., lupus erythematosus). Finally, there are diagnostic categories that cannot be clearly categorized as diseases because they are so common that they may be considered "normal" (e.g., nevocellular nevi, photoaging, and interdigital tinea pedis), even though they represent a deviation from some concepts of ideal cutaneous health.

For these reasons, global assessments of the burden of skin disease are plagued with ambiguities. It can be argued that such global assessments

Table 1 Number of Deaths from Selected Skin Diseases, United States, 1990

Melanoma	6420
Chronic skin ulcer	2407
Nonmelanoma skin cancer[a]	2170
Vulvar malignancies	607
Cellulitis and abscess of the skin	630

[a] Approximately 1000 of these deaths are misclassified and are attributable to squamous cell carcinomas arising on mucosal surfaces in the head and neck region (4,21).
Source: Ref. 1.

are generally not worthwhile. However, there is an obvious need for assessments of the impact of individual skin diseases and of more restricted and sharply defined groups of skin disorders.

MORTALITY

Any assessment of the scope of skin disease must start with mortality. Registration of the underlying cause of death is mandatory in the United States, and the certification of this cause serves as the basis for our understanding of cause-specific mortality. Statistical analysis of cause of death by the United States government uses the International Classification of Diseases, 9th revision (ICD-9), which includes a definition of diseases of the skin and subcutaneous tissues (ICD-9 codes 680–709) (1). Large categories of disorders that involve the skin, including neoplasms and many infections, are excluded from the ICD-9 definition of skin disease, despite the fact that they primarily effect the skin and are within the purview of the dermatologist. Mortality from selected categories of skin disease (including malignancies not included in the ICD-9 definition of skin disease) is shown in Table 1.

For some causes, such as melanoma, these mortality statistics appear to be quite accurate (2,3). However, for others (including nonmelanoma skin cancer) they are known to be quite inaccurate due to ambiguities in the identification, description, or coding of the underlying cause of death on death certificates (4). The tabulated data indicate that melanoma is the leading cause of death among skin conditions in the United States under any reasonable definition.

Table 2 Crude Prevalence (per 1000 persons) of Selected Skin Disorders in the United States, 1992

Sebaceous skin cyst	6.1
Acne	26.1
Psoriasis	11.6
Dermatitis	40.8
Dry itching skin	22.2
Chronic ulcer	2.7
Ingrown nails	25.9
Corns and calluses	20.7
Benign neoplasm of skin	4.5
Malignant neoplasm of skin	16.8

Source: Based on 1992 National Health Interview Survey, National Center for Health Statistics, Hyattsville, MD.

PREVALENCE

For many skin diseases, the most important measure of frequency of occurrence is not incidence (the rate at which new cases arise), but prevalence (the proportion of the population with the disorder). In general, the prevalence of skin conditions is not known. However, population-based data for certain common disorders was assessed in the National Health Interview Survey (5). Table 2 provides crude prevalence estimates for 10 selected cutaneous disorders. These estimates must be interpreted with caution because they were based on self-reports in a stratified sample of the United States population and are not adjusted for age, race, or gender.

VISITS TO PHYSICIANS

An alternative and complementary measure of the scope of skin disease are visits to physicians for these disorders. The U.S. government regularly surveys a sample of physicians to determine certain features of medical visits. This effort, the National Ambulatory Medical Care Survey (NAMCS), provides an important alternate source of information regarding the public health burden of disease, although it also has important limitations (6). Among these limitations are its restriction to nonfederal office-based physicians and its sample size, which allows reliable inference only for rather common disorders. This survey, its limitations, and its implications for the assessment of skin disease have been the subject of several published reports (7–11).

Table 3 Visits of Nonfederal Office-Based Physicians for Selected Skin Diseases, United States, 1993

	Number of visits[a]	Proportion to dermatologists (%)
Eczematous dermatitis	7.8	39
Acne vulgaris	6.5	73
Actinic keratosis	4.2	86
Skin cancers	4.2	51
Warts	4.0	56
Benign skin neoplasm	2.5	67
Fungal infections	2.1	31
Psoriasis	1.5	96
All disorders	717.2	4

[a] In millions.
Source: Adapted from Ref. 12.

Skin disease is primarily an outpatient disorder, so the cost of visits to physicians is a substantial portion of the overall cost of these disorders, as well as an indicator of their morbidity. A representative tabulation is displayed in Table 3 (12). It should be noted that the eight listed disorders alone represent a significant proportion (5%) of all visits to physicians in the United States.

MALIGNANT MELANOMA

Any discussion of the scope of skin disease must include a discussion of the descriptive epidemiology of the disorders in question. This includes not only the overall incidence, prevalence, and mortality, but also the distribution of occurrence by person (i.e., age, race, gender), place (i.e., geographic distribution), and time (e.g., secular trends) (13). Special risk groups and risk factors complete this aspect of the scope of disease. From the epidemiologic point of view, among the best studied of cutaneous disorders is malignant melanoma. It can be used to illustrate some of the relevant issues in defining scope.

Mortality from malignant melanoma is significant. An estimated 7300 Americans died from melanoma in 1996 (14). The mortality rate has been increasing for many decades and appears to follow a cohort pattern of increase (15). Among the youngest cohorts, mortality appears to have peaked (16). Nevertheless, melanoma remains among the most rapidly increasing causes of cancer mortality.

Melanoma incidence has been increasing faster than melanoma mortality over the past several decades, although there are now signs that incidence of invasive melanoma has stabilized for younger cohorts. Approximately 38,000 cases of invasive melanoma were diagnosed in the United States in 1996 (14). It is more common among Americans 25–29 years of age than any noncutaneous malignancy (17).

The discrepancies between mortality and incidence are determined by the case-fatality rate, which has been in steady decline since systematic measures were first obtained (17). This decline appears to be primarily due to an increased proportion of thin lesions among invasive melanomas, presumably due to early detection.

Melanoma is primarily a disorder of light-skinned racial groups. In the United States, melanoma is more than 10 times more common among whites than among blacks. In white populations, melanomas occur most commonly at sites that are intermittently exposed to intense sunlight, such as the trunk and extremities. Indeed, intermittent intense sun exposure, particularly during childhood and early adult years, appears to be the major avoidable risk factor. However, melanomas that occur in dark-skinned populations most commonly occur on the sole of the foot, also commonly occur on the palms or nail beds, and have not been linked to any form of sun exposure. At least in part because of this variation in anatomic site, the case-fatality rate also exhibits a pronounced racial gradient, with worse prognosis among dark-skinned populations, although the overall mortality rate among blacks remains about one-sixth the rate among whites. The differences in patterns appear to be primarily a direct function of the concentration of pigment in the skin (17–20).

Geographic variation in melanoma rates is primarily determined by skin color, as described above, and by proximity to the equator, with relatively low incidence among similarly pigmented peoples in more polar climates. The incidence among migrants tends to resemble the incidence of the population living at the location in which the migrant resided during childhood (15,16,18,20).

Future trends in melanoma cannot be reliably predicted. Changes in factors that cause melanoma will not be reflected in melanoma mortality for decades due to the latent period of the disease. Ozone depletion and possibly increased use of indoor tanning devices may tend to increase melanoma morbidity and mortality. However, these may be more than counterbalanced in the future by increased use of sunscreens, clothing, and shade, as well as other efforts to minimize exposure to intense sunlight. Increased awareness of melanoma warning signs and efforts at early detection will more rapidly effect melanoma morbidity and mortality, but these effects are also difficult to predict with certainty. The extent to which mortality can be decreased by these measures is unclear, since there appears to be a subgroup of melanomas that are quite difficult to detect early and a subgroup of the population who have great difficulty engaging in effective early detection. The effect on morbidity is even more complex, since early detection efforts may increase morbidity among these needlessly worried or intervened upon for this purpose. Improved treatment in the future may decrease mortality, but its effect on morbidity is uncertain.

CONCLUSION

Population-based assessment of the scope of skin diseases, including their impact on quality of life and costs, requires an understanding of the relevant epidemiological features. It is difficult to quantify overall skin disease impact, in part because skin disease itself is difficult to define reasonably. Mortality is a key parameter in general, but a relatively small proportion of cutaneous disorders are fatal. Other measures such as incidence, prevalence, and visits to health care providers can be monitored to inform judgments regarding quality of life and costs. However, limited data are available with respect to these parameters for skin disorders. Efforts to systematically gather epidemiological data on skin disorders will serve as a key support for estimates of quality of life and cost impact.

ACKNOWLEDGMENTS

The author receives support from the National Institutes of Health grants AR43051 and CA50087 and from the Department of Veterans Affairs.

REFERENCES

1. National Center for Health Statistics. Vital Statistics of the United States 1990. Volume II—Mortality, Part A. Hyattsville, MD: Public Health Service, 1994.
2. Percy C, Stanek E, Gloeckler L. Accuracy of cancer death certificates and its effect on cancer mortality statistics. Am J Public Health 1981; 71:242–250.
3. Swerdlow AJ. Interpretation of England and Wales cancer mortality data: the effect of enquiries to certifiers for further information. Br J Cancer 1989; 59:787–791.
4. Weinstock MA, Bogaars HA, Ashley M, Litle V, Bilodeau E, Kimmel S. Inaccuracies in certification of nonmelonoma skin cancer deaths. Am J Public Health 1992; 82:278–281.
5. Benson V, Marano MA. Current estimates from the National Health Interview Survey. National Center for Health Statistics. Vital Health Stat 1994; 10:1–13.
6. Schappert SM. National Ambulatory Medical Care Survey: 1992 Summary. Advance Data from Vital and Health Statistics; No. 253. Hyattsville, MD: National Center for Health Statistics.

7. Nelson C. Office Visits to Dermatologists: National Ambulatory Medical Care Survey, United States, 1989–90. Advance data from vital and health statistics; No. 240. Hyattsville, MD: National Center for Health Statistics.
8. Fleischer AB, Feldman SR, Bradham DD. Office-based physician services provided by dermatologists in the United States in 1990. J Invest Dermatol 1994; 102:93–97.
9. Krowchuk DP, Bradham DD, Fleischer AB. Dermatologic services provided to children and adolescents by primary care and other physicians in the United States. Pediatr Dermatol 1994; 11:199–203.
10. Stern RS. Acne therapy: medication use and sources of care in office-based practice. Arch Dermatol 1996; 132:776–780.
11. Stern RS. Managed care and the treatment of skin diseases: dermatologists do it less often. Arch Dermatol 1996; 132:1039–1042.
12. Weinstock MA, Boyle MM. Statistics of interest to the dermatologist. In: Sober AJ, Fitzpatrick TB, eds. Year Book of Dermatology, 1996. St. Louis: Mosby, 1996:7–23.
13. MacMahon B, Pugh TF. Epidemiology: Principles and Measures. Boston: Little, Brown and Company, 1970.
14. Parker SL, Tong T, Bolden S, Wingo PA. Cancer statistics, 1996. CA 1996; 46:5–27.
15. Weinstock MA. Skin cancer I: melanoma and nevi. In: Williams HC, ed. The Challenge of Dermatoepidemiology. Boca Raton, FL: CRC Press, Inc., 1997:187–204.
16. Weinstock MA. Epidemiology of melanoma. In: Nathanson L, ed. Current Research and Clinical Management of Melonoma. Boston: Kluwer Academic Publishers, 1993:29–56.
17. Ries LAG, Miller BA, Hankey BF, Kosary CL, Harras A, Edwards BK, eds. SEER Cancer Statistics Review, 1973–1991 (NIH Pub. No. 94–2789). Bethesda, MD: National Cancer Institute, 1994.
18. Armstrong BK, Kricker A. Skin cancer. In: Weinstock MA, ed. Dermatoepidemiology. Philadelphia: W.B. Saunders Company, 1995:583–594.
19. Weinstock MA. Ultraviolet radiation and skin cancer: epidemiologic data from the United States and Canada. In: Young AR. Björn LO, Moan J, Nultsch W, eds. Environmental UV Photobiology. New York: Plenum Press, 1993:295–344.
20. Elwood JM, Koh HK. Etiology, epidemiology, risk factors, and public health issues of melanoma. Curr Opin Oncol 1994; 6:179–187.
21. Weinstock MA. Nonmelanoma skin cancer mortality in the United States, 1969 through 1988. Arch Dermatol 1993; 129:1286–1290.

2

Evolution of Quality-of-Life Assessment

Lynda C. Doward and Stephen P. McKenna *Galen Research, Manchester, United Kingdom*

OVERVIEW

Recognition of the importance of the "quality" of human life is not new. The question of how life gains its quality has been raised by philosophers throughout history. However, the twentieth century has seen an increased interest in the concept of quality of life (QoL). Questions of definition, methods, and motives have been hotly debated by social scientists, psychologists, moral philosophers, and, more recently, clinical researchers and physicians.

Advances in medical technology and improvements in public health have eradicated, or reduced the significance of, many life-threatening infectious diseases in the developed world. Western health and social care systems are now increasingly concerned with the treatment of chronic, disabling conditions associated with an aging population. In addition, patients' perception of the impact of treatment is being given greater consideration, as it is recognized that patients have ultimate responsibility for major decisions taken in connection with their own health. Where medical interventions and health care programs are designed to make life more comfortable rather than to cure, interest now focuses on QoL outcomes.

While there is no generally accepted definition of QoL, several approaches to its assessment can be identified. These include the health-related quality-of-life approach (focusing on the individual's role in society), the needs-based approach (derived from theories of human motivation), and the individualistic approach (which emphasizes the perception of the individual).

The evolution of these three approaches will be described and an assessment made of their importance and value to outcome assessment.

INTRODUCTION

> We should set the highest value, not on living, but on living well.
>
> Socrates (1)

The question of how life gains its quality has been raised by philosophers throughout history. As early as the fourth century B.C., Socrates declared that there were some things he feared more than death and that it is not life itself but the quality of that life that counts most. For Socrates, facing the death sentence at the Athenian court, it was moral merit that gave "quality" to his life (2). Other eminent philosophers, including Aristotle (3), Bentham (4), More (5), and Royce (6), have debated whether there are "universal goods" that improve the life of all people and who should be the judge of such improvements (2).

The last quarter of the twentieth century has seen a dramatic increase in interest in QoL. It is now difficult to identify a sphere of life or an area of academic study where the term QoL is not used. For many western societies, QoL has become an accepted colloquialism used in everyday language (7). Within the academic arena, questions of definition, methodology, and motives for its measurement have been heatedly debated from the perspectives of a variety of disciplines. Aiken (8) observes that the popularity of QoL in contemporary debates has crossed diverse areas such as medical ethics, environmental ethics, moral issues in law, and social justice. Häyry (9) and Bubolz et al. (10) report on the divergent interests in QoL of social scientists, psychologists, economists, moral philosophers, environmentalists, and political scientists. In particular, Häyry (9) reports that social scientists and psychologists are predominately interested in definitions and methods, while moral philosophers have concentrated on the motives for defining and measuring human QoL and on the ethical questions that arise from such measurement.

Within the health care sector, interest in QoL has increased steadily since the late 1940s and particularly over the past 20 years. During that time, QoL has developed from an imprecise concept into a topic of scientific enquiry (11,12). The first clinical publications incorporating the term

QoL appeared in the 1960s. Wider acceptance was gained when QoL was introduced as a heading on MEDLINE in 1975 and accepted as a concept by Index Medicus in 1977. The number of MEDLINE publications using QoL as a keyword has grown exponentially since then. Between 1965 and 1974 only 64 MEDLINE publications used the term. This increased to 5083 publications between 1981 and 1990, with 8136 published between 1991 and 1996.

The vast interest in QoL belies the fact that the construct is still beset by theoretical disagreement. Definitions of QoL, where they are presented, vary widely. Methods of assessment and the quality of investigation are subject to similar variation. In many cases, the term is applied inappropriately, without theoretical foundation. This has led some authors to conclude that current disagreements on the meaning of QoL are indicative of a lack of direction rather than of a healthy diversity of opinion (7). However, in reality the situation is not as bleak as such opinions suggest. The current chapter reviews the three main approaches to the measurement of QoL; the functional-based health-related quality of life (HRQL) approach, the needs-based approach and the individualistic approach. A fourth, the existentialist approach, will not be considered. Existentialist QoL is largely concerned with questions of ethics and as such, forms part of a wider debate that is outside the remit of this chapter. The evolution of the three main approaches is described and their value to outcome assessment in health care is considered.

WHY MEASURE QUALITY OF LIFE?

> There is no value in survival as such—the quality of the prolonged life is always a factor in any evaluation of medical procedures.
>
> Häyry, 1991 (9)

In developed countries, changes in medical technology and improvements in public health have eradicated, or reduced in significance, many life-threatening diseases. Advances in diagnostic procedures, surgical techniques, therapies, and drugs have revolutionized the treatment of previously fatal conditions (13). With the major exception of AIDS, medical attention has shifted away from life-threatening infections towards the alleviation of chronic conditions such as neurological, rheumatological, pulmonary, dermatological, oncological, and cardiovascular diseases (14).

Read (14) believes that changes to the basic ground rules by which physicians are guided in their actions have been a further stimulus to the importance of QoL. He asserts that there has been a shift from "First Do No Harm" (in the preantibiotic era), through "Be Complete" in the 1960s (when the primary emphasis was placed on reliance on technical procedure), to "Give Value for Money" in the 1980s. The last approach is the result of pressure from health care funders, who now demand that alternative treatments (particularly competing pharmaceutical products differing little in clinical impact) should show some clearly demonstrable benefit (15). In the clinical field, three main roles for QoL have been identified: to facilitate clinical decision making, to assist patients in autonomous decision making, and to aid in the allocation of scarce medical resources (9,14). Parmenter (12) identifies four interest groups for which QoL evaluations are relevant: patients, medical practitioners, the pharmaceutical industry, and politicians. For the patient and the clinician, assessment of QoL should improve the effectiveness of care by allowing the benefits of alternative therapies to be evaluated. For the pharmaceutical industry, QoL assessments are used to demonstrate the greater effectiveness of a certain drug compound than a competitor's product and (increasingly) to accelerate the approval process for new drugs. Finally, politicians can use QoL data to determine the allocation of health resources.

From a medico-ethical viewpoint, the value of QoL assessment is seen in the justification or nonjustification of, for example, treatment, abortion, and euthanasia. Ethical issues relating to QoL assessment have largely centered on "who should be the judge" of what is "good" or "poor" QoL (2,8, 16–18).

WHY ASK THE PATIENT?

> One must always respect the autonomy of the patient. The patient's views and priorities must always be paramount.
>
> Parmenter, 1994 (12)

It is to be hoped that progress has been made since Morgan (19) asserted that "the subject's own opinion of his condition is not to be relied upon." Morgan, in his attempt to measure happiness, observed that some persons "enjoy being miserable," whereas others "maintain that they are always happy, when observation belies their statements" (19).

Prior to the seventeenth century, medicine relied on the triad of observation, introspection (on the part of the clinician), and dialogue (between clinician and patient) (12). However, the advent of natural science in the seventeenth century lessened the credibility of the "nonobjective" components of the clinical interview (12). According to Engel (20), the subjective components (introspection and dialogue) were relegated to a nonscientific status. In striving for the rigorous application of the Scientific Method, medical research began to view the subjective assessment of outcome by the patient with scepticism (12).

The advent of the World Health Organisation's 1947 definition of health as "a state of complete physical, mental and social well-being and not merely the absence of disease or infirmity" (21,22) marked a turning point in the evaluation of treatment outcomes. The tide had turned and, once again, it became acceptable to consider outcome parameters beyond the traditional clinical indicators.

It is now generally recognized that the utilization of health services is more closely linked to how people feel than to their clinical condition (15, 23). Guyatt et al. (24) points out that two patients sharing identical clinical criteria can have dramatically different responses to their condition. Whether or not individuals seek medical attention is less dependent on the "objective" presence of symptoms than on their response to these or to their general perception that something is amiss (25). Such differences affect utilization of health services to the degree that one individual may seek medical advice while another may not. Compliance with treatment regimes is also largely dependent on the patient's perception of their effectiveness and on how the treatment affects his or her well-being (15,26).

It is no longer considered acceptable for medicine to operate a "beneficence model" of health care, whereby it is assumed that health professionals are best placed to determine what promotes or protects the best interests of the patient (12). Research suggests that there are wide discrepancies between clinicians and patients in their views of the best form of treatment (27,28) and the efficacy of the treatment they receive (27,29,30). It is not uncommon for patients to feel marked benefits from a treatment that the physician considers to have had little impact. Conversely, the physician may be satisfied that the patient has improved, but the patient may feel little benefit or may even feel worse (15). This raises the distinction between subjective outcomes (such as QoL benefits) and objective outcomes (e.g., changes in blood pressure or improvements in functional status as rated by a clinician). Improvements in functioning following treatment might result in a patient being able to return to work (a beneficial outcome from the clinician's viewpoint). However, the significance of rates of return to work has been questioned, especially for patients in late middle age. Return to work may or may not be seen as a good outcome by such patients (31).

Challenging the paternalistic patient-doctor relationship has led to a call for greater autonomy by patients. Several authors, acknowledging that patients can provide the best information about what is in their interests, view QoL assessment as a means of opening up a dialogue between physician and patient. In this way, the patient is given an opportunity to take a more proactive role in health care decision making (9,32).

It is now generally accepted that where interventions are designed to make life more comfortable rather than to cure, the only valid source of information is the patient (33). Fitzpatrick et al. (34) assert that QoL represents a general striving towards a more holistic view of the individual. Therefore, the emergence of QoL as an indication of outcome reflects the growing awareness by health care practitioners of the importance of evaluating the benefits of therapeutic interventions from the patient's viewpoint (17).

THE IMPORTANCE OF THEORY

Any instrument designed to assess QoL must be based on a stated model or theory of the construct. Unfortunately, this requirement is often neglected. There is a tendency for investigators to refer to any patient-completed outcome measure as a QoL instrument, even where it was designed for a different purpose. In their critical appraisal of the quality of QoL measures, Gill and Feinstein (17) found that the investigators had defined QoL conceptually in only 15% of the 75 articles reviewed. This raises two related problems. First, unless investigators explicitly identify what they mean by QoL, it is not possible to determine whether their definition is reasonable. Second, and perhaps more fundamental, without a testable underlying model, it is not possible to establish that an instrument has construct validity (35).

Unfortunately, even where a conceptual model of QoL is presented, the adequacy of the model can often be questioned. The common misuse and abuse of the term QoL has led some authors to suggest that it be dropped altogether (36). However, such an opinion undermines the progress that has been made in developing QoL models and in refining measurement techniques.

APPROACHES TO QUALITY-OF-LIFE MEASUREMENT

Philosophical and political interest in QoL has continued throughout history. The ancient Greek philosophers were concerned with the conditions or goods necessary for achieving fulfilment and, hence, the "upper limits" of life quality (what has been termed the "good life"). In the early nineteenth century concern with equality and freedom led the Liberals to focus on the lower limits of life quality necessary to live a minimally human existence (8).

Approaches to QoL assessment in the twentieth century have been influenced by these philosophical and political debates. The general lack of consensus on what constitutes QoL results, primarily, from the existence of different schools of thought (7). Parmenter (12) argues that it is evident from the literature that a tension exists between those who advocate the biomedical aspects of disease as a focus (the objective group) and those who take a broader approach, seeking to open up the dialogue between the clinician and the patient (the subjective group).

It is possible to identify three main approaches to the measurement of QoL: (1) the health-related quality-of-life approach, (2) the needs-based approach, and (3) the individualistic approach. In order to understand the different types of assessments, it is important to be aware of the theories underpinning them.

The Health-Related Quality-of-Life Approach

The advent of the functionalist approach to QoL grew out of the work of Durkheim in the late nineteenth century. Durkheim (37) analyzed social and cultural phenomena in terms of the functions they perform in a sociocultural system. The basis of this approach was the model of organic systems found in the biological sciences.

Early attempts to develop QoL measurement instruments were strongly rooted in the functionalist tradition. For example, in 1949, Karnofsky and Burchenal (38) outlined criteria for the evaluation of new therapeutic agents that included performance states, mood, and well-being, together with traditional indicators such as survival. Function-based measures appeared particularly attractive to a medical world that was still reluctant to embrace subjective elements in outcome assessment. Function-based tools appeared to offer an ideal solution by allowing a subjective judgment (where instruments were patient-completed) of questions that were still primarily objective (such as the presence or absence of symptoms or the degree of limitation to "normal" functional ability).

The concept was developed further by Parsons (39), who defined health as "the state of optimum capacity for the effective performance of valued tasks." In this system, illness only becomes a problem when it affects role performance and health is the most valued state of existence (40,41). Thus, functionalist definitions of health focus on the main social roles considered "normal" for people in western societies.

The recent adoption of the term health-related quality of life (HRQL) has grown out of the functionalist approach to QoL. Patrick et al. (42) define HRQL as the capacity to perform the daily activities appropriate to a person's age and major social role. The role could be paid employment, school, housework, or simply self-care (42). Deviation from normality results in a reduced QoL. Patrick and Erikson (43) also defined HRQL as "the value assigned to duration of life as modified by the impairments, functional states, perceptions and social opportunities that are influenced by disease, injury, treatment or policy." Kaplan et al. (44) emphasizes that the focus of HRQL is on the qualitative dimension of functioning and can be defined as the impact of treatment of disease on disability and daily functioning.

HRQL requires two basic assumptions: that health is the most important influence on QoL and that there are no significant interrelations between health and other determinants of QoL. There is general agreement that the concept is multidimensional. However, there is less agreement about the specific dimensions that make up HRQL. Van Dam (45) suggests that HRQL may refer to a variety of issues such as physical complaints, psychological complaints, sexual functioning, activities of daily living, and feelings of well-being. Wenger (46) proposed a three-dimensional approach (functional capacity, perceptions, and symptoms) that can be broken down into nine further subdimensions. Patrick and Bergner (47) assert that HRQL covers five broad categories: duration of life, impairments, functional status, health perceptions, and opportunities. They argue that these are "health-related" insofar as they are influenced by disease, injury, treatment, or health policy. Torrance (48) argues that it is inappropriate to include

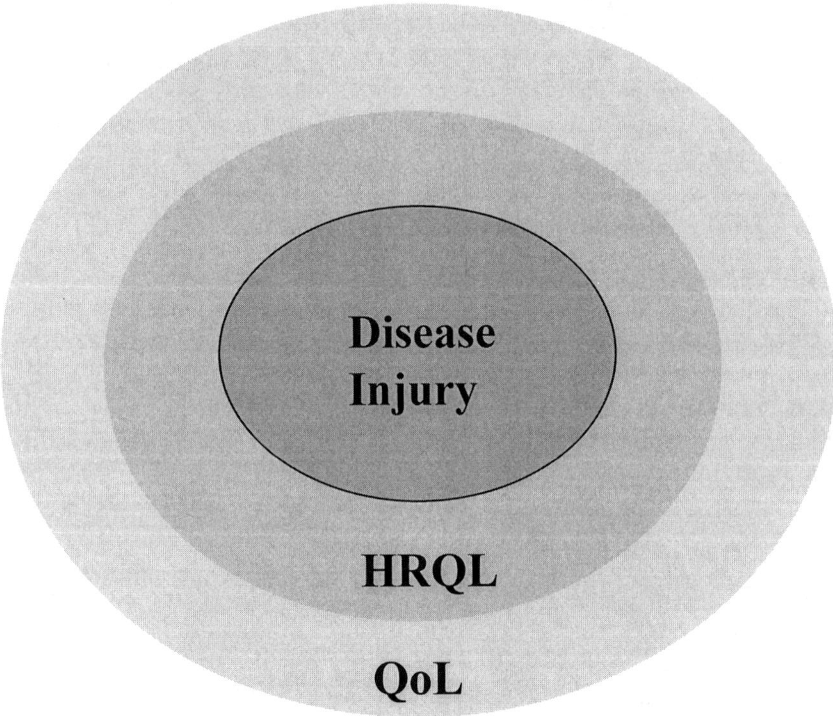

Figure 1 The functionalist conception of quality of life.

social functioning as a dimension of HRQL as it is "beyond the skin." This is in direct contrast to Spilker (49), who lists five major domains of HRQL: physical status and functional abilities, psychological status and well-being, social interactions, economic and/or vocational status, and religious and/or spiritual status. In doing so he goes beyond the accepted range of HRQL concerns, arguing that as individual researchers include only some of these domains, they cannot be said to have investigated the full range of HRQL characteristics. However, as there is no clear consensus on the "full range" of HRQL domains, it can never be proven that the concept has been measured adequately. Some researchers address this issue by suggesting that certain domains are irrelevant to some studies (49). Certain studies have been criticized for using a single variable of human behavior, such as employment, happiness, or sexual functioning, as ad hoc indicators of HRQL (50).

Recently, clear distinctions have been made between the HRQL dimensions and QoL (51–53). HRQL instruments tend to focus on symptoms and disability (in functional terms) and, as such, provide information about the level of impairment of disability experienced by the patient. However, it is argued that they do not inform as to the impact of the condition on the patient's QoL. For example, the salience of limited mobility is dependent on environmental, employment, and social factors. Tennant and McKenna (51) argue that QoL goes beyond the impairment, disability, handicap continuum by asking what the patients' health prevents them from doing and also about their emotional response to these restrictions. HRQL can be seen as equating to health status, and the terms are often used interchangeably (24, 47). Indeed, almost any measure that assesses some aspect of health status may be referred to as a HRQL instrument.

The Needs-Based Approach

One of the early advocates of the importance of needs to QoL was Thomas More (5). In 1516 More argued that human life quality is dependent on the satisfaction of certain basic needs, for example, those for health, mobility, adequate nutrition, and shelter (5). In the nineteenth century the radical utilitarianist and socialist reformers supported the Liberal view that equality of freedom was a prerequisite for an acceptable QoL. However, they also argued that liberty alone did not ensure this. Instead, they emphasized the need for equal distribution of material and social goods, stressing that an acceptable QoL could only be achieved if members of a society received the basic goods required to satisfy their physical needs. These included food, clothing, shelter, health resources, employment, mobility, and public education.

Major advances in needs theory in the 1940s and 1950s resulted from investigations into human motivation. Researchers in this field proposed that individuals are driven or motivated by their needs (54,55). The relation between needs and QoL continued to be explored within the social indicators movement (56).

The needs-based approach to QoL measurement draws on these theories. Its application to QoL measurement has developed in Europe and is now being adopted by researchers in the United States. Hunt and McKenna's (15) model, which is the most widely implemented, arose during the development of a QoL instrument specific to depression. Recognizing the importance of deriving the content of an instrument directly from relevant patients, the researchers began by interviewing patients about the impact of depression on their lives. Analyzing the interview transcripts, they noticed that the respondents described their experiences in terms of needs that were, or were not, being met rather than in functional terms. Patients who had recovered from their illness referred to needs that they had become able to satisfy as their health improved.

Proponents of the needs-based approach postulate that life gains its quality from the ability and capacity of the individual to satisfy their needs (either inborn or learned during socialization processes) (15,57). Functions such as employment, hobbies, and socializing are important only insofar as they provide the means by which these needs can be fulfilled. It is taken as axiomatic that QoL is high when most human needs are fulfilled and low when few needs are being satisfied.

Advocates of the needs-based approach view QoL as a distinct construct, separate from function and health status. Gill and Feinstein (17) argue that QoL, rather than being a description of a patient's health status, is a reflection of the way in which patients perceive and react to their health status and to other nonmedical aspects of their lives. Similarly, health is not necessarily the most important factor in QoL, although it may increase in importance during severe illness. Many other factors can affect QoL, as shown in Figure 2. In certain cultures, religion and spirituality may also play an important part. Furthermore, these areas interact with each other and with health to influence QoL (58).

The Individualistic Approach

The basis of the individualistic approach to QoL is the work of the American philosopher Josiah Royce (6) during the early twentieth century. Royce believed that humans are best viewed as lives lived with some degree of coherence (6). Thus, a human being could be thought of as a life lived according to a human plan. Certain qualities advance the "life plan" (such

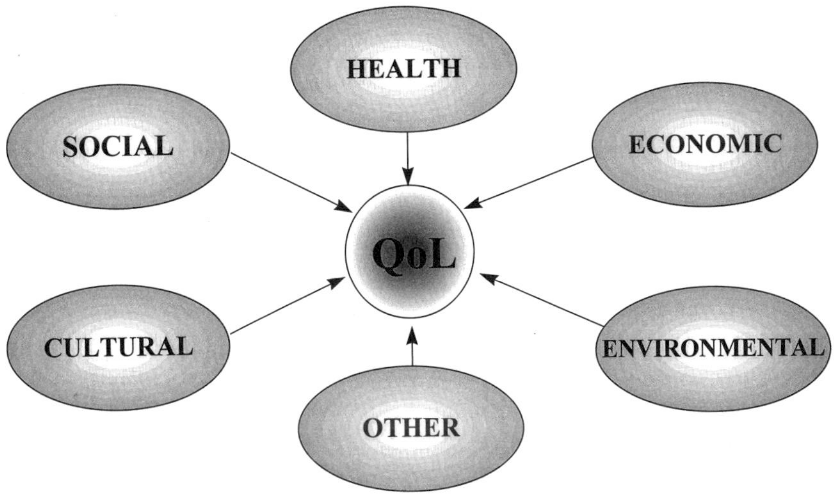

Figure 2 The needs-based conception of quality of life.

as intelligence, mobility, stamina "the pursuit of one's vocation" and "the practice of one's art"), and other features hinder its advancement (including confinement to bed, mental instability, fear, and pain) (2).

Royce's work was developed in the 1980s by Cohen (2), who argues that, when considering QoL, it is necessary to address the issues of importance to the lives whose qualities we are concerned about. Cohen asserted that treatment should be evaluated not merely from a biological standpoint but also in terms of its affect on the "life plan"—how far the treatment facilitates or hinders pursuit of the life-plan. He termed this the "life-plan approach" to QoL.

Similar views were expressed by Calman (59), whose study of the QoL of cancer patients led him to suggest that QoL can only be described and measured in individual terms. He asserts that QoL is high when the hopes and expectations of the individual are fulfilled by experience. Thus, he believes that QoL can be conceived of as the gap between hopes/expectations and achievements. Improvements in QoL occur when treatment narrows this gap. This approach allows a comparison of present state against the gold standard of the patient's expectations. However, Calman has been criticized for asserting that it is justifiable to improve a person's QoL by *reducing* his or her expectations (9).

The importance of the individual's views of QoL were further highlighted by Joyce (60,61), who argues that QoL should be defined as "what the individual says it is." He believes that existing methods of assessing QoL impose an external value system on individuals, rather than allowing them to describe their lives in terms of those factors that they consider to be most important. Following from this, McGee et al. (62) argue that even where the content of instruments is derived from patients, the items and the responses to them do not represent the free choice of the individual.

As with the needs-based approach, the individualistic approach considers that health is not the main determinant of QoL and that there are wider influences that can have a major impact on the QoL of the individual.

INSTRUMENTS DEVELOPED FROM THE THREE APPROACHES

HRQL Instruments

Functionalist theory had a major impact on the development of health status instruments in the 1970s. Measures such as the Sickness Impact Profile (63) and the RAND 36-Item Health Survey 1.0 (64) assess the individual's ability to perform specific tasks or functions. This approach, later termed health-related quality of life, became particularly popular in the medical outcomes field in the 1980s.

The most widely used HRQL instrument is the Short-Form 36 (SF-36) (65). The SF-36, although identical in content to the original RAND measure, has been separately copyrighted and employs a different scoring algorithm (66). The content of the RAND/SF-36 was adapted from longer instruments completed by patients participating in the Medical Outcomes Study (an observational study of variations in physician practice styles and patient outcomes in different systems of health care delivery) conducted in the early 1970s as part of the RAND Health Insurance Survey (64,67). Items for the original longer instruments were drawn from existing questionnaires that had been in use for up to 30 years. The content of these instruments was not derived from empirical research but reflects areas considered to be important by the developers.

The RAND/SF-36 instrument is a generic measure of health status covering eight domains-physical functioning, bodily pain, role limitations due to physical health, role limitations due to personal or emotional problems, emotional well-being, social functioning, energy/fatigue, and general health perceptions. In addition, it includes one item indicating perceived change in health.

The Sickness Impact Profile (SIP) was developed in the 1970s as a measure of perceived health status. The intention was to provide a descriptive profile of the changes in a person's behavior due to sickness (63). "Sickness" was defined as an individual's experience of illness perceived through its effect on daily activities, feelings, and attitudes (68). The content of the SIP was derived from professionals, interviews with healthy and ill lay people, and a review of the literature.

The Quality of Well-Being Scale (QWBS) (69,70) has also been widely used. The measure was developed in the 1970s as a component of the General Health Policy Model to assess "wellness." The QWBS and its associated decision models were designed to be used for policy analysis in determining current and future requirements for health care resources (71). The instrument assesses level of functioning in three areas: mobility, physical activity, and social activity. In addition, mortality, symptoms, and problems are assessed. The authors claim that this allows health, disability, and death to be placed on a single scale, although this procedure has been questioned (72). The content of the QWBS was derived from previous questionnaires rather than from lay individuals.

Condition-specific instruments developed using the HRQL approach often consist of a generic measure (generally the SF-36) with several additional questions seen by the investigators as being relevant to the patient group concerned. For example, the Epilepsy Surgery Inventory (ESI-55) (73) contains the SF-36, 13 additional items taken from the RAND Medical Outcomes Study (MOS) (5 taken directly and 8 adapted), one Dartmouth Co-op Chart (74), an item on patient preference (75), and 4 additional items. The process of combining and supplementing questionnaires in this way is of questionable validity.

Needs-Based QoL Instruments

The development of measurement tools based on the needs approach has gained particular credence in the 1990s. This is largely due to a dissatisfaction with HRQL instruments developed in the 1970s and 1980s and the recognition of the need to develop instruments based on the perceptions of patients. Furthermore, as was seen above, the theory underpinning needs-based measures predates the functional approach.

Although needs-based models have been discussed by many researchers (particularly in Scandinavia) over the last 20 years, it was not until the 1980s that attempts were made to develop needs-based measures of QoL for medical outcomes assessment (57,76). In the 1990s, the needs-based QoL model proposed by Hunt and McKenna (15) has formed the basis of several condition-specific QoL instruments developed by researchers in the United Kingdom and in the United States. These include measures for depression, adult growth hormone deficiency, recurrent genital herpes, migraine, rheumatoid arthritis, and male erectile dysfunction (15,77–84) (see Chapter 30 in this volume). The content of each of these instruments was developed from interviews with relevant patients. Consequently, the items reflect the concerns of the patients rather than the investigators. The measures are easy to administer and complete and are well accepted by both investigators and respondents. All language versions of the instruments developed have better psychometric qualities than HRQL instruments. For example, all 11 language versions of the Quality of Life in Depression Scale display test-retest reliability values above 0.90. Where they have been used in research studies, instruments based on this model have been shown to have high responsiveness (77).

Instruments Developed Using the Individualistic Approach

In the present decade, researchers have attempted to develop measurement techniques that consider QoL in terms of advancement or frustration of the life plan. Joyce's definition (60,61) formed the basis for the development of the Schedule for the Evaluation of Individual Quality of Life (SEIQoL) (62), the first instrument that operationalizes the individualistic approach to QoL measurement. The method of assessment used for the SEIQoL is based on judgment analysis, a technique derived from social judgment theory. The SEIQoL is administered in a standardized semi-structured interview, in which patients are asked to identify and rate the relative importance of the five most important aspects of their lives at that moment (85). In recognition of the impracticality of the SEIQoL for routine clinical situations, the SEIQoL-direct weighting (SEIQoL-DW) has been produced (86). This is reported to be a simpler procedure for assigning weights to patient-nominated life areas.

THE VALUE AND LIMITATIONS OF THE THREE APPROACHES TO QUALITY-OF-LIFE MEASUREMENT

Value and Limitations of the HRQL Approach

As has been seen, HRQL focuses on those aspects of life that are considered to be the province of health professionals. The emphasis is on the measurement of symptoms and functions. Consequently, the main value of HRQL measurement is in the assessment of health status: levels of impairment (losses or abnormalities at the organ level), disabilities (excesses or deficiencies of customarily accepted activity, performance, and behavior for the individual), and, to a lesser extent, handicap (disadvantage preventing fulfillment of a role that is normal for that individual) (87). Such information is often valuable to clinical assessment of outcome.

However, HRQL cannot be considered to be equivalent to QoL. Justification for this assertion lies in the two fundamental assumptions of HRQL—that health is the major influence on QoL and that there is no interaction between health and other determinants of QoL. Research has shown that health is only one (often a minor) influence on QoL (13,88). Limiting consideration of QoL to "health-related" aspects fails to take into account patients' response to ill health and treatment. Lipowski (89) argues that how a person experiences the pathological process, what it means to him or her, and how this meaning influences his or her behavior are all integral components of disease viewed as a total human response. Similarly, Spilker (49) asserts that "we are as much concerned with the patient's view of the importance of the dysfunction as with its existence."

Many researchers have recognized the importance of the wider influences on QoL. For example, Parmenter (12) argues that QoL encompasses much more than the status of one's health. He adds that the most fruitful approaches to QoL research are those that recognize the interaction between the person with the disease and his or her environment. Draper (7) believes that the HRQL approach "reflects a fractured perception of human being, lacking both coherence and significance." Rosenberg (16) argues that the approach should be called "multidimensional evaluation" of treatment outcome and not QoL assessment.

There are a number of additional problematic issues in the functionalist approach. The focus on fulfillment of "normal" roles (i.e., roles considered normal for a certain age and sex within a given culture) creates problems for societal groups that deviate from the "norm." Certain groups, such as unemployed or disabled individuals, are automatically devalued under this approach. The emphasis on physical functioning found in HRQL instruments determines that disabled people cannot have a high QoL, a fact not necessarily borne out by experience.

The instruments developed to assess HRQL have a number of limitations. First, the methods of generating instrument items is not consonant with the currently accepted view that QoL instruments should reflect the concerns of the patient. HRQL is viewed by its proponents as patient-based. However, a distinction must be made between instruments that are patient-*derived* and those that are patient-*completed*. Although HRQL questionnaires are completed by the patients, where the content of instruments was written by "experts" or researchers, the answers reflect *their* interests rather than those of the respondents. As has been seen above, there is seldom overlap between "experts" and patients' views of what is important to their QoL.

Function-based measures attempt to overcome the problem of limiting "QoL" to health-related influences by asking respondents to attribute their loss of function to their illness(es). However, such attributions are difficult at best and probably impossible in most cases. For example, the SF-36 requires respondents to say whether they have accomplished less at work as a result of their physical health and then as a result of emotional problems. This requires levels of insight and expertise beyond the capacity of many respondents.

In addition, because role performance is dependent on the ideology and culture of the society in which the measure is developed, instruments based on this approach are heavily ethnocentric. Consequently, the content of instruments developed in, for example, the United States may not be relevant to patients in Europe. This makes adaptation of instruments for use in other cultures rather difficult. A good example of this is the SF-36 item: "Does your health now limit you in . . . vigorous activities, such as running, lifting heavy objects, participating in strenuous sports?" A majority of people in most European countries (and many in the United States), *never* engage in vigorous activities of any kind. The latest survey of leisure activities in the United Kingdom found that fewer than 10% of the population took part in sports requiring more than low-level physical activity (58). Consequently, a response of "no" to this question is difficult to interpret, as it could imply either that an individual is not limited or that they do not take part in such activities. Asking irrelevant questions can alienate respondents and lead to high levels of missing responses.

Chronically ill people adapt their lives in order to undertake activities (functions) that they can manage. In this way they are able to maintain their QoL. Function-based measures are unable to cope with such adaptation. Consequently, they make it difficult for severely ill or disabled patients to show improvement, even following effective intervention. Hill and Harries (90) found that the SF-36 was unable to show the benefits of cataract operations for elderly patients, even though interviews with the patients suggested that their lives had actually been greatly improved.

A further important consideration is the age of the most common HRQL instruments. The most widely used instruments (SIP, SF-36, and QWBS) were developed in the early 1970s. However, the way in which patients conceptualize their problems and the terms in which they express themselves can change in a generation (91). Moreover, certain issues may become less important with time. For example, lack of mobility may be compensated for by advances in technology. Furthermore, the generic health status instruments have not benefited from improvements in test-construction methodology and scaling techniques. Consequently, their reliability and responsiveness fall far short of that required for instruments included in clinical trials (92).

Value and Limitations of the Needs-Based Approach

Proponents of the needs-based approach argue that QoL encompasses more than just those influences within the jurisdiction of the health services.

Consequently, the approach allows consideration of all aspects of life that may be influenced by ill health and its treatment. HRQL researchers argue that an assessment of all possible influences on QoL is impractical. However, such an argument could only be applied to generic QoL instruments. With careful development, all relevant influences on QoL can be included in a manageable condition-specific instrument.

The needs-based conception of QoL has a number of positive advantages for measurement. Rather than asking directly about a function, it is possible to inquire about the needs that could be satisfied by that function. This is helpful, as the function in itself may not be important. For example, questions about sexual performance are frequently left unanswered on questionnaires. By focusing on needs it is possible to ask about needs for intimacy, touch, and sharing with another person outside the context of a sexual relationship. The needs-based approach avoids irrelevant questions and considerably reduces the number of missing responses (93).

The needs approach also copes well with patient adaptation to illness. A chronically ill person can maintain a reasonable level of QoL by mastering independence and by the use of aids and/or assistance. With this approach, patients who have physical functional limitations can still be shown to have a good quality of life, as the concern here is the degree to which they can meet their needs, irrespective of how this is achieved. Similarly, an objectively healthy individual can be dissatisfied with his or her situation and have a relatively poor QoL.

A further advantage of this approach is that needs are, on the whole, culture-free, although the degree to which self-actualization needs become important may vary between extremes of culture. Consequently, instruments based on this approach are far more amenable to adaptation for use in other countries and for use with cultural minority groups within a society.

Instruments developed using Hunt and McKenna's needs-based model (15,77–84) are patient-based, thus fulfilling a basic requirement for QoL instruments. They do not contain predetermined components, rather, the content is derived from in-depth qualitative interviews conducted with relevant patients. As instruments reflect the concerns of the patient group, their acceptability to respondents is maximized and missing data reduced to a minimum. Response rates are also consistently high. Furthermore, enquiring about need fulfillment rather than function means that severely ill or disabled people can be shown to improve by these instruments.

Studies have also shown that needs-based instruments are highly responsive, that is, able to detect changes in QoL associated with a change in the condition of the patient. Moreover, as these instruments were developed relatively recently, the latest scaling techniques have been applied during their development. Recent evidence shows that the instruments are unidimensional, providing an index of QoL that is essential for use in pharmacoeconomic studies.

The main disadvantages of needs-based instruments is that, being condition-specific, direct comparisons cannot be made between patient groups. Furthermore, the same instrument cannot be used with different diagnostic groups. However, evidence now suggests that such comparisons cannot be made with generic instruments, as items appear to work in different ways with different patient groups (94).

Value and Limitations of the Individualistic Approach

Like the needs-based approach, the individualistic approach rejects the prescriptive restriction of QoL to those factors that are within the control of health professionals. An advantage of the life plan approach is that it emphasizes the importance of the views of the patient. Proponents argue that because human beings are individuals, the relevance of instruments developed using grouped data for individuals could be questioned (13). Such instruments have been criticized for imposing external value systems on individuals, containing information on behaviors or functions that are not relevant to all, and omitting functions that are relevant to specific individuals (13).

There is also recognition that an outcome that increases the QoL of one individual may not necessarily produce similar benefit for another. An example of this is the ability to return to work following surgery. As Cohen (2) observes, return to work is often a direct function of personality type or the need for income, rather than of the impact of surgery on the patient's health. This suggests that it is not *functions* that advance or hinder life plans but the fulfillment of *needs*.

A further merit of this approach is that it seeks to empower patients and to allow them to participate in decision making as to the management of their condition. The importance of this is highlighted by Rosenberg (16), who asserts that the dialogue between the clinician and the patient is one between peers in an existential rather than technical sense. From an ethical standpoint, patients have a right to participate in decision making about their treatment if they so choose. Consequently, the main advantages of this approach are in the clinical setting.

The main limitation of the individualistic approach lies in the measurement techniques devised to assess individual QoL. Although the theories underlying this approach recognize the importance of the fulfillment of needs for advancement of the life plan, the measurement tools developed have a particular focus on functioning. Despite the focus on the concerns of the individual, the underlying emphasis of the approach is on the "goods" that improve life quality. The interpretation of these is still largely functional, and as has been seen above this presents many problems. O'Boyle (13), reporting on the SEIQoL, asserts that "a valid measure of QoL should quantify the level of functioning of each individual in those areas of life that he or she considers to be most important." There appears to be no reason why an individualistic approach could not focus on needs rather than on functions.

Although the SEIQoL has been used in a number of studies (62,85), the psychometric values obtained with it are rather lower than desirable. Furthermore, the requirement for a trained interviewer and the complexity of the instrument [as acknowledged by the authors (86)] render the technique impractical for most clinical situations.

The authors of the SEIQoL-DW argue that it has a potentially important role to play in the consultation process, providing a means by which the health care team can formulate and monitor therapeutic plans (86). The value of the instrument for clinical trials is not proven, as little information is available on its effectiveness. No data have yet been published on the psychometric properties of this SEIQoL-DW. These would need to be established before its use could be considered.

CONCLUSIONS

Increased longevity per se is no longer a sufficient justification for treatment. The efficient and cost-effective management of any disease requires that competing interventions be evaluated in terms of their ability to both control the disease and improve the QoL of patients. Accurate and valid QoL instruments are essential to this evaluation, and this has led to an exponential growth of interest in the construct and its measurement.

Since the 1970s, numerous studies have claimed to incorporate an assessment of QoL. However, the popularity of the term belies the fact that many of these studies have used instruments designed to assess very different constructs. Too often, any instrument completed by the patient is referred to as a QoL measure. Moreover, many studies incorporate "QoL" instruments that have inadequate psychometric and scaling properties. Parmenter (12) argues that one of the most serious omissions in the development of scales is the paucity of studies that have tested their construct validity against a sound theoretical base.

Since the 1970s three clear approaches to QoL measurement have emerged: the functionalist (HRQL) approach, the needs-based approach, and the individualistic approach. Although the needs and individualistic approaches have enjoyed a much longer philosophical tradition than functionalism, up to the late 1980s measurement was dominated by function-based (predominantly generic) health status instruments.

HRQL measures have a number of drawbacks, including poor psychometric and scaling properties. Their emphasis on generic rather than condition-specific measurement also appears misplaced. There is growing evidence that generic instruments do not allow comparisons between different disease groups, their only apparent advantage over specific measures (94).

The 1990s has seen a resurgence of interest in the needs-based and individualistic approaches to QoL. Instruments for assessing QoL based on these approaches are now available. Research on needs-based measures is concentrating on methods of developing condition-specific instruments that allow comparisons across disease groups. Such work involves the application of new statistical models that identify weaknesses in the traditional psychometric approach.

These are exciting times for QoL research. Advances in measurement techniques are rapid, leading to the development of more sensitive and responsive tools. The advent of this new generation of QoL instruments will improve the precision with which the outcomes of clinical interventions can be assessed. The greatest barrier to advancement in the field is the desire to continue using measures that, despite their wide use and familiarity have, nevertheless, outgrown their usefulness. Of particular concern is the practice of working parties recommending the most appropriate instruments for use in evaluation of specific diseases. Such recommendations are often based on questionable assumptions and inadequate evidence. This can lead to outcome measures being used simply because they have been widely used in previous studies. This approach stifles new advances in QoL measurement and deprives future studies of the most useful outcome measures. It is now time to give the old generic health status instruments, such as the Nottingham Heath Profile, SF-36, SIP, and QWBS, a peaceful retirement. Although they have proved useful workhorses during the development of the science of QoL measurement, much more is now demanded of outcome measure, and suitable new instruments are already available to researchers.

REFERENCES

1. Plato. In: Church FJ, trans. Euthyphro, Apology, Crito. New York: Bobbs-Merrill, 1956: 57.
2. Cohen C. On the QoL: some philosophical reflections. Circulation 1982; 66 (suppl III): III-29-III-33.
3. Aristotle. In: Ostwald M, trans. Nicomachean Ethics, New York: Bobbs Merrill Company, Inc., 1962.

4. Bentham J. In: Goldworth A, ed. Deontology: Together with a Table on the Springs of Action and Article on Utilitarianism. Oxford: Clarendon Press, 1834 (1983).
5. More T. Utopia. London: Chatto & Windus Publishers, 1516 (1908).
6. Royce J. The Philosophy of Loyalty, Lecture IV, Section 4. New York: Macmillan, 1908.
7. Draper P. Quality of life as quality of being: an alternative to the subject-object dichotomy. J Adv Nurs 1992; 17:965–970.
8. Aiken W. The quality of life. Appl Philos 1982; 1:26–36.
9. Häyry M. Measuring the QoL: Why, how and what? Theor Med 1991; 12:97–116.
10. Bubolz M, Eicher JB, Evers SJ, Sontag MS. A human ecological approach to QoL: conceptual framework and results of a preliminary study. Soc Indic Res 1980; 7:103–136.
11. Bech P. Measuring quality of life: the medical perspective. Nordic J Psychiatry 1992; 46:85–89.
12. Parmenter TR. Quality of life as a concept and measurable entity. Soc Indic Res 1994; 33:9–46.
13. O'Boyle CA. Assessment of quality of life in surgery. Br J Surg 1992; 79(May):395–398.
14. Read JL. The new era of quality of life assessment. In: Walker SW, Rosser RM, eds. Quality of Life Assessment: Key Issues in the 1990s. London: Kluwer Academic Publishers, 1993:3–10.
15. Hunt SM, McKenna SP. The QLDS: a scale for the measurement of quality of life in depression. Health Policy 1992; 22:307–319.
16. Rosenberg R. Health-related quality of life between naturalism and hermeneutics. Soc Sci Med 1995; 41(10):1411–1415.
17. Gill TM, Feinstein AR. A critical appraisal of the quality of quality of life measurements. JAMA 1994; 272(8):619–625.
18. Stensman R. Severely mobility-disabled people assess the quality of their lives. Scand J Rehab Med 1985; 17:87–89.
19. Morgan AE. An attempt to measure happiness. Int J Med Ethics 1934; 44:271–274.
20. Engel GL. On looking inward and being scientific. A tribute to Arthur H Schmale, MD. Psychother Psychosom 1990; 54:63–69.
21. World Health Organisation. Constitution of the World Health Organisation. Geneva: WHO, 1947.
22. World Health Organisation. Official Records of the World Health Organisation. No. 2. Geneva: WHO, 1948:100.
23. Cella DF. Quality of life: concepts and definition. J Pain Symptom Manage 1994; 9(3):186–192.
24. Guyatt GH, Feeny DH, Patrick DL. Measuring health-related quality of life. Ann Intern Med 1993; 118:622–629.
25. Mechanic D. The concept of illness behaviour. J Chronic Dis 1962; 17:18[illegible]–194.

26. Coronary Drug Project Research Group. Influence of adherence to treatment and response of cholesterol on mortality in the coronary drug project. N Engl J Med 1983; 303:1038–1041.
27. Jachuck SJ, Brierly H, Jachuck S, Wilcox PM. The effect of hypotensive drugs on the quality of life. J Roy Coll Gen Pract 1982; 32:103–105.
28. Sugarbaker P, Barnofsky I, Rosenberg S, Gianola F. Quality of life assessment of patients in extremity sarcoma clinical trials. Surgery 1982; 91:17–23.
29. Orth-Gomer K, Britton M, Rehnqvist N. Quality of care in an out-patient department: the patient's view. Soc Sci Med 1979; 13A:347–351.
30. Thomas MR, Lyttle D. Patient expectations about the success of treatment and reported relief from low back pain. J Psychosom Res 1980; 24:297–301.
31. Mayou R. Quality of life in cardiovascular disease. Psychother Psychosoma 1990; 54:99–109.
32. Pearlman RA, Jonsen A. The use of quality of life considerations in medical decision making. In: Walter JJ, Shannon TA, eds. Quality of Life: The New Medical Dilemma. New York: Paulist Press, 1990:93–103.
33. Parmenter TR. An analysis of the dimensions of quality of life for people with physical disabilities. In: Brown RI, ed. Quality of Life for Handicapped People. London: Croom Helm, 1988:1–36.
34. Fitzpatrick R, Fletcher A, Gore S, Jones D, Spiegelhalter D, Cox D. Quality of Life measures in health care: in applications and issues in assessment. Br Med J 1992; 305:1074.
35. Streiner D, Norman G. Health Measurement Scales. Oxford: Oxford University Press, 1989.
36. Annas GJ. Quality of life in the courts: Earle spring in fantasyland. In: Walter JJ, Shannon TA, eds. Quality of Life: The New Medical Dilemma. New York: Paulist Press, 1990:319–324.
37. Durkheim E. Suicide. In: Spaulding JA, Simpson G, trans. New York: The Free Press, 1897 (1951).
38. Karnofsky DA, Burchenal JH. The clinical evaluation of chemotherapeutic agents in cancer. In: McLoed CM, ed. Evaluation of Chemotherapeutic Agents. New York: Columbia University Press, 1949:191–205.
39. Parsons T. Definition of health and illness in the light of American values and social structure. In: Gartly JE, ed. Patients, Physicians and Illness: A Sourcebook in Behavioural Science and Health. New York: Free Press, 1958:165–187.
40. Rokeach M. The Nature of Human Values. New York: Free Press, 1973.
41. Kaplan RM, Feeny D, Revicki DA. Methods for assessing relative importance in preference based outcome measures. Qual Life Res 1993; 2:467–475.
42. Patrick DL, Bush JW, Chen MM. Methods for measuring levels of well-being for a health status index. Health Services Res 1973; 8:228–245.
43. Patrick DL, Erikson P. Health Status and Health Policy. Oxford: Oxford University Press, 1993.
44. Kaplan RM, Anderson JP, Wu AW, Matthews WC, Kozin F, Orenstein D. The Quality of Well-Being Scale. Applications in AIDS, cystic fibrosis and arthritis. Med Care 1989; 27:S27–S43.

45. Van Dam F. Quality of life: methodological aspects. Cancer Bull (Paris). 1986; 73:607–613.
46. Wenger NK, Mattson ME, Furberg CD, Elinson J. Assessment of Quality of Life in Clinical Trials of Cardiovascular Therapies. New York: LeJacq, 1984.
47. Patrick DL, Bergner M. Measurement of health status in the 1990's Ann Rev Public Health 1990; 11:165–183.
48. Torrance GW. Utility approach to measuring health-related quality of life. Chronic Dis 1987; 40:593–600.
49. Spilker B. Introduction. In: Spilker B, ed. Quality of Life Assessments in Clinical Trials. 2nd ed. New York: Raven Press, 1996:11–23.
50. Levine S, Croog SH. The primary care physician and the patient's quality of life. Qual Life in Cardiovasc Care 1984; 5–19.
51. Tennant A, McKenna SP. Conceptualising and defining outcome. Br J Rheumatol 1995; 34(10):899–900.
52. Heinemann AW, Whiteneck GG. Relationships among impairment, disability, handicap and life satisfaction in persons with traumatic brain injury. J Head Trauma Rehabil 1995; 10:54–63.
53. Whiteneck, GG. Measuring what matters: key rehabilitation outcomes. Arch Phys Med Rehabil 1994; 75:1073–1076.
54. Maslow AH. Motivation and Personality. New York: Harper & Row, 1954.
55. McCelland DC. Personality. New York: William Sloane, 1951.
56. McCall S. Quality of life. Soc Indic Res 1975; 2:229–248.
57. Hörnquist JO. The concept of quality of life. Scand J Soc Med 1982; 10:57–61.
58. McKenna SP. Commonly used measures of health status in European clinical trials. In: Doward LC, McKenna SP, Hunt SM, Mackenzie Davey K, eds. Quality of Life Assessment in Clinical Trials. The Practical, Theoretical and Cross-Cultural Issues. Br J Med Econ 1993; 6C:3–15.
59. Calman KC. Quality of Life in cancer patients—an hypothesis. J Med Ethics 1984; 10:124–127.
60. Joyce CRB. Psychological benefits. In: Walker SW, Asscher W, eds. Medicine and Risk Benefit Decisions. Lancaster: MTP Press, 1987:99–109.
61. Joyce CRB. Quality of life: the state of the art in clinical assessment. In: Walker SW, Rosser RM, eds. Quality of Life Assessment and Application. Lancaster: MTP Press, 1988:169–179.
62. McGee HM, O'Boyle CA, Hickey A, O'Malley KM, Joyce CRB. Assessing the quality of life of the individual: the SEIQoL with a health and a gastroenterology unit population. Psychol Med 1991; 21:1–11.
63. Bergner M, Bobbit RA, Kressel S, Pollard WE, Gilson BS, Morris JR. The Sickness Impact Profile: conceptual formulation and methodology for the development of a health status measure: Int J Health Services 1976; 6(3):393–415.
64. Brook RH, Ware JE, Davis-Avery A, Stewart AL, Donald CA, Rogers WH, Williams KN, Johnston SA. Overview of adult health status measures fielded in Rand Health Insurance Study. Med Care 1979; 17(7 suppl):iii-x, 1–131.
65. Ware JE, Sherbourne CD. The MOS 36-Item Short-Form Health Survey (SF-36). Med Care 1992; 30:474–483.

66. Hays RD, Sherbourne CD, Mazel RM. The RAND 36-item health survey 1.0. Health Econ 1993; 2(3):217–227.
67. Hays RD, Shapiro MF. An overview of generic health-related quality of life measures for HIV research. Qual Life Res 1992; 1:91–97.
68. Gilson BS, Gilson JS, Bergner M, Bobbitt RA, Kressel S, Pollard WE, Vesselago M. The Sickness Impact Profile: validation of a health status measure. Med Care 1975; 65:1304–1310.
69. Fanshel S, Bush JW. A health status index and its application to health-services outcomes. Oper Res 1970; 18:1021–1065.
70. Kaplan, RM, Bush JW, Berry CC. Health status: types of validity and the Index of Well-Being. Health Services Res 1976; 11:478–507.
71. Kaplan RM, Atkins CJ, Timms R. Validity of a quality of well-being scale as an outcome measure in chronic obstructive pulmonary disease. J Chronic Dis 1984; 37(2):85–95.
7. McDowell I, Newell C. Measuring Health: A Guide to Rating Scales and Questionnaires. Oxford: Oxford University Press, 1987.
73. Vickrey BG, Hays RD, Graber J, Rausch R, Engel J, Brook RH. A health-related quality of life instrument for patients evaluated for epilepsy surgery. Med Care 1992; 30(4):299–319.
74. Nelson EC, Landgraf JM, Hays RD, et al. The Coop Function Charts: a system to measure patient function in physician's offices. In: Lipkin M, ed. Functional Status Measurement in Primary Care: Wonca Classification Committee. New York: Springer-Verlag, 1990.
75. Hadhorn D, Hays RD. Multi-trait-multimethod analysis of health related quality of life preferences. Med Care 1991; 29:829–840.
76. Hörnquist JO. QoL: concept and assessment Scand J Soc Med 1989; 18:69–79.
77. McKenna SP, Hunt SM. A new measure of quality of life in depression: Testing the reliability of construct validity of the QLDS. Health Policy 1992; 22:321–330.
78. Hunt SM, McKenna SP, Doward LC. Preliminary report on the development of a disease-specific instrument for assessing quality of life of adults with growth hormone deficiency. Acta Endocrinol 1993; 128(suppl 2):37–40.
79. Holmes SJ, McKenna SP, Doward LC, Shalet SM. Development of a questionnaire to assess the quality of life of adults with growth hormone deficiency. Endocrinol Metab 1995; 2:63–69.
80. McKenna SP, Doward LC. Measuring quality of life in recurrent genital herpes. Eur Rev Appl Psychol 1995; 45:289–295.
81. McKenna SP, Patrick D. The development of a migraine-specific quality of life measure for multi-national clinical trials. Cephalalgia 1995; 15(suppl 14):280.
82. Whalley D, McKenna S, de Jong Z, van der Heijde D. Quality of life in rheumatoid arthritis. Br J Rheumatol 1997; 36.
83. de Jong Z, van der Heijde D, McKenna SP, Whalley D. The reliability and construct validity of the RAQoL: a rheumatoid arthritis-specific quality of life instrument. Br J Rheumatol 1997; 36.

84. Wagner TH, Patrick DL, McKenna SP, Froese MA. Cross-cultural development of a quality of life measure for men with erection difficulties. Qual Life Res 1996; 5:443–449.
85. O'Boyle CA, McGee H, Hickey A, O'Malley K, Joyce CRB. Individual quality of life in patients undergoing hip-replacement. Lancet 1992; 339:1088–1091.
86. Hickey, AM, Bury G, O'Boyle CA, Bradley F, O'Kelly FD, Shannor W. A new short form individual QoL measure (SEIQoL-DW): application in a cohort of individuals with HIV/AIDS. Br Med J 1996; 313:29–33.
87. World Health Organisation. The International Classification of Impairments, Disabilities and Handicaps. Geneva: WHO, 1980.
88. Fuhrer MJ. Subjective well-being: implications for medical rehabilitation outcomes and models of disablement. Am J Phys Med Rehabil 1994; 73(5):358–364.
89. Lipowski ZJ. Psychosocial aspects of disease. Ann Intern Med 1969; 71(6):1197–1206.
90. Hill S, Harries U. Assessing the outcome of health care for older people in community settings: Should we use the SF-36? Outcomes Briefing 1994; 4(August):26–27.
91. McKenna SP. Generic vs. specific measures in clinical trials. In: Doward LC, McKenna SP, Hunt SM, Mackenzie Davey K, eds. Quality of Life Assessment in Clinical Trials. The practical, theoretical and cross-cultural issues. Br J Med Econ 1993; 6C:17–25.
92. Dixon P, Heaton J, Long A, Warburton A. Reviewing and applying the SF-36. Outcomes Briefing 1994; 4(August):3–25.
93. McKenna SP. Quality of life assessment in the conduct of economic evaluations of medicines. Br J Med Econ 1995; 8:33–38.
94. Whalley D. Recent advances in the evaluation of the scaling properties of health status and quality of life instruments. J Econ Med 1996; (Oct.):73.

3

Psychometric and Related Considerations in Dermatological Assessments of Health-Related Quality of Life

Roger T. Anderson *Bowman Gray School of Medicine of Wake Forest University, Winston-Salem, North Carolina*

Ron D. Hays *University of California, Los Angeles, and RAND Health Program, Los Angeles, California*

Dennis Revicki *MEDTAP International, Bethesda, Maryland, and School of Public Health, University of North Carolina, Chapel Hill, North Carolina*

INTRODUCTION

Not long ago there were few health-related quality-of-life (HRQL) instrument developed for use with dermatological diseases. Today much has changed, as several assessment tools intended for clinical and research use alike are available, and new instruments targeted to specific dermatological diseases are under development. Selecting the most appropriate or psychometrically sound HRQL instrument, however, is not a simple task. The user must consider several things, including (1) the conceptual framework used to develop the instrument and its concordance with the disease or condition of interest (1,2), (2) how the instrument is to be used, either in the clinic to identify benefits or complications associated with treatment or in clinical trials to evaluate and compare treatments, and (3) the instrument's reliability and validity under circumstances that closely resemble those faced by the investigator. Much of the needed technical and empirical evidence about the instruments may be difficult to obtain from a single source in the literature. Even if a source is found, the information may be incompletely described or missing in the literature or the instrument's user's manual. Generally, the interested researcher is faced with the prospect of conducting a thorough review of the literature, carefully collecting the requisite information, and proceeding to compare the results against accepted psychometric standards for reliability and validity. This chapter is intended as a brief technical guide for the clinical investigator to the process of evaluating and interpreting psychometric properties of HRQL instruments published in the literature. While this chapter is general in scope as far as assessing quality of life, where possible, special consideration has been given to dermatological applications.

SOME PRELIMINARY CONSIDERATIONS

The scientific concepts of reliable and valid measurement are neither universal nor absolute. An instrument shown to possess an adequate level of sensitivity to detect benefits from treatment for acne vulgaris compared to no treatment at all may not necessarily be as sensitive to similar contrasts involving other diseases, such as in persons with psoriasis or contact dermatitis. Thus, it is uncertain whether an instrument developed and validated for one cutaneous disease will have comparable validity for another. Even within the same disease group, our hypothetical HRQL instrument may fail to show treatment effects between two active treatments that produce small but clinically important differences in treatment effectiveness.

Another consideration in evaluating the soundness and sensitivity of HRQL measurement is its applicability across respondents. Is the instrument's performance robust across demographic characteristics of the population of interest (3,4)? Desired role activities, occupational responsibilities, interpersonal relationships, socialization, and thus definitions of usual functioning may vary across age or gender and could affect how or to what extent appearance-altering skin diseases may affect HRQL. Smith et al. (see Chapter 9) describe effects of acne on quality of life from a developmental perspective, focusing on the psychological and social lives of adolescents and young adults as contexts for understanding how acne may affect their life quality. Another condition, alopecia, can be expected to affect men and women, young and old, differently, in part because of social norms governing appearance and personal appraisals of attractiveness or expectations.

For some diseases, the severity, history of recurrence and duration, and pathogenesis of skin disease may vary substantially according to the subject's age. This variability could have implications for the types of irritations experienced, their tolerability, and resultant functioning (5).

In order to organize the scientific process of collecting information about the various impacts of dermatological disease upon patients' lives, it is important to begin with a theoretical model that states the potential or expected HRQL effects of treatment as well as what factors may modify or mediate these effects (1,6). Thus, the first guidepost is that the HRQL instrument selected should closely resonate with the theoretical model held valid by the investigator.

The required complexity or specificity of the theoretical model needed may depend upon the motivation for collecting the HRQL information. Exploratory HRQL research may be broad based enough to rely upon general models of quality of life to document outcomes associated with skin disease or its treatment. Evaluative research, in contrast, seeks to demonstrate treatment effects using explicit hypotheses derived from a specific theoretical model or conceptual framework from dermatology. For example, it may be demonstrated that acne vulgaris affects HRQL primarily in terms of self-perceptions and physical symptoms. These effects, in turn, limit social functioning and increase general psychological distress. In this example, a newly developed instrument that fails to find such a profile may require further testing and development. Alternatively, a new medication, studied with a well-validated instrument, that showed significant improvement only in physical symptoms when compared to controls would likely be ineffective.

As another consideration, the conceptual model should specify not only what must be measured by the HRQL instrument, but what aspects or indicators are valid (i.e, depression and anxiety may be unique dimensions of general distress) and which levels of measurement can be used to represent the construct (e.g., reports of behaviors vs. subjective experiences) in self-report instruments.

Once the model is specified, the selected instrument must also cover an adequate range of the concepts or dimensions of HRQL. Too limited a range will affect the discriminant ability of the instrument to detect treatment effects or the magnitude of impact on HRQL within the patient population of interest. Related to this issue is the question of whether only negative components of HRQL should be assessed. Do the hypotheses about HRQL effects from treatment include more than just the absence of negative effects? Could positive experiences result from treatment?

Once one or more theoretically sound instruments have been identified, the next task is to review the technical considerations of their psychometric properties, including reliability, validity, and the generalizability of that evidence to the specific dermatology population of interest. Also of interest is the ease of completing the questionnaire by respondents, as this will influence measurement error and completeness of the data obtained.

A final consideration has to do with how the information will be used. Clinical uses of HRQL information requires briefer measures, self-administered, including information familiar to health care providers and demonstrated to predict level or duration of need for health services. Research uses, such as for clinical trials, may have different emphases, including discriminability of treatment effectiveness relative to a comparison group. This will require highly reliable measures, perhaps more comprehensive in scope, and with proven responsiveness to change. Clinical applications with individual patients may require higher levels of reliability than group comparisons, a specification made more difficult by an additional desire for a brief measure.

RELIABILITY OF MEASUREMENT

Reliability refers to the extent to which the measure yields the same number or score each time it is administered, all other things being equal (i.e., no true change in the attribute being measured has occurred). Reliability is a necessary measurement characteristic of a scale because it provides evidence of its stability over different repeated measurements. Thus, it is important to evaluate the reliability of a quality-of-life scale before its widespread use in clinical trials and health outcome studies.

From classical test theory, observed HRQL scores include a true score component, a systematic error component, and a random error component. A true score for an individual is assumed to be invariant on repeated measurements. If no random error is present, the reliability is 1.0. Reliability approaches zero as the relative amount of random error increases. Both the true score component and the systematic error contribute to the reliability of the measure because they derive the observed score for an individual towards a consistent value. However, systematic error leads to bias in measurement, because it causes the score to be consistently too high or too low relative to the true score. Systematic errors include social desirability responding (reporting in such a way as to minimize the presentation of undesirable and maximize the presentation of desirable characteristics), acquiescent responding (agreement with statements regardless of content), and observational bias (such as halo effects, whereby a single positive feature colors the general impression and ratings of another). Relatively few HRQL instruments have examined these or other sources of systematic error. Since skin disease may have substantial effects on appearance and self-image, Anderson and Rajagopalan (7) examined systematic error in the Dermatologic Specific Quality of Life questionnaire (DSQL) scores for social desirability and found little or no bias from this source. These results, however, cannot be generalized to other instruments or other patient populations.

Reliability involves examining agreement between an individual's score on two measurements. There are four basic categories of reliability estimation, each reflecting somewhat different ways by which random error of measurement is estimated: interrater, equivalent forms, test-retest, and internal consistency reliability.

Interrater Reliability

This form of reliability refers to a comparison of scores assigned to the same target (either patient or other stimuli) by two or more raters. Although it is widely accepted that HRQL information should be obtained from the patient's perspective using self-report measures, physician or expert ratings of disease severity are often used to aid in the interpretation of HRQL data. For this case, interrater reliability would be of interest. Both rater selection and intraindividual response variability influence random error in this case. For example, a clinician rating of severity of skin disease may consist of a lesion count with acne, differentiating between morphological types of lesions, or assessing percent of psoriasis body area involved, such as in the Psoriasis Area Severity Index (PASI) (8). Reliability coefficients for the different ratings estimate the reliability for the average of multiple assessments. The intent is to measure how well different raters (level of agreement between raters), using a scale, assign the same score to the same patient. An intraclass correlation coefficient estimates the corresponding reliability for a single assessment (one rater). In interrater reliability evaluations one is most likely interested in the reliability of multiple ratings. The intraclass correlation would be of interest if the reliability of a single rater was of concern.

Equivalent Forms Reliability

Equivalent forms reliability refers to the agreement between an individual's score on two or more versions of the same instrument designed to measure the same attribute. Both item selection and intraindividual response variability contribute to random error in this method of estimating reliability. If the forms are truly equivalent in terms of item content, then the correlation between scores provides a good estimate of their reliability. However, it is difficult to devise equivalent forms of the same instrument, and intervening events or practice effects can distort the results from this method of reliability assessment. The same formulas used for interrater reliability can be used to estimate equivalent forms reliability, with the different forms substituted for multiple raters.

Test-Retest Reliability

This form of reliability is the relationship between scores obtained by the same person on two or more separate occasions and is more commonly found in the HRQL literature then equivalent forms reliability. Here, intraindividual response variability is used to estimate random error in test-retest assessments. Several factors may influence the reliability of a measure between test dates, such as the conditions of administration, testing effects, change in health status, specific factors affecting the participants in their daily lives, or the length of time between administrations. The assessment of reliability is further complicated, on the one hand, by the fact that too short a time period may result in learning effects whereby subjects recall how they previously answered each item, and, on the other hand, by changes in the attribute being measured that may have occurred between administrations from too long a time period. The time period is particularly important with skin diseases that undergo varying intensities or are episodic in terms of impact upon HRQL. A low test-retest correlation may therefore reflect not the reliability of the test, but a less-than-optimal design for assessing reliability. Generally, test-retest assessments become most useful when there is evidence that real changes did not occur between the first and second assessment of the attribute being measured.

Internal Consistency Reliability

The internal consistency reliability of a scale is a function of the number of items and their covariation and models random error due to item selection. Cronbach's (9) alpha is the coefficient commonly used to estimate the reliability of HRQL instrument based on internal consistency. Generally, one is most interested in the reliability of the average of the items (rather than the intraclass correlation, or estimated reliability of a single item). Formulas for computing the significance of difference between alpha coefficients are provided elsewhere (10). Guttman scales are a special case of internal consistency. A Guttman scale consists of dichotomous items that adhere to a strict deterministic response model related to the prevalence of item endorsement (11). If observed data fit the Guttman scale model, then individuals with same total scale score also tend to exhibit the same pattern of response to each item in the scale. Thus, by knowing a person's scale score it is possible to predict with good accuracy his or her answer to every item in a Guttman scale.

STANDARDS FOR RELIABILITY

For clinical trials, the standard for reliability of measures is less stringent than it is for individual assessment. Because different groups of people (e.g., patients who do or do not receive patch-testing after unsuccessful treatment for contact dermatitis) are compared rather than individuals, a 0.70 standard is appropriate for clinical trials (12). A reliability level of 0.90 was advocated by Nunnally (12) as a minimum standard for measurement designed for interpretation of scores at the individual level. This recommendation stems from the fact that the standard error of measurement is about one third of the measure's standard deviation if it has a reliability of 0.90 (standard error of measurement is estimated by the product of the measure's standard deviation and the square root of the difference between 1.0 and the reliability of the measure). Confidence intervals around an individual's estimated true score are wide at reliabilities below this recommended cut point. Despite the rationale for the 0.90 reliability standard for individual assessment, in practice it may be too stringent, particularly since clinic constraints may favor briefer measures. To achieve this level of reliability requires several items per scale. Many highly regarded instruments fail to meet these standards. For example, only two of the eight subscales (physical functioning and emotional well-being) in the SF-36 satisfied the 0.90 reliability standard in the Medical Outcomes Study (MOS) (13,14). Test-retest reliabilities (24-hour) for widely used clinical measures may not meet this standard either. For example, systolic and diastolic blood pressure reliabilities were 0.87 and 0.67, respectively (15). In dermatology, the interrater reliability of many of clinical ratings of disease severity, such as physician's global evaluations like the Acne Severity Rating (16) and the psoriasis area severity ratings (PASI) (8), have not been extensively tested and reported in the literature. Even if the measure falls short of the 0.90 reliability level, obtaining this information is preferred to not doing so. Although the confidence interval around an individual patient's score is wider than one might like, the interval is still tighter than that based on no information at all. Clinicians need to be aware of the extent of unreliability in all of their measures and interpret them with appropriate caution. However, as noted above, reliabilities exceeding 0.70 are acceptable for group comparisons in randomized clinical trials and other clinical studies.

VALIDITY OF MEASUREMENT

Validity of a scale reflects how well it measures what it is intended to measure. The distinction between reliability and validity is important because a measure may be reliable (i.e., always yield the same score for the same patient), but it may be consistently measuring the wrong thing. While demonstrating reliability in measurement is essentially accumulating evidence of the existence of a stable property over repeated measurement, validity is an estimation of the extent to which an instrument measures what it was intended to measure. The key question for validity evidence is whether the scale is valid for a particular application and a specific population.

The assessment of validity normally begins with an assessment of content validity and then proceeds with an evaluation of construct validity and responsiveness of the scale to clinically meaningful changes in HRQL. Construct validity and responsiveness are key psychometric criteria for measures used in clinical trials. Ongoing accumulation of research evidence regarding a scale's validity is important for demonstrating the scale's usefulness. For the developer and users of a quality-of-life scale, the accumulation of evidence of the scale's validity is continuous.

Content Validity

Content validity is the extent to which a measure samples a representative range of the behavior under study, viewed according to the conceptual model of HRQL. In interpreting content validity, questions regarding item sufficiency and patient population should be addressed carefully. For example, the range of items needed to adequately assess impacts from psoriatic arthritis or chronic vulvar dermatoses (see Chapter 18) may be too gross for application to persons with less severe and debilitating forms of skin disease. Thus, a clear idea of what aspects of a concept are to be measured and what hypotheses should be tested is essential. Content validity evaluations tend to be fairly subjective, but ideally include a systematic comparison of a measure with existing standards, well-accepted definitions, expert opinions, and interviews with individuals for whom the measure is targeted (17). Often in the development of a new scale a content map is created and items are constructed to cover the dimensions of interest. In dermatology, the content validity of HRQL instruments has advanced in recent years from sole reliance upon measures of severity, such as the PASI for psoriasis, to a broader conceptual framework including respondent's reports of psychological, social, and physical well-being (18) as is described in numerous chapters in this volume.

Construct Validity

Construct validity is evaluated by hypothesizing how HRQL measures should "behave" and confirming or disconfirming these hypotheses (19).

Hypotheses are stated regarding the direction (and sometimes the strength) of relationships that might be expected, and validity is supported when the associations are consistent with hypotheses. Construct validation is iterative by its very nature, with empirical results feeding into revision of measures, retesting, and further revisions, if necessary. Convergent and discriminant validity are two fundamental aspects of construct validity. Convergent validity refers to the extent to which different ways of measuring the same construct intercorrelate with one another. One difficulty with this approach is that a well-validated dermatology-specific HRQL instrument must be available for the comparison. Alternatively, if generic HRQL measures are correlated with disease-specific measures, impacts on HRQL detected with the former may be quite broad and include effects not related to dermatological conditions. This could act to reduce the size of the correlation with the disease-specific measure, for example, when a person experiences little HRQL impact from acne but has significant limitations from chest pain. The two measures will tend to not agree because they are measures different sources of HRQL impact.

Discriminant validity involves demonstrating that a measure does not correlate too strongly with measures that are intended to assess a different construct. As mentioned above, HRQL instruments relevant to dermatology should measure something distinct from traits or factors that may regulate the disclosing of information about physical appearance or the revealing of embarrassment or negative life impacts. Some considerations include psychological constructs of social desirability, neuroticism, introversion/extroversion, and denial. Other considerations are aging and social support. When two or more constructs (traits) are assessed using more than one method of assessment, convergent and discriminant validity can be assessed using multitrait-multimethod (MTMM) analytical methods (20). Procedures for implementing the MTMM methodology have been developed based on zero-order correlations among measures (21) and confirmatory factor analysis (22).

Criterion Validity

This form of validity can be viewed as a special case of construct validity in which stronger hypotheses are made possible by the availability of a criterion or gold standard measure. For example, the PASI is completed by clinicians to record the extent of the body surface affected psoriasis from key properties of the disease including erythema, induration, and desquamation. As an widely accepted standard psoriasis severity, this index served as a "gold standard" for the recently developed self-reported PASI (SAPASI), which is based solely on patient responses (23). It should be noted that although some agreement may be reached about disease severity in terms of its morphological characteristics, absolute gold standard measures do not exist for the broader construct of quality of life. Instead, quasi–gold standards may be found for distinct components of HRQL. For example, performance-based measures of daily activities, such as fastening buttons and grasping objects, can be used to validate self-reported activities of daily living.

A quality-of-life measure developed to assess the impact of skin disease across a range of severity should discriminate patient groups with mild disease from those with moderately severe or severe disease. Evaluation of the extent to which this holds can be considered a variant of quasi–gold standard validation. This "known-groups" strategy typically involves evaluating an instrument in relation to clinical measures-of-disease status (17). Relative validity calculations (between group ANOVA F-ratios) can be used to evaluate the sensitivity of different HRQL measures to known groups differences. Relative validities are determined by dividing the F-statistic for each measure by the F-ratio of a designed reference measure. The relative validity of the reference measure is thereby set to 1, by definition (24). These relative validates are equivalent to the ratio of sample sizes that would be required to detect the known group difference using one measure versus the other. When a dichotomous criterion is used, it is possible to perform standard contingency table analysis, examining sensitivity and specificity of the HRQL measure at designated cutpoints. To minimize the effects of a specific cut point, receiver-operator characteristic (ROC) methods can be employed. Hanley and McNeil (25) reported a practical method of estimating the area under a ROC using the Wilcoxon statistic. They also developed a nonparametric method for comparing ROC curves from the same sample (26). The area under ROC curves, their standard errors, and the significance of difference between areas for different measures can be calculated.

Responsiveness

The validity of a measure may be supported by cross-sectional analyses; however, the measure may not perform well at detecting small, but clinically meaningful, changes over time. A final indicator of validity that is important in clinical trials is responsiveness (27). Responsiveness refers to the ability of a measure to reflect underlying change (28,29). Although reliability and cross-sectional validity studies have been conducted on the widely used HRQL measures, there is very little information about their responsiveness. Quality-of-life changes can be compared to change in clinical status, intervening health events, interventions of known or expected efficacy, and direct reports of change by patients or providers (27,31,32).

Three statistics used to index responsiveness are effect size (32), *t*-test comparisons (24), and the responsiveness statistic (27). The formulas for these statistics are as follows:

$$\text{Paired } t\text{-statistic} = \frac{\text{D}}{\text{SE}}$$

$$\text{Effect-size statistic} = \frac{\text{D}}{\text{SD}}$$

$$\text{Responsiveness statistic} = \frac{\text{D}}{\text{SD\#}}$$

where D is the raw score change on measure, SE is the standard error of the difference, SD is the standard deviation at time 1, and SD# is the standard deviation of D among stable (those whose true status is constant over time) subjects.

The paired *t*-statistic is best suited to pre-post assessments of interventions of known efficacy. Relative validity calculations (ratios of the squares of paired *t*-statistics—see earlier discussion) for alternative measures can be used to compare their responsiveness to the intervention. The effect-size statistic relates change over time to the standard deviation of baseline scores. The responsiveness statistic looks at HRQL change relative to variability for clinically stable respondents. The effect-size statistic ignores variation in change entirely, the *t*-statistic ignores information about variation in scores for clinically stable respondents, and the responsiveness statistic ignores information about variation in scores for clinically instable respondents. When the results of a clinical trial comparing an intervention of known clinical efficacy with a control group are available, the most useful measure of responsiveness is a between-groups *t*-statistic for change scores (see below). This *t*-statistic allows for direct determination of the sample size needed to detect a given clinical effect for a particular HRQL measure.

$$\text{Between-groups } t\text{-statistic for change} = \frac{\text{D1} - \text{D2}}{\text{SE}}$$

where D1 is the raw score change for intervention group, D2 is the raw score change for control group, and SE is the standard error of the difference between group means.

Although not enough attention was given to the responsiveness of HRQL measures previously, investigators are increasingly providing this information. Evidence on responsiveness is provided in this volume for the Dermatology Life Quality Index (Chapter 7), and is available for the Dermatology Specific Quality of Life instrument (see Chapter 8) from its developers. Additional work is needed to calibrate the meaning of the responsiveness statistics themselves and how they relate to one another. If one statistic suggests one conclusion about relative scale performance and a second statistic suggests a different conclusion, which one is to be believed? It is always important to evaluate validity of a measure by considering all of the evidence collected in the areas pertaining to its content, construct, and responsiveness taken together.

SUMMARY

There is a need for psychometrically sound measures of HRQL for different applications in dermatology, such as comparing treatments in randomized controlled clinical trials, monitoring health of patients over time, and understanding the impact of skin diseases on patient functioning and well-being. Presently there is a dearth of literature describing the psychometric properties of such measures in clinical trials of skin disease treatments. It is not all that unusual to find that a measure viewed as "validated" is considered so simply because it has been used by other investigators, was published in a scientific journal, or has met only basic measurement criteria (e.g., internal consistency reliability). The concepts of reliability, validity, and responsiveness to change are important and should be presented for each instrument under consideration under varying research conditions. Thus, the process of validation is ongoing across populations, treatments, and study conditions. Consistent performance of a measure with regard to the stated psychometric properties is more important than single reports of positive or negative findings.

Many HRQL instruments specific to skin disease presently available were only recently developed and have just begun to establish an appreciable amount of evidence on validity and reliability. With this in mind, it is important that developers of new HRQL instruments carefully document the initial psychometric properties and update that information periodically in the literature for the benefit of interested researchers. A user's manual including technical data is another means of documenting this important information. Users of current instruments should carefully examine the psychometric properties of HRQL instruments, taking care to document the reliability and validity of the particular instrument in their own studies. An obstacle toward greater precision in measurement is the lack of refined theoretical models of HRQL applicable to skin diseases. Though there is rich clinical feedback about the benefits of dermatological treatments for patients' lives, there are few systematic descriptive reports in the literature (33). One important issue for consideration is whether several skin diseases share a sufficiently common framework of HRQL to be measured by a general dermatology HRQL instrument, or whether some diseases impose a unique profile of impact on daily life and well-being, requiring an independent focus. This should be the focus of future validation studies.

Much has been accomplished toward developing and refining HRQL instruments in dermatology. This positive trend signals the growing recognition more broadly within medicine and health policy of the need for HRQL information to evaluate care and to manage patients. This chapter hopefully supports this trend in its description of aspects of measurement that are standards for clinical studies and as a guidepost to help investigators select from among a growing array of HRQL measures.

REFERENCES

1. Wilson IB, Cleary PD. Linking clinical variables with health-related quality of life. JAMA 1995; 273(1): 59–65.
2. Anderson RT, McFarlane M, Naughton M, Shumaker SA. Conceptual issues and considerations in cross-cultural validation of generic health-related quality of life instruments. In: Spilker B, ed. Quality of Life and Pharmacoeconomics in Clinical Trials. 2d ed. Philadelphia: Lippincott-Raven, 1996: 605–612.
3. Shumaker SA, Anderson RA. The selection of heath-related quality of life measures for older patients with cardiovascular diseases. In: Walters PJ, ed. Coronary Bypass Surgery in the Elderly: Ethical, Economical and Quality of Life Aspects. Dordrecht: Kluwer Academic Publishers, 1995: 145–154.
4. Dimenäs E, Carlsson G, Glise H, Israelsson B, Wiklund I. Relevance of norm values as part of the documentation of quality of life instruments for use in upper gastrointestinal disease. Scand J Gastroenterol 1996; 31(suppl).
5. Baldor RA, Lapidus CS, Weinreb LF. Effective management of acne: considerations for the adult patient. J Clin Outcomes Manage 1996; 3(5): 9–20.
6. Tsevat J, Weeks JC, Guadagnoli E, Tosteson ANA, et al. Using health-related quality-of-life information: clinical encounters, clinical trials, and health policy. J Gen Intern Med 1994; 9: 576–582.
7. Anderson RT, Rajagopalan R. A profile of patients with contact dermatitis with suspected allergy (history, physical characteristics and quality of life). J Am Acad Dermatol 1997; 37: 41–50.
8. Fredriksson T, Pettersson U. Severe psoriasis—oral therapy with a new retinoid. Dermatologica 1978; 157: 238–244.
9. Cronbach LJ. Coefficient alpha and the internal structure of tests. Psychometrika 1959; 16: 297–334.
10. Feldt LS, Woodruff DJ, Salih FA. Statistical inference for coefficient alpha. Appl Psychol Measure 1987; 11: 93–103.
11. Goodenough WH. A technique for scale analysis. Ed Psychol Measure 1944; 4: 179–190.
12. Nunnally J. Psychometric Theory. 2d ed. New York: McGraw-Hill, 1978.
13. Hays RD, Sherbourne CD, Mazel RM. The RAND 36-Item Health Survey 1.0. Health Econ 1993; 2: 217–227.

14. Ware JE, Sherbourne CD. The MOS 36-Item Short-Form Health Survey (SF-36). I. Conceptual framework and item selection. Med Care 1992; 30:473–483.
15. Prisant LM, Carr AA, Bottini PB, Thompson WO, Rhoades RB. Repeatability of automated ambulatory blood pressure measurements. J Fam Pract 1992; 34:569–574.
16. Allen BB, Smith JG Arch Dermatol 1982; 118:23–35.
17. Stewart AL, Hays RD, Ware J. Methods of validating MOS health measures. In: Stewart AL, Ware JE, eds. Measuring Functioning and Well-Being: The Medical Outcomes Study Approach. Durham, NC: Duke University Press, 1992.
18. Jowett S, Ryan R. Skin disease and handicap: an analysis of the impact of skin conditions. Soc Sci Med 1985; 20(4):425–429.
19. Cronbach LJ, Meehl PE. Construct validity in psychological tests. Psychol Bull 1955; 52:281–302.
20. Campbell DT, Fiske DW. Convergent and discriminant validation by the multitrait-multimethod matrix. Psychol Bull 1959; 56:81–105.
21. Hayashi T, Hays RD. A microcomputer program for analyzing multitrait-multimethod matrices. Behav Res Methods Instruments Computers 1987; 19:345–348.
22. Kenny DA, Kashy DA. Analysis of the multitrait-multimethod matrix by confirmatory factor analysis. Psycho Bull 1992; 112:165–172.
23. Feldman SR, Fleischer AB, Reboussin DM, Rapp SR, et al. The Self-Administered Psoriasis Area and Severity Index Is Valid and Reliable. Soc Invest Dermatol 1996; 183–186.
24. Liang MH, Larson MG, Cullen KE, Schwartz JA. Comparative measurement efficiency and sensitivity of five health status instruments for arthritis research. Arthritis Rheumatol 1985; 28:545–547.
25. Hanley JA, McNeil BJ. The meaning and use of the area under a receiver operating characteristic (ROC) curve. Radiology 1982; 143:29–36.
26. Hanley JA, McNeil BJ. A method of comparing the areas under receiver operating characteristic curves derived from the same cases. Radiology 1983; 148, 839–843.
27. Guyatt G, Walter S, Norman G. Measuring change over time: assessing the usefulness of evaluative instruments. J Chronic Dis 1987; 40:171–178.
28. Hays R, Hadorn D. Responsiveness to change: an aspect of validity, not a separate dimension. Qual Life Res 1992; 1:73–75.
29. Kazis LE, Anderson JJ, Meenan RF. Effect sizes for interpreting changes in health status. Med Care 1989; 27:S178–S189.
30. Chambers LW, Haight M, Norman G, MacDonald L. Sensitivity to change and the effect of model of administration on health status measurement. Med Care 1987; 25:470–480.
31. MacKenzie CR, Charlson ME, DiGioia D, Kelley K. Can the sickness impact profile measure change? An example of scale assessment. J Chronic Dis 1986; 39:429–438.
32. Kazis LE, Anderson JJ, Meenan RF. Effect sizes for interpreting changes in health status. Med Care 1989; 27:S178–S189.
33. Rajagopalan, R, Anderson RT. Am J Contact Dermatitis 1997; 8:26–31.

4

Philosophical and Conceptual Issues in the Assessment of Quality of Life in Patients with Skin Disorders

John Koo *University of California, San Francisco Medical Center, San Francisco, California*

John Siebenlist *University of Texas Health Science Center, San Antonio, Texas*

INTRODUCTION

Over the years, quality-of-life assessments have been conducted for many different types of medical conditions. However, with regard to patients with skin disorders, the importance of qualitatively and quantitatively documenting quality of life has only recently gained widespread recognition. Consequently, even though there are numerous types of skin disorders ranging from acne to eczema, only for psoriasis does there exist a reasonably accepted instrument to measure quality of life, namely, the Psoriasis Disability Index (1). There are no universally accepted quality-of-life instruments for other skin conditions such as acne, eczema, vitiligo, alopecia, etc. This, in some ways, reflects the fact that psychodermatology, which focuses on the interface between the mind and the skin, has, until recently, received relatively little attention in the dermatology community in the United States. However, the recent changes in the health care system in the United States have resulted in increased interest in the dermatology community in assessing and more scientifically documenting quality-of-life issues among patients with skin disorders. In many ways, this came about as an indirect result of "belt-tightening" measures by the government and insurance companies restricting the resources devoted to health care. With every medical specialty competing for a cut of the same and limited financial pie, each field in clinical medicine, including dermatology, has developed an increased interest in "outcomes research" to better document the benefits resulting from our therapeutics.

With the enhanced awareness of the importance of conducting outcomes research, it became more apparent to dermatologists that it is important to develop a quality-of-life scale that is reliable, sensitive, and validated. However, in venturing into this new field, it is important to recognize that there are issues relatively unique to the assessment of skin patients as compared to the assessment of other medical conditions such as hypertension or cardiac disease. First, traditional outcome measures used in most areas of medicine, such as survival data or measurable changes in laboratory values, are most often not available to assess outcomes among skin patients because the threat of death is rare in dermatology practice and also many common skin conditions such as psoriasis do not have easily measurable laboratory data to document the status of the disease. On the other hand, patients with skin disorders can be greatly affected by disfigurement. Because skin disorders are frequently visible to others, the patient's quality of life may be devastated because of his or her body image or the reaction of others to his or her disfigurement (2–4). In other words, as one ventures into this new field of assessing quality-of-life issues in skin disease patients scientifically and quantitatively, understanding the underlying philosophical and conceptual issues involved so that one does not inadvertently "bark up the wrong tree" is very important. In this chapter, various issues pertaining to assessing quality of life in patients with skin disorders will be discussed, with an emphasis on those aspects unique to the application of quality-of-life assessment in the skin patient.

RELEVANT PARAMETERS FOR QUALITY-OF-LIFE ASSESSMENT IN SKIN PATIENTS

"Quality of life" is a somewhat vague and abstract term. To be able to assess quality of life quantitatively and scientifically, it is important to define all of the relevant parameters defining the term. In defining "quality of life," it is important to make the assessment as comprehensive as possible, encompassing the psychological, social, and occupational impact of a disease as well as its physical impact. Because most physicians, including dermatologists, have very limited training in the field of psychology or mental health, there is a natural tendency among some dermatologists to emphasize (or *exclusively* emphasize) the physical aspects of skin disease, such as the physical symptoms or limitations. Such a tendency is understandable, since most dermatologists will probably feel more comfortable discussing quality of life in physical terms and will intentionally or unintentionally avoid the more unfamiliar arena dealing with the psychosocial and occupational aspects of a disease. However, if the definition of "quality of life" is skewed this way, the inadvertent consequence seriously compromises understanding the full impact of skin disorders on the quality of life of patients and also devalues the benefits of dermatological therapy. As stated previously, unless the patient has the worst case of a skin condition, such as erythrodermic eczema or generalized pustular psoriasis, observable physical limitations such as the inability to ambulate would not be an issue. For the great majority of dermatological patients, the most important negative impacts on quality of life are appearance-related. Skin disorders rarely totally physically disable a patient, but they frequently disfigure them. Consequently, the psychosocial and occupational consequence of disfigurement is much more relevant for dermatological patients than are the purely physical limitations. In other words, if one were to leave out or deemphasize the psychosocial and occupational impact of disfigurement, one could easily trivialize dermatological interventions and minimize the documentable benefits in an outcome study (5).

In order to assess the full impact of skin disorders on a person's quality of life, it is important to consider at least four different aspects of the skin disorder: physical aspects, psychological impact, social impact, and occupational impact. The physical aspect has two subcomponents, namely, physical symptoms and physical (i.e., functional) limitations. "Physical symptoms" refers to the presence and intensity of symptoms such as itching, irritation, pain, etc. "Functional limitations" refers to observable, objective limitations on the part of the patient, such as the inability to use the hands or to ambulate due to the presence of a painful skin condition on the palms or soles.

Psychological impact refers to purely subjective, experiential factors such as the impact of the skin disease on self-esteem and body image, as well as the presence or absence of various subjective symptoms such as depression, anxiety, anger, embarrassment, self-consciousness, etc., which can compromise the patient's quality of life, even if nobody else seems to notice the presence of this intrapsychic distress in the patient. Social impact refers to the impact a skin disorder has on social functions such as courtship, sexual relationships, relationships with family members, etc. Finally, occupational impact refers to the impact of the skin disease on the types of occupation the patient can engage in, promotion or rejection in the workplace, etc.

For each of these aspects, one can assess both the patient's purely subjective discomfort and the "objective" assessment of how the skin disease has actually prevented the patient from participating in various activities. For instance, some patients may feel uneasy about dating because of their psoriasis, but this may not be enough to prevent one patient from dating, while another may shy away from such activity altogether. The impact of the skin disease on daily activities can be broken down into specific types of activities, such as swimming in public pools, going to beaches, participating in gym activities, going to hairdressers, clothing choice (to conceal the skin disorder), etc.

STRATEGY FOR VALIDATING A PSYCHOMETRIC INSTRUMENT DESIGNED TO MEASURE QUALITY-OF-LIFE ISSUES IN SKIN PATIENTS

Since the specific investigation of the impact of skin disorders on quality of life has just begun, there is a need to develop a validated psychometric instrument to quantitatively assess this aspect of skin disease. However, in developing any such psychometric test, it is important to have a clear understanding of how those instruments can be validated—what "gold standard" one can use to verify the fact that these instruments are accurate and useful. In the field of mental health, such validation of a new psychometric instrument is usually accomplished by showing a good correlation with existing, validated, and well-accepted psychometric tests such as the Minnesota Multi-Facet Personality Inventory (MMPI). However, this usual mode of validation may not be possible for a quality-of-life instrument to be used for skin disease patients for two reasons. First, the existing, validated psychometric tests are designed to measure global psychological functions rather than the psychosocial or occupational impact of a particular aspect of the subject's life, such as having eczema. Second, the use of existing, validated psychometric tests on skin patients may be inappropriate since most of the psychometric tests are designed to assess psychopathology in mental patients, and most patients with skin disorders do not have a diagnosable psychiatric condition.

Well-validated psychometric instruments such as the MMPI, Brief Symptom Inventory, Hopkin's Check List, etc. are designed to measure the overall psychological functioning of a person with special attention paid to assessing the presence of absence of certain psychiatric symptomatology. Using regular psychometric tests, if a subject is found to have "low self-esteem" or "depression," there is no logical reason to assume that such symptoms necessarily result from the presence of the skin disease. For example, a particular individual with "depression" may be feeling depressed because of financial problems, difficulties with a mother-in-law, being sued by a neighbor, or some other psychosocial stressor that happens to be active at the time the test is taken. Therefore, it is totally unpredictable whether such a global finding will correlate with the specific psychosocial impact indicated by the patient with the new instrument in relationship to the presence of a specific skin disorder. Even in cases where a certain correlation might be found between the result of these validated psychometric tests and the new instrument designed to assess quality of life in skin patients, one can never be sure whether such a correlation might have been fortuitous rather than indicating a real relationship between the results of the two instruments.

Elaborating on the second point, the majority of the psychometric tests that are well accepted and validated are designed to assess psychopathology in the psychiatric population. Therefore, they frequently contain questions about homicidal ideation, suicidal ideation, paranoid delusions, auditory hallucinations, etc. If the investigator is interested in developing another instrument to assess psychopathology, the use of a correlation between the new instrument with the existing, validated psychometric instruments is valid. However, for skin patients, most of whom are not "mental cases," the use of these instruments as validating tools is not appropriate; the types of questions as stated above are more likely to confuse and confound the findings.

If it is conceptually invalid to use existing psychometric instruments to validate a new questionnaire to assess quality-of-life issues in skin patients, one needs an alternative method of validation to be confident that the issues being assessed are relevant to the skin condition in question. Conceptually, it would make more sense to validate a particular physical, psychosocial, or occupational issue by demonstrating a good correlation between these quality-of-life factors and the severity of the skin disease. With regard to a particular item being assessed, whether it is physical, psychological, social, or occupational, if the patient indicates the same intensity of distress whether he or she has a severe skin disease or no skin disease (i.e., the skin disease in question is in complete remission), one can conclude that particular item has no relevance with regard to the quality-of-life impact of that skin disorder. On the other hand, if another item shows a good correlation between the intensity of the distress indicated by the patient and the severity of the skin disease, despite the presence of natural variation in the patient's subjective experiences, then one can be reasonably assured it is valid to include that item in an assessment of the quality-of-life impact of the skin disease in question.

ASSESSING OBJECTIVELY AND QUANTITATIVELY THE SEVERITY OF SKIN DISEASE

In order to make the most reliable validation, it is important for patients to be quantitatively assessed with regard to the severity of their skin disease. It would be ideal if patients were objectively evaluated by a dermatologist using a well-accepted method of assessing the severity of the skin disease, such as the Psoriasis Area and Severity Index (PASI). If this is not feasible, a compromise approach may be to use some form of the patient's own assessment that is quantitative, such as drawing in areas of involvement on a standardized figure of human skin surfaces, for example, a self-assessment PASI score.

GENERATING RELEVANT QUALITY-OF-LIFE ISSUES

Before any questionnaire designed to assess quality-of-life issues can be constructed, it is critical to generate the right type of questions to assess the most relevant issues experienced by the patient population. Since it is not practical to assess every conceivable physical, psychological, social, or occupational issue, one must first ascertain which questions are likely to be most relevant and important for the largest number of patients with regard to the quality-of-life impact of their skin disease. For example, in the realm of psychological impact, is it more important to ask about low self-esteem, depression, or social phobias? With regard to day-to-day activities, is it more important to ask about inhibitions regarding going to the gym, going to the beach, or going to the hairdresser? Rather than the investigator arbitrarily limiting the types and numbers of issues to be explored by the way he or she constructs the first draft of the questionnaire, a more scientific and conceptually superior approach would be to give the patient an opportunity to express the most important ways the skin disease affects his or her life in a free, unstructured setting with minimal interference by the investigators. This can be accomplished by having randomly selected subjects talk freely about their experiences into a tape recorder in private, without the presence of an investigator or any other individual. These responses can be analyzed and a list can be formulated of the most frequently mentioned psychological issues and activities of daily living impacted by the skin disease. Once such a "master list" of relevant issues and activities is generated, one is in a much better position to construct a questionnaire with the highest probability of accurately documenting the impact of the skin disease on quality of life.

SELECTING THE MOST APPROPRIATE PATIENT POPULATIONS TO BE STUDIED

In the process of creating an accurate instrument to assess quality-of-life issues, it is critical that such an instrument be tested on a statistically balanced patient population rather than a sample of convenience. Such a population needs to be well balanced with regard to demographic characteristics such as gender, severity of the disease, ethnic background, etc. If the sample population upon which the instrument was based turns out to be excessively skewed toward severe cases, the resulting instrument may only be valid in assessing other severe cases. For example, the Psoriasis Disability Index (PDI), which was developed in England, heavily emphasizes the assessment of physical disability while minimizing the assessment of the psychological impact of psoriasis. In England dermatologists do not have ready access to mild to moderate psoriasis patients, since they are mainly followed by primary care physicians. Therefore, an instrument was developed based on patients with severe disease hospitalized in British hospitals. When such an instrument is applied to totally different populations such as the average mild to moderate psoriasis cases seen by dermatologists in the United States, many of the issues explored in the instrument, such as physical disability, become irrelevant, while the more relevant psychological issues remain unassessed. This is clearly illustrated in a recently published epidemiological study on psoriasis with emphasis on quality-of-life issues where the data was derived from statistically balanced population samples from the entire United States (6). In the psychiatric literature, it is also well known that women tend to be more open about reporting psychosocial distress than are men. Also, certain ethnic populations such as first-generation Chinese-Americans and Hispanics are also known to have a tendency toward emphasizing physical complaints while minimizing psychological, subjective complaints (7–9). Because of these issues, it is critical to develop a questionnaire regarding quality-of-life issues based on a well-balanced patient population.

CONCLUSION

Even though dermatologists may have had a tendency to emphasize the purely physical assessments such as morphology and the extent of skin disease in assessing outcomes of treatments or clinical research, patients have always recognized quality-of-life issues as being of critical importance in how they perceive the effectiveness of dermatological therapy. Because of the advent of health care reform and the managed care "revolution" in the United States, there has been an enhanced recognition by the dermatological community of the importance of documenting the impact of skin disorders on patients' quality of life and understanding how they are modified by therapeutic interventions. However, because this is a relatively new field of endeavor for the dermatology community, before one attempts to develop reliable, validated instruments to more quantitatively and scientifically document the impact of skin disease and therapy on patients' quality-of-life, it is important to make sure that the philosophical and conceptual understanding of this subject matter is well grounded. In this chapter, many of the relevant conceptual issues were discussed, including the importance of comprehensiveness in assessing quality of life, the pitfalls of using existing psychometric tests for validation, a suggestion regarding validating future quality-of-life instruments using a positive correlation with the severity of the skin disease as the "gold standard," the importance of ascertaining relevant issues in a nonstructured environment, and the importance of testing questionnaires on a well-balanced, statistically validated population sample. With these conceptual guidelines, one can maximize the chance of developing reliable and accurate questionnaires in assessing quality-of-life issues among dermatological patients, which will be the critical first step in our effort to more comprehensively document the outcomes of dermatological therapeutic interventions.

REFERENCES

1. Finlay AY, Khan GK, Luscombe DK, Salek MS. Validation of Sickness Impact Profile and Psoriasis Disability Index in psoriasis. Br J Dermatol 1990; 123:751–756.
2. Gupta MA, Gupta AK, Haberman HF. Psoriasis and psychiatry: an update. Gen Hosp Psych 1987; 9:157–166.
3. Ginsberg IH Link BG. Feeling of stigmatization in patients with psoriasis. JAAD 1989; 20:53–63.
4. Ben-Tovim DI, Walker MK. Body image, disfigurement and disability. J Psychosom Res 1995; 39(3):283–291.
5. Jowett S, Ryan TJ. Skin disease and handicap: an analysis of the impact of skin conditions. Soc Sci Med 1985; 20:425–429.
6. Koo JYM. Population-based epidemiological study of psoriasis with emphasis on quality of life assessment. Dermatol Clinics 1996; 14(3):485–496.
7. Farooq S, Gahir MS, Okyere E, Sheikh AJ, Oyebode F. Somatization: a transcultural study. J Psychosom Res 1995; 39(7):883–888.
8. Escobar JI. Cross-cultural aspects of the somatization trait. Hosp Commun Psych 1987; 38(2):174–180.
9. DuAlba L, Scott RL. Somatization and malingering for workers' compensation applicants: a cross-cultural MMPI study. J Clin Psychol 1993; 49(6):913–917.

5

Sexually Transmitted Disease

Implications of This Diagnosis for Patients' Lives

Melissa McPheeters and Peggy Clarke *American Social Health Association, Research Triangle Park, North Carolina*

INTRODUCTION

A diagnosis for a sexually transmitted disease (STD) can generate an intense emotional reaction in many patients. The way the infection is acquired, as well as its anatomical site, distinguishes this diagnosis as one that calls for unique communications between patients and their health care professionals. While clinicians are logically focused on the physical nature of infections, patients with STDs may be more concerned with the personal, interpersonal, and sexual aspects of their condition. For some patients, the diagnosis may trigger feelings of low self-esteem, immediate concerns about their sexual relationship(s), and a preoccupation with how and when the infection was contracted (1,2). With viral STDs, such as genital herpes, external genital warts, and other HPV infections, the additional knowledge that the infection is likely incurable—albeit manageable—can be distressing.

In educating and counseling patients who are newly diagnosed with a viral STD, focusing on the physical manifestations of the infection to the exclusion of the emotional and personal aspects of the conditions is counterproductive. It may leave patients dissatisfied with their level of care, confused about their reactions, and unsure about how to manage their condition. Achieving a balance between educating patients about their physical condition and counseling them about the emotions that may accompany the diagnosis can be difficult. In addition, providing anticipatory guidance on protective sexual behavior and the need to communicate the infectious status to sexual partners can make the counseling process potentially complicated and possibly daunting to the providers faced with the task.

Some barriers to counseling issues include an added burden in terms of time and resources, particularly in busy clinic and office settings, and clinician skill and comfort in communicating to the patient receiving psychoeducational material. Clinicians in medical practice have recounted that the emotional reaction to a genital herpes diagnosis, for example, is sometimes disproportionate to the medical significance of the infection, and some are concerned that the response can block patient understanding of treatment or management advice due to the high levels of stress at time of diagnosis.

BACKGROUND

The majority of the literature on STD counseling to date focuses on counseling individuals with HIV infection (3–5). While this is not surprising, given the virulence of HIV infection and the need to address urgent counseling issues due to the life-threatening nature of the infection, clinicians wishing to appropriately counsel patients with other STDs have little guidance in their efforts since most of the HIV-counseling guidelines are less applicable to patients with other STDs. In comparison with HIV, the medical significance of a diagnosis with HSV and the vast majority of HPV infections is clearly slight and the counseling needs are decidedly and dramatically different. But from the perspective of the patient who often lacks a global view of the medically trained profession, diagnosis with this clinically benign infection can be extremely traumatic.

In this chapter, the implications of a diagnosis with viral sexually transmitted disease will be presented from the patients's viewpoint based on survey data and experiences recounted by patients who have called the National STD hotline and the National Herpes Hotline, both operated by the American Social Health Association (ASHA). With that as background, the chapter will include a suggested counseling approach with particular concentration on the anticipatory guidance for newly diagnosed individuals.

PRACTICAL INFORMATION PATIENTS NEED TO KNOW

Herpes

One in four Americans is estimated to be infected with genital herpes infection, with perhaps two thirds of that population being unaware of their infection. (3). With such high prevalence and an apparent increase in the spread of herpes simplex virus (HSV) in this country, the number of patients presenting with HSV lesions will continue to rise. With new information about the benefits of antiviral therapy and expanded treatment options, more demand for patient counseling should be expected.

Nature of the Infection

Patients need to understand that herpes is a viral skin condition that is transmitted sexually. It is caused by one of two viruses: herpes simplex type 1 (HSV-1) and herpes simplex type 2 (HSV-2). While the symptoms of a herpes outbreak can be treated, the disease itself is not curable. The virus remains latent in the body, producing periodic outbreaks. The first episode of a herpes outbreak, which tends to be much more pronounced than later outbreaks, usually occurs within 2 weeks after the virus is transmitted. On the other hand, some people's first episode is so mild they don't even notice it. The episode that brings them to a physician may be a reactivation that is first noticed months or years after they contracted the virus (6).

Signs and symptoms of genital herpes vary greatly and include skin irregularities, itching, or the "classic" blisterlike lesions that crust over. In recurrent herpes, healing generally takes less than half the time as for first episodes. It is possible for the virus to be active, or transmissible, in the absence of recognizable symptoms either because the symptoms are so mild that the patient does not notice them or through asymptomatic shedding.

Herpes is spread through direct skin-to-skin contact, including sexual contact when there are no recognized symptoms. Herpes is often transmitted by people who are unaware that they are infected or by people who don't recognize that their herpes infection is in its active phase.

Treatment

The treatments available for genital herpes address the discomfort associated with the symptoms and promote healing, but they do not cure the disease itself. A patient may use acute therapy, in which medication is taken only during outbreaks, or suppressive therapy, in which medication is taken every day to control HSV. The decision to follow a particular course of treatment must be made by the physician and patient while considering the frequency, duration, and intensity of symptoms as well as cost and convenience. Patients should understand that they remain infectious while taking antiviral medicine.

Of more than 3000 respondents to an ASHA survey of people with herpes, 78.6% had taken oral acyclovir for genital herpes, but many had not submitted insurance claims although they were eligible for reimbursement.

Three fourths of respondents said they were sure their insurance covered all or part of prescription drugs, but only half had submitted a claim to cover the costs of oral acyclovir. (Only 12.7% said their health insurance did not cover prescription drugs; 6.2% were not sure, and 3.8% did not currently have health insurance.)

The survey did not ask why people with the option of filing did not submit claims. However, anecdotal experience from ASHA's Herpes Resource Center indicates that at least some patients are concerned about confidentiality if they file a claim.

Human Papillomavirus

One of the most common STDs, human papillomavirus (HPV), affects between 20 and 40 million Americans. Some estimates indicate that as many as 1 million people are infected annually. HPV is often asymptomatic, although some strains of the virus cause genital warts or cervical dysplasia (7).

Nature of the Infection

HPV is a potentially persistent viral infection that is most often sexually transmitted. HPV is implicated in both genital warts and cervical cancer, but the viral types of HPV likely to cause warts are not the same types that are linked to cancer. HPV and genital warts are usually spread by direct, skin-to-skin contact during vaginal, anal, or oral sex with someone who has this infection. Warts on other parts of the body, such as the hands, are caused by different types of HPV. Contact with these warts does not seem to cause genital warts. Warts may appear within several weeks after sexual relations with an infected person, or they may take months to appear, or they may never appear. This makes it difficult, if not impossible, to trace the infection to a source partner. Very little is known about the duration of infectiousness or the transmission of subclinical HPV (8).

Treatment

Health care providers should explain the rationale for treating vs. not treating genital warts or cervical dysplasia, as well as the treatment failure and recurrence rates. Patients should understand that some treatments require multiple applications before they are effective. Some treatments can cause scarring or have side effects or may simply be more uncomfortable than is warranted by the severity of the infection. In terms of follow-up, patients should be instructed about time to healing and about the potential need to refrain from sex until tissue is fully healed.

PERSONAL IMPLICATIONS OF AN STD DIAGNOSIS: LISTENING TO PATIENTS' CONCERNS

Through the operation of the National STD Hotline and the National Herpes Hotline, as well as the management of the Herpes Resource Center, the ASHA provides education and counseling services to an estimated 160,000 people concerned about herpes each year. Because ASHA had little data available beyond their vast experience regarding the impact of herpes infection on people's lives, the organization conducted a systematic survey of a group of 5000 people with genital herpes. (9) The sample was randomly selected from the readership of ASHA's quarterly newsletter, *the helper*, which is written for individuals with genital herpes. While this is clearly a highly specialized group and caution must be taken in interpreting the results for any other population, this is the largest survey of patients on this sensitive topic area, and the results may be instructive to providers who are assessing or planning their counseling practices.

A greater than 60% response rate was achieved for this survey, which included over 200 questions, indicating a high degree of interest and concern. A majority of respondents (65%) were male; 80% were over 30 years of age, 92% were Caucasian, and 70% reported having graduated from college. Ninety percent of the respondents had experienced at least one outbreak in the 12 months prior to the study, and 55% had experienced their first genital herpes outbreak 6 or more years prior to the study.

Initial diagnosis had a dramatic effect on many people. When asked to recall their reactions to the initial diagnosis with genital herpes, most reported feeling depressed (82%) and isolated (69%). They also feared rejection (75%) and discovery (55%), and more than a quarter (28%) reported self-destructive feelings at the time of diagnosis.

Over time, negative feelings about a diagnosis with genital herpes infection appeared to decrease, indicating adjustment or management by many. When asked to reflect on their reactions to their herpes infection during the recent 12 months, 36% reported feelings of isolation and 28% feared discovery. However, 52% reported recent feelings of depression due to their infection and 52% still feared rejection.

Individuals who are notified that they have an STD are often concerned about how it will affect their social and sexual relationships. In ASHA's herpes study (9), 89% expressed concern about transmitting their infection to a partner, 69% feared rejection by a new partner, and 20% had, in fact, experienced rejection related to their infection.

IMPLICATIONS OF AN HPV DIAGNOSIS

To better understand the psychosocial issues that affect people with HPV, ASHA surveyed 837 individuals who receive *HPV News*, ASHA's quarterly newsletter about HPV. A total of 454 surveys were completed and analyzed (10). Most (77%) respondents were female, and 76% were at least 30 years of age. Ninety-two percent had attended college, with 70% having graduated. Most (72%) were in a relationship, with 45% currently married or living with a partner. Almost all (98%) were heterosexual. Nearly half of the respondents had had HPV for at least 3 years, and the majority (60%) reported having had visible warts at some time.

Like the respondents to the herpes survey, individuals with HPV reported a number of negative feelings when they were diagnosed with their infection. Their initial reactions included anger (78%), depression (76%), isolation (70%), fear of rejection (70%), shame (66%), and guilt (60%). These feelings did tend to decrease dramatically over time.

Respondents also had significant concerns about how HPV would affect their relationships, with 72% feeling sexually less desirable due to their infection and 68% enjoying sexual contact less. In addition, two thirds were concerned that their infection would cause them to be rejected by a potential sexual partner. Nineteen percent reported that they had been rejected by a sexual partner due to their infection.

In terms of how they felt about the care provided by their practitioners, most respondents were dissatisfied. Nearly 60% rated their providers either "poor" or "fair", and the highest levels of dissatisfaction were noted regarding providers failing to offer advice on emotional issues surrounding the infection (84%) and failing to ask questions about sexual practices to provide the best health care (75%).

COUNSELING ISSUES

ASHA's research clearly demonstrates that appropriate counseling is important to patients upon diagnosis of a sexually transmitted disease and that assistance in dealing with the psychosocial ramifications of the diagnosis is deemed beneficial by patients. However, discussing sexual matters can be difficult for practitioners, who are often not taught appropriate methods for broaching the subject, and for patients, who are concerned that their clinician may judge them negatively if they want to discuss sexuality.

Other studies have also shown need for improvement in the area of communication and counseling around an STD diagnosis. For example, a 1992 national survey by the Centers for Disease Control and Prevention of primary care physicians in the United States found that only 49% asked new adult patients about STDs, 31% about condom use, 27% about sexual orientation, and 22% about the number of sexual partners. By comparison, 94% asked these same patients about cigarette smoking behavior (11). One review of practice in five health departments found that, although almost all patients were diagnosed with an STD, about a quarter of the patients did not receive any information about treatment or prevention, and only slightly more than half were given complete information about their condition.

Of course, providing appropriate counseling is not easy. Communication between provider and patient is subject to the same constraints as are other interpersonal relationships. These include verbal mismatches, in which the provider and patient differ in their levels of communication skills, or differing personality styles. Cultural, experiential, or other outlook differences can be a barrier, as can differing demographic characteristics, such as gender, race, or age. Finally, the physical environment (noise, privacy, etc.) and the type of relationships the provider has with the patient (first encounter, long-term patient) can influence communication.

Another barrier may be that providers prejudge whether or not taking a sexual history is appropriate for specific patients. They may not want to bring up sexual matters with patients who they perceive to be at low risk of sexually transmitted disease, even in the face of an STD diagnosis (12, 13).

Even without these barriers, the traditional patient/provider relationship, in which the provider is the authority over the patient, can itself be intimidating. The patient may wait for the provider to broach the subject of sexual health, assuming that the provider will do so if it is important, and the provider may assume that the patient will bring it up if need be (14). In particular, with an infection like herpes or HPV, the provider and patient may have extremely different views on the importance of the infection in the patient's life. The provider may view the infection as medically benign, and therefore not terribly important. For the patient, the fact that the discomfort accompanying the infection is mild may be overshadowed by emotional turmoil.

ASHA COUNSELING MODEL

ASHA worked with an advisory panel of medical experts to design tools that might assist health care providers with counseling patients in a clinical setting. The resultant counseling model (Fig. 1), combined with numerous patient education materials, helps physicians counsel patients on all aspects of sexual health and educate the patient (15).

The counseling model consists of four discrete stages. Stage One, prescreening counseling, is based on a complete sexual health history that examines personal risk-taking behaviors and clinical symptoms in the patient and partner(s). In Stage Two, the clinician determines whether STD screening for the patient is indicated. If screening is elected, counseling should include a discussion of reasons for the screening, what the procedure will

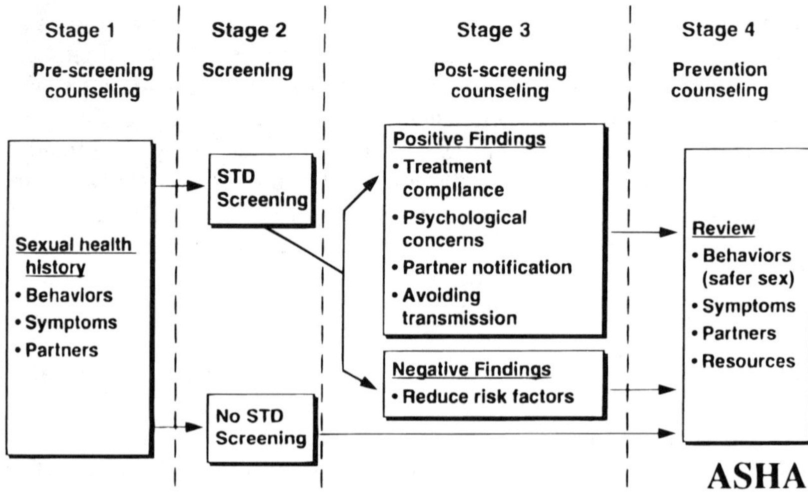

Figure 1 American Social Health Association STD counseling model.

entail, and any associated cost considerations for the procedure. If screening is not elected, the patient receives the counseling associated with Stage Four, prevention counseling.

Stage Three, for patients who receive screening, addresses postscreening considerations. If a patient tests positive, it is important to discuss several topics relevant to the specific diagnosis. These topics include a review of both the short-term and long-term implications of the infection, a discussion of the treatment options and compliance concerns, partner(s) notification and follow-up requirements, and a discussion of infection-control strategies. For patients with negative screening results, discussion includes the limitations of such results.

Stage Four of the model addresses prevention counseling. All patients need to understand fundamental concepts of STD prevention, including safer sex practices, clinical signs and symptoms, and partner considerations. They also need to know where they can turn for further information and emotional support related to STDs.

In Stage One, a careful sexual history should be taken, using nonjudgemental, assumption-free questions. Questions about the number and gender of sexual partners—and the likelihood that a partner has other sexual partners—should be asked as tactfully as possible. Generally, open-ended questions that permit the patient to explain an answer are better than questions that can be answered in one word. While eliciting information about sexual history, it is important to watch carefully for verbal and nonverbal cues of confusion, misinformation, or anxiety. Using straightforward terms for sexual behavior and body parts facilitates comfort and honesty with responses.

The screening counseling that takes place in Stage Two is relatively short and consists mainly of explaining the decision to screen to the patient. Discussion about clinical concerns or suspicions of STD provides the physician with an opportunity to educate the patient about STDs. Another component of Stage Two counseling is a description of the procedure involved in screening, including associated costs.

The counseling that takes place after screening obviously depends on the screening results. For patients who receive negative results, the possibility of a false-negative test should be reviewed. In addition, negative results provide an opportunity to reevaluate personal practices and consider lifestyle modifications. Patients should also be reminded that screening for any one STD is not universal; it is possible to test negative for one infection and still asymptomatically harbor another infection.

Patients with positive findings require more detailed counseling. Applying this stage to a patient with genital herpes or HPV, the health care provider should discuss several key topics. A full explanation of the implications of infection should begin the discussion. This would include a description of the natural history of the disease. Patients should also be informed about available treatment regimens. As the ASHA surveys demonstrate, people with genital herpes or HPV often have psychological concerns at the time of first outbreak and diagnosis. It is important that health care providers acknowledge the negative emotions a patient may feel and provide anticipatory guidance on emotional issues. Simply acknowledging that negative feelings at the time of diagnosis are normal or common may help patients understand that the feelings will pass and help them handle their own emotions.

People recently diagnosed with herpes or HPV are often concerned about identifying the sexual partner who transmitted the infection to them or about letting current or future partners know about the disease. It is important to acknowledge that the patient may not be able to identify the person from whom they contracted the infection. In addition, they need to be able to explain their diagnosis and how it will affect their sexual activity to their current and future partner(s). Written instructions for partner notification are often helpful.

Finally, counseling should include referrals for more information and emotional support. By openly discussing STDs during all routine visits, and by providing support to those diagnosed with incurable, viral STDs, in particular, clinicians help their patients become more comfortable discussing sexual health, and increase their awareness and practice for preventive behaviors.

CONCLUSION

Counseling patients diagnosed with an STD, particularly a viral STD, is clearly an important part of patient care. However, it is understandably a difficult undertaking for many physicians. There are few guidelines for the practice of this type of patient counseling, and in our society, addressing issues of sexuality can be uncomfortable under any circumstances. To help address this problem, ASHA conducted surveys to better understand patients' emotional issues, the results of which were presented in this chapter. Patients are clearly concerned about much more than the physical implications of their diagnosis, and most would like their clinicians to address the psychosocial and psychosexual issues they face. To assist with this process, ASHA also developed the counseling model presented here. By following this model, clinicians can be more comfortable that they are addressing the range of issues their patients are facing and are guided in their approach to these very difficult, sexual issues.

REFERENCES

1. VanderPlate C, Aral SO. Psychosocial aspects of genital herpes virus infection. Health Psychol 1987; 6: 57–72.
2. Catotti D. Survey shows how we live HPV. HPV News 1993; 3(2): 4–8.
3. Centers for Disease Control. 1991 Division of STD/HIV Prevention Annual Report. Atlanta: Center for Prevention Services, Centers for Disease Control, 1992: 167.
4. Department of Health and Human Services. Coping with AIDS: Psychological and Social Considerations in Helping People with HTLV-III Infection. Washington, DC: U.S. Government Printing Office, 1986.
5. World Health Organization. Report from Consultation on Psychological Research Needs in HIV Infection and AIDS. Geneva: World Health Organization, 1987.
6. Ebel C. Managing Herpes: How to Live and Love with a Chronic STD. Research Triangle Park, NC: American Social Health Association, 1994.
7. CDC, 1993.
8. AMA Consensus Conference on External Genital Warts, Palm Springs, CA, 1997.
9. Catotti DN, Clarke P, Catoe KE. Herpes revisited. Sex Trans Dis 1993; 20(2): 77–80.
10. Clarke P, Ebel C, Catotti DN, Stewart S. The psychosocial impact of human papillomavirus infection: implications for health care provides. Int J STD AIDS 1996; 7: 197–200.

11. Loft J, Marder W, Bresolin L, Rinaldi R. HIV prevention practices of primary-care physicians—Unites States, 1992. MMWR 1994; 42(51, 52): 988–992.
12. Ende J, Rockwell S, Glasgow M. The sexual history in general medicine practice. Arch Intern Med 1984; 144: 558–561.
13. Lewis CE, Freeman HE. The sexual history-taking and counseling practices of primary care physicians. West J Med 1987; 147(2): 165–167.
14. Alexander L, Clarke P. Effective STD counseling. In: STD Counseling and Treatment Guide. Research Triangle Park, NC: American Social Health Association, 1995.
15. Alexander L, Clarke P. The ASHA STD counseling model. In: STD Counseling and Treatment Guide. Research Triangle Park, NC: American Social Health Association, 1995.

6

Personal Impact of Chronic Skin Disease

One Patient's Perspective

Curtis S. Phinney *Herndon, Virginia*

INTRODUCTION

The incidence of genital herpes is rapidly reaching pandemic proportions worldwide. Genital herpes has become the most common cause of genital ulceration, with an estimated 107 million people infected worldwide. The condition is generally considered to be underdiagnosed, with only about one in five of the seropositive population having recognized symptomatic expression of their infection. Even this population is often undertreated, with less than one in three having taken a course of antiviral therapy. A number of consumer issues have arisen as a result of this situation. Patients are unhappy with the management of their condition overall. This has led to a rethinking of control strategies by the medical profession. The need is recognized to better address patient concerns with regard to genital herpes natural history, sequelae, and treatment options. Understanding and investigating the patient's point of view and including it in the development of a practical control strategy is now seen as essential in addressing that need.

HERPES SIMPLEX VIRUS—AN OVERVIEW

Infection with some member of the herpes virus group is, in fact, quite common. One or both of the two types of herpes simplex virus will have infected the majority of Americans by the time that they reach adulthood. Herpes simplex virus type one (HSV-1) has infected approximately 80% of adults in the United States. In 1978, herpes simplex virus type two (HSV-2) was estimated to have infected 16% of the population in the United States between the ages of 15 and 74 years (1). By 1991, HSV-2 seroprevalence had increased to 22% in the same age group (2). The rates of acquisition of new, primary infection are estimated to be about 2–4% per year.

HSV-1 is often referred to as "oral herpes" or "cold sores." This strain generally, but not always, infects the areas around the mouth. HSV-2 or "genital herpes" generally is associated with the genitalia as the site of infection. Obviously, many individuals are infected with both strains.

Patients who are symptomatic and seropositive for HSV-2 virtually all experience recurrence within 2 years of their primary outbreak. Genital expression if HSV-1 has a much lower recurrence rate. Typing (IgG, IgM, or Western blot) for which strain a patient has at first presentation therefore is of some predictive value to the physician. The focus of this discussion is primarily with the physical and psychosocial implications of recurrent HSV-2 (or HSV-1) in the genital area.

The first, or primary, clinical manifestation of genital herpes is often associated with illness, often resembling flu symptoms. In addition, one may experience redness, itching, burning, and the formation of blisters in the genital area. The blisters are, at first, small and white in appearance. They are covered by a fragile layer of tissue, and often appear in clusters, or clumps. The fragile covering is often subsequently broken away, leaving clusters of weeping red pitted sores. This area eventually scabs over and heals. Symptoms may vary widely from this description, however, or the infection may be entirely asymptomatic.

Asymptomatic viral activity at the surface of the skin, or "shedding," is believed to be a major route of HSV-2 transmission. Asymptomatic shedding of HSV-2 may occur in measurable amounts about 1 day out of 25, during the first year following a primary infection. The frequency of shedding seems to decrease after the first year, to about 1 day in 100. The frequency of subclinical shedding for HSV-1 is much lower, even if the clinical expression is in the genital area.

Medical complications of herpes infections are infrequent, but potentially severe. Infections of the fingers (herpetic Whitlow) and eyes (ocular herpes) are reported. An individual may be at higher risk for these types of infections via autoinoculation during primary clinical manifestations of the disease. This may be due to the generally high severity of a first outbreak, the lack of a conditioned immune response, and patient unfamiliarity with the condition. Ocular herpes is most often caused by HSV-1 and may resemble conjunctivitis. Herpetic infection can also occur in the cornea (keratitis) or the iris (iritis). Uncommon complications of HSV infection include viral meningitis and neuralgia of the type often associated with shingles infections. Active outbreaks, particularly primary outbreaks, are hazardous from the standpoint of infecting infants during vaginal delivery. Infant infections also infrequently occur prior to birth, in the uterus, or after birth by direct infectious contact.

Psychological and Social Adjustment

The natural history of psychosocial adjustment to herpes infections has received considerable attention. In one such study, subjects with multiple episodes of genital herpes participated (3) in a questionnaire-based investigation to investigate the causal relationship between stress and outbreaks of HSV. Stress was reported as a factor by 78% of the individuals who completed the study. Over half the study participants cited being physically run down as a factor. They frequency of patient sexual activity had not changed significantly, and the majority had told their partners of their infection. Most people were found to be able over time to adjust to the psychosocial changes associated with managing herpes, but a significant minority did not. Easing the adjustment process and identification and treatment of these patients could have the benefit of improving life quality for the patients and lowering the incidence of transmission to others. The patients had a mean age of 34, were single (63%), and generally were well educated and from the middle to upper social classes. Almost half the respondents had at least one other STD. This was a highly sexually active population overall. The study showed that the severity of symptoms beared no relation to "postrecovery" sexual activity. Reduced sexual activity during the first 6 months was common, however.

While 68% of respondents said that they would tell a future sexual partner, 11% said outright that they would not and 21% would not commit. This subpopulation is much more likely to transmit the condition to an uniformed partner by accident or by design. Patients who avail themselves of herpes-specific social support (see below) are more able to face the challenges associated with confiding in a potential partner, thereby allowing partners to make informed choices with regard to managing their risk of infection.

Women in this study were more apt to feel less desirable sexually, have lowered self-confidence, feel dirty, and suffer anxiety over their general health and future outbreaks. However, they were less likely to harbor bitterness and resentment toward the person they felt was responsible for infecting them. In general, distressed individuals reported a reduced capacity for intimacy, interest in sex, ability to climax, and overall enjoyment of sex. They reported improved relationships with family, while relationships with friends and partners worsened.

Those individuals in a relationship reported *increased* levels of interest in sex and heightened enjoyment. This may be the result of arriving at a new self-perception of one's sexuality, thereby reassessing the role of sex relations in one's life.

Relation of Stress and Depression on Symptoms

Recent studies have suggested that the oft-mentioned relationship between stress and outbreaks may not be as strongly correlated as patients seem to feel. Stress was the most commonly indicated cause of recurrences of HSV in the study by Brookes et al. (3). Almost 8 out of 10 patients associated stress with outbreaks. However, Zorilla et al. found clinical recurrence to have a stronger correlation with depression than with stress (4). This study suggests that certain individuals may be more prone to clinical manifestation of the virus as a response to stressors or depression than the majority of subjects. Even in the case of depression, the statistical correlation was of "marginal predictive value."

Reconciling these academic observations with my own personal experience is challenging. It certainly has been my observation, both during outbreaks and after careful thought, that my own outbreaks were directly related to stressful periods in my life. This was particularly clear during the period prior to initiating suppressive antiviral therapy. Do stressful life events predispose some of us to depressive conditions? Could those conditions actually be the causal factor in triggering outbreaks? If so, it is certainly a connection that is not readily apparent to many patients, myself among them. There was a tendency on my part to start to dread the possibility of an outbreak during stressful situations. Rather than mentally projecting the onset of a severe recurrence, coping with the possibility of symptoms on a day-to-day basis would certainly have left me in a better position to deal with the stressor event itself. Ideally this sort of acceptance-based mind set would forestall the "stress-related" outbreak entirely. Similarly to when a patient tells a friend or potential partner about HSV, the patient may have some control over the degree to which emotional distress and the associated immunological changes are associated with stressors.

Herpes infection is often of minor consequence or even entirely subclinical. Of those infected with HSV-1 in the oral area, clinical expression manifests itself in about one third of the population. Only 1 individual out of 12 will suffer frequent (more than three episodes per year) expression. For individuals infected with genital herpes, HSV-2, about one in three is effectively asymptomatic. A similar number may have mild, unnoticed, or ignored recurrences, presumably infrequently. Finally, there is a minority of the infected population that suffers noticeable recurrent outbreaks of viral activity in the genital area. I am a member of this subset of the HSV-2–seropositive population, and I attempt to describe patient's concerns from that perspective herein.

ONE PATIENT'S PERSPECTIVE

Chronic diseases of the skin have been a powerful force in my life for many years. I have based many life decisions—some that have shaped the definition of whom I am—on skin disease management. During my adolescence and early adulthood chronic cystic acne plagued me. This condition did not succumb to treatment until I was well into my thirties. Some years afterwards I was first diagnosed with genital herpes, presumably HSV-2. This made it certain that I would be dealing with chronic skin disease management for the rest of my life. Thus, chronic diseases of the skin have, to varying degrees, been influential in shaping many of my personal, social, and health-management strategies. The coping strategies that I have developed for the management of my ego, fears, self-perception, and personal relationships are all intertwined with the actual or perceived condition of my skin. Some of these concerns have in themselves led to the development of recovery-management strategies.

One of the issues of greatest immediate concern to HSV patients is, interestingly enough, transmission to others. Considerable effort is often devoted to protecting partners. Others may wish to conceal the physical manifestations of the condition during an outbreak. Therefore, those factors that trigger an outbreak of genital herpes are very important to the patient. While there is debate with regard to most of these real or perceived "factors," several are commonly enough voiced by patients to warrant mention here. Evidence suggests that illness, stress, fatigue, menstruation, poor nutrition, ultraviolet (UV) light, and physical irritation can all have some correlation with recurrent physical manifestation of HSV. Animal studies have implicated skin irritation, nerve trauma, a variety of toxic xenobiotics, and UV radiation as trigger factors to one degree or another. While there is considerable debate among patients and the statistical correlation in study groups appears weak, stress is the most common single factor reported by patients as a trigger.

Management of outbreaks tends to become more sophisticated and personalized over time. Management strategies that address certain trigger actors include relaxation, guided imagery exercises, and social support. Herpes-specific social support (HSSS) has been shown to be a particularly effective management strategy. Areas that HSSS addresses include stress reduction, reduction in the frequency of outbreaks, and the establishment of perspective regarding the condition or its clinical manifestation. Perspective is quite important because for many HSV patients, genital herpes is the first chronic, incurable illness that they have to cope with. The trauma associated with infection can be very much involved in the sequelae of triggering recurrent outbreaks. HSSS is also helpful in the development of acceptance, a process that can take years.

Maintenance of generally good health is often a heightened priority in HSV patients. Rest, exercise, and a balanced diet are all undoubtedly helpful. Diet and herbal therapies have some proponents. The use of lysine, garlic or its components, and capsicum have all been credited with some degree of benefit. Effective, highly selective prescription antiviral medications are providing some patients, myself among them, with considerable relief. Disease management by some combination of these approaches gives patients control over their infection, as well as a heightened quality of life.

Clearly, herpes infections can manifest themselves in a variety of ways. The clinical expression of one's symptoms undoubtedly affects the degree to which one is challenged to develop coping strategies. It is not surprising that for genital herpes sufferers, each individual's recovery is as unique as the expression of the condition itself. Each person's path to recovery is guided by both the severity and site of clinical expression and the manifold social, medical, and psychological choices that are made with regard to them.

IMPACT OF HERPES ON PERSONAL DOMAINS

Physical Symptoms and Diagnosis

My initial diagnosis for HSV took place about 3 years ago. The symptoms of my primary episode looked to me like acne at first. I thought I was seeing evidence of the return of a dormant nemesis. Initially, my reaction was one of total unacceptance. I attacked the site of activity with unproductive and unfulfilling squeezing. Next, I made every effort to simply put the tiny white "pimples" out of my mind. That weekend a cluster of lesions had formed that defied denial and was frighteningly unfamiliar. An appointment with my family doctor was a priority for the following Monday.

Almost immediately upon seeing the sores on my genitals, my doctor said "That's herpes. I know you don't want to hear that, but I've seen a lot of this." I stood in shocked silence. Suddenly, I felt cold and faint. I was starting to lose my balance, but my pants were down around my ankles and prevented me from moving my feet. Fortunately, there was a chair immediately behind me. I half sat, half fell into it. Subsequently, my doctor took a culture and explained the existence of antiviral treatments. Shocked, I said that I was an unlikely candidate for HSV infection. I told him that I was in a relationship that I had assumed to be committed and monogamous. Explaining that I was actually quite typical demographically of new HSV patients, my doctor went on to say that he had heard variations of my story many times before. Shaken, angry, and frightened, I left the office in a state of shocked disbelief.

Early Management Strategy

Having had some experience with group psychotherapy, I set out to find if a support group existed for people suffering from genital herpes. Meanwhile, I had to cope with a shattered self-perception of my sexuality. I felt dirty, unlovable, and untouchable. I had been divorced some years earlier and had been active in the tumultuous world of adult dating in the 1990s. Suddenly, what had been a difficult situation had become impossible. The certainty that I was now "damaged goods" would no doubt prevent me from ever having a mutually satisfying relationship with anyone again.

Anger toward the person that we presumed to be was the source of our exposure may lend itself to development of feelings of resentment or revenge. This trap occupied me with resentments that temporarily blocked the development of acceptance and its associated physical and emotional benefits. The moment that I was able to release myself from resentment towards that person was a pivotal moment in my own recovery.

I tried at first to withdraw totally from the pursuit of an expression of my sexuality. In so doing, I attempted to focus on my career, hobbies, and the like. However, nothing seemed to be fully effective. I started to consider alternative approaches to my expression of sex and sexuality, but found nothing that I was really willing to pursue. It eventually became apparent that efforts aimed at the total suppression of my sexuality in response to contracting HSV were not going to work. Apparently, I had no choice but to find a way to continue on and live with my condition.

COPING STRATEGIES

The impact of learning one has genital herpes affects ones self-image, personal relationships, and social functioning to one degree or another. A failure of acceptance of the diagnosis is common initially. Anger at the (ex) partner blamed for the infection follows, along with frustration with friends who are perceived as judgmental or unable to be of any substantial help. A great deal of energy is often spent mourning the perceived loss of the ability to pursue partners. A symptom-based self-perception of sexuality places severe restrictions on pursuing the development of sexual expression. The positive side of this difficult period in one's recovery is that it may predispose the patient to seek help.

The open-minded, knowledgeable patient will start to integrate the physical changes and the knowledge he or she has gained into a redefined and evolving self-perception that is based less and less on clinical symptoms of HSV. The patient who chooses to remain injured and angry is unlikely to undergo this type of emotional evolution. Depression and social isolation often persists for years and cuts the patient off from that which would allow him or her to grow and recover, i.e., active participation in one's own recovery and social support.

Avoidance of development of an effective and open expression of sexuality resulting in a dishonest or uncontrolled physical sexual expression is a victory for the virus. I have seen example after example of attractive, desirable people avoiding relationships for years because of an inability to overcome fear related to telling a partner, or anyone else, about their condition. To avoid this situation, social support is critical, but it requires taking the risk of disclosure. Nondisclosure blocks support, promotes conditions that are conducive to the establishment of new infections, and promotes the stress associated with dishonesty and guarding secrets. The development of a supportive emotional environment and alternate forms of sexual expression, e.g., without involving penetration, is certainly not immediate, but has no doubt caused the strengthening of many relationships.

Disclosure

The temptation to succumb to dishonesty and denial is one of the virus's greatest allies with regard to infecting others and an ineffective recovery. Telling a present or potential sexual partner is one of the first and most difficult problems that a patient must face. This person must face the possibility of rejection and social stigma and risks vulnerability. Effectively dealing with this challenge, however, sets the patient on the path to recovery. This exercise is important for several reasons. First, the chance of transmission to a partner is considerably lower if both partners are aware of the condition. In addition, the infected partner is relieved of the stressful burdens of fear of discovery, guilt, and secrecy. The uninfected partner is allowed to accept a degree of responsibility by way of making an informed choice and by accepting some of the risk associated with transmission.

Honesty, openness, and a willingness to accept change are important to telling a partner successfully. The patient has a considerable amount of control over how the partner will receive the news. Self-acceptance of one's condition is of paramount importance for acceptance by others. Emotional trauma over herpes infections is quite as contagious as the virus itself. A well-informed, confident delivery can lend considerably to the chances of a positive response by the other person. One cannot expect a partner to be confident and assured if they are frightened and questioning themselves. Self-acceptance of one's condition and the impact on one's sexuality is a precondition to the development of healthy relationships after contracting HSV. It is very difficult for newly diagnosed HSV patients to disconnect their self-image, particularly regarding their sexuality, from the virus itself. This must be overcome if one wants to project a positive image of one's sexuality to another person. Becoming informed about herpes before telling a partner is important, as one can certainly expect questions. Herpes support groups or telephone information lines are very effective in the development of a patient's personal information base. It is essential to have trust in a (potential) partner in order to make these kinds of personal disclosures. Making this type of personal disclosure is in itself an expression of trust that is often received in a very positive light by the other person. Patients now have the need to know potential partners well before taking the risk of disclosure.

This kind of behavioral change is, in itself, conducive to the establishment of long-term relationships, with an associated reduction in the number of potential exposures. The development of a mutual expression of physical intimacy that considers the infected partner's herpes can lead to the development of a well-rounded and fulfilling sexuality. This is in marked contrast to the difficulty that stereotypes or the patients own initial perceptions may have placed on the prospect of developing a fulfilling sexuality with HSV-2. With some form of sexually transmitted disease affecting one in five American adults, persons challenged to find a fulfilling partnership with one or both partners having a STD are not a small minority.

Recovery

How did I start my recovery from HSV-2? Honesty, an acceptance of my condition and the associated responsibilities to myself and others. Openness, the release of anger and resentment, allowing me to become teachable. Willingness, a deliberate effort to *actively participate* in my own recovery. A healthy, well-balanced approach to HSV-2 is indeed transmissible to others. I cannot assume the responsibility for, nor control the outcome of, disclosure to others. I had to be willing to allow time for others to adjust, just as I needed time to adjust myself. The willingness to participate in my own recovery was fundamental in breaking the emotional cycle of stress-induced outbreaks, as well as preparing me for breaking the physical cycle of frequent recurrences with suppressive oral antiviral therapy.

As a result of early participation in HSSS, as well as a very successful response to suppressive antiviral therapy, my emotional condition had improved dramatically during the first year. As evidence of this, an excerpt from a letter that I sent to my primary care physician follows:

> *Dear Dr. H—,*
>
> *It has been 1 year today since my dismal diagnosis with HSV-2. I am writing this short note to express my thanks for your enlightened attitude and support with regard to this condition.*
>
> *In the year that has passed, my condition has changed from one of dismal resignation to one of optimistic enthusiasm. I have responded remarkably well to suppressive drug therapy, and I have become active (no pun) in HELP of Washington and the Amer. Social Health Assoc. (ASHA). Through these associations, I have developed effective techniques to address both the physical and mental challenges associated with a chronic STD. In fact, this situation may, in a back-asswards sort of way, be the vehicle by which I find myself finally able to find a stable, safe, and long-term expression of my sexuality.*

This letter may be the most compelling testimony for actively participating in one's own recovery (from genital herpes) that I can offer.

Challenges

Some degree of stigmatization by both overt and indirect reinforcement of stereotypes occurred in my case at first. often, I did not get the desired response from people to whom I disclosed my condition, no matter how carefully I tried to select them. There was sometimes a degree of inadvertent victim-blaming mixed in with their responses, i.e., that some aspect of my behavior prior to infection was to blame for my becoming infected. Participation in the area herpes support group was very helpful in restoring perspective to that situation.

The self-perception that I had a condition that was severe and recurrent enough to warrant suppressive antiviral therapy was also a very difficult one for me to accept. I did not want to have herpes. I certainly did not want to have a severe case of herpes. I was unwilling to bear the fact that I had a condition that was both severe in its clinical manifestation and recurred frequently enough to warrant daily therapy. I resisted my physician's first efforts to prescribe oral antiviral therapy, based in part on my perception that this treatment regimen was reserved for the worst cases. However, I was to discover that the regimen was both easily tolerated and very effective. Stressful events that would surely have triggered an outbreak earlier passed without any indication of new activity. Suddenly, I felt once again at liberty to pursue life goals and activities that I had previously considered too risky. The physical cycle of stress-induced outbreaks was broken at last. Almost immediately, the emotional cycle, i.e., causing stress by worrying about outbreaks under stressful circumstances, was broken as well.

This new confidence allowed the development of a whole new, qualitatively different, array of coping strategies. I finally felt like I was in control of my life again, and the connection between the self-perception of my own sexuality and clinical symptoms of HSV was broken.

Personal Medical History

Neither I nor any of my past partners was aware, to my knowledge, of any exposure to HSV. However, my symptoms were classic and were confirmed by culture. Although no treatment was prescribed during my first visit to the doctor, a resurgence of my initial outbreak prompted episodic antiviral treatment, to which I responded well. Within 4 months I had established a pattern that involved having outbreaks when challenged by stress, under eating, dating anxiety, and the like. Having about one episode a month, on the average, prompted my physician to strongly recommend daily suppressive therapy. Under protest, I agreed to try it. I went almost a full year without any activity at all, weathering some significant stressor events without the associated outbreak that had characterized my condition prior. When I did have a mild recurrence of symptoms, it felt like it was more on my terms, as I had been physically challenged and lax in my dosage regimen. Afterwards, I returned to my suppressive regimen, paying closer attention to making my daily dose. Eventually, I became courageous enough to titer down my dose, finding the minimum where I started to have mild "breakthrough." Now, over a year later, I have had no activity at all and feel that I have control by use of the antiviral drug that I so vigorously resisted at first. As of this writing, my experience with this drug has been characterized by the total absence of noticeable side effects. In addition, during the time that has elapsed without any outbreaks, I have developed a number of coping strategies and personal associations that take the fear and self-loathing out of the clinical manifestation of my condition.

Patient Advocacy

As a member of the local HSSS group, I heard stories from other patients regarding their infection, management strategies, and relationships. It soon became apparent to me that the secrecy and stigma associated with HSV was of little benefit to patients. This burden of shame and secrecy prevents us from being able to be honest and open with sexual partners. Some feel that they were actually given the virus with forethought and malice by persons who succumbed to anger and resentment over having the disease themselves. As a result of these personal observations, I volunteered to join a small group of individuals who were willing to break their anonymity with regard to having genital herpes. Some time later, I was contacted by the producer of a nationwide talk show and asked to participate in an episode based on "STDs other than AIDS/HIV." The message that other HSSS group members and I tried to tell was simply that there is help and information available to herpes sufferers and that information and support had enabled us to enjoy life, love, and relationships after herpes. The interest that the show sparked was remarkable. The phones at the American Social Health Association and Herpes Hot Line were jammed for days. There is an unfulfilled demand for information and support that exceeds the resources available to the general population of herpes sufferers.

This talk-show activity indirectly led to my participation in a U.S.-based interview video of a number of patients, which is intended for HSV patient education and health care providers. Some time later, I was fortunate enough to be asked to participate in an international forum of herpes patients and health care providers held in Montreux, Switzerland. Patients from Europe, Australia, and the United States met with physicians, advisors, and facilitators. Our goal was to attempt to develop training materials and guidelines, emphasizing patients's concerns and management needs. Ultimately, we wanted to present a patient's perspective on care strategy for health care providers to follow when diagnosing and treating genital herpes.

It was soon evident that there was tremendous variation in the development of treatment and support regimens among the countries represented. One patient was simply assured that his condition had been cured! Another patient had been advised to apply chloroform to his lesions. No herpes support or information-distribution system existed in several of the countries represented. It was this very disparity in herpes information and treatment that the meeting aimed to address.

Similarly, the following year I was asked to participate in a meeting of the International Herpes Management Forum (IHMF). This workshop addressed the increasing incidence of HSV worldwide, patient and physician perceptions of HSV, clinical and asymptomatic manifestations, and management issues. Once again, considerable emphasis was placed on investigating the patient's perspective in an effort to keep the guidelines understandable, pertinent to the issues, and effective.

This sort of material and guidelines could have significant impact on a patient's first visit. In Montreux, we developed an outline of primary diagnosis–management strategy that was later presented to a group of 300 European physicians, presumably mostly dermatologists. In addition, some of us had volunteered to participate in making a "training video," we were asked to respond to questions about our initial diagnosis and subsequent recovery. The emotional implications of this exercise was apparent to the audience. The auditorium was silent, and the doctors repeatedly referred to the video in an extremely positive light throughout the remaining sessions. Hopefully it will be a powerful motivator for health care professionals to reconsider the way they manage genital herpes.

In the following sections, I attempt to describe some of the observations and opinions that were voiced at these meetings, particularly those that address concerns from a patient's perspective.

Patient Desires

The primary concern of newly diagnosed patients is trying to understand enough about the disease so that they will know when they are likely to transmit the condition to others. It is very reassuring to know that effective treatment is available that may also reduce the risk of subclinical shedding and transmission.

An ideal treatment regimen would achieve reduction of pain, shortened duration and frequency of attacks, prevention of impending or future attacks, and prevention of conditions that would lead to transmission. A complete cure and vaccination against the disease tops the "wish list" of this group of patients.

TREATMENT GUIDELINES

First Diagnosis

Providers need to be aware of the fact that when they tell a new patient that he or she has genital herpes, it could be the worst news they have ever heard. Directing the new patient to accurate information and emotional support is as important as taking a culture or prescribing a treatment. In the United States, immediate support is available through the National Herpes Hotline or the National STD Hotline, managed under the auspices of the American Social Health Association.

Patients need to be allowed to describe their perception of the condition. This enables the health care provider to dispel misconceptions and to address specific symptoms effectively. Ideally, this discussion should be conducted in person, with the patient in an uncompromised position, e.g., not in stirrups or partially dressed. Patients need to understand the limitations and implications of any testing or typing, as well as the results.

The primary episode of genital HSV-2 is thought to be highly effective at transmission, even in subclinical or asymptomatic stages. It is therefore important to raise transmission issues, to the extent possible, during first presentation. Providers should also be willing to prescribe an appropriate course of antiviral therapy on the basis of a presumptive diagnosis.

Providing written information is helpful and empowers the patient to come to informed decisions on his or her own. As the patient is often quite overwhelmed, there is a limit to how much information can be taken in during the first visit.

The fact that a lot is known about the condition is comforting to patients. The sheer number of diagnosed cases is helpful to the patient in dispelling feelings of self-pity or entertaining notions of self-inflicted bodily harm. While the provider cannot be expected to provide peer counseling, a discussion of relevant sexuality and relationship issues at this point could be important in limiting behavior that could lead to the infection of others. This is particularly important during a vigorous primary outbreak. The temptation to indulge in dishonest behavior is already present and should be strongly discouraged. Many such behaviors, e.g., nondisclosure or lying, are very difficult for the patient to recover from after the fact.

Follow-Up

The patient should be strongly encouraged to make a follow-up appointment at once. Otherwise, they may drop out of the care system. Patients should be seen for a second visit within 2 weeks of first presentation. This allows for assessment of lesion healing, test results, and the course of subsequent treatment. The emphasis should be on the *treatability* of this chronic illness. Overt or unintentional judgment of the patient should be avoided. A positive conceptual outlook on life after genital herpes is important for the provider to convey. In general, subsequent management of the condition is most successful when the patient has speedy access to the provider, is encouraged to make regular visits, develops a personalized base of information and support, and is encouraged to lead a generally healthy lifestyle.

ACTION STEPS

More impact is needed from the control strategies that exist at present. Immediate suppressive therapy for a duration of one year could allow patients to develop coping mechanisms without the anguish of repeated, severe, or unexpected outbreaks. They would then have the ability to choose whether to remain on suppressive therapy, as I have, or manage their outbreaks in an episodic fashion. The temptation to deny the existence of the condition or lie to partners would be greatly diminished. In addition, the period of highest symptomatic and subclinical viral shedding would be past, reducing the chance of traumatic transmission to a partner. Oral antiviral therapy would be useful during periods that are challenging to the patient, such as dating, pregnancy, periods of high disease activity, and the tumultuous first year of infection. While valid arguments exist for continuation of the conservative approach to prescribing oral antiviral therapy, the undisputed existence of 500,000 new cases a year underscores the urgency of developing a new, proactive approach to the management of this disease.

CONCLUSION

Understanding the patient's point of view in coping with genital herpes has come to be regarded as essential for developing a coherent and practical management strategy. An effective, patient-sensitive management strategy will encourage high patient compliance. That in turn will stimulate recovery and reduce the probability of inadvertent transmission. In light of the worldwide prevalance of genital herpes, the psycosocial factors that lend themselves to underdiagnosis and undertreatment of the condition have to be identified and corrected.

I have found the experience of recovery from genital herpes to be characterized by a variety of choices. Patients are almost immediately called upon to choose one of two paths. One path is acceptance of the condition and the associated responsibilities. This predisposes the individual to developing the honesty, openness, and willingness necessary to enjoy life, love, and happiness *after* genital herpes. The other choice, suppression and denial, shuts the infected individual off from growth, information, and support. These individuals are less likely to develop healthy, effective techniques for coping with their own condition and managing relationships with others. All too often other people are drawn into the vicious cycle of bitterness, resentment, and anger caused by transmission of this virus.

Similarly, health care providers have choices to make when called upon to treat new cases of genital herpes. They can choose to simply treat the lesions on an ad hoc basis and leave the psychosocial implications of the condition up to the patient. The other approach available to health care providers is to take an active role in the patient's development of coping strategies. The provider can provide a better climate for recovery by being accessible, prescribing antiviral therapy where indicated, encouraging regular visits, and promoting a generally healthy lifestyle. Addressing the psychological component of this approach, i.e., promoting acceptance and honesty, and directing the patient to social support and information can positively affect not only the patient's recovery, but the health and well-being of others as well.

REFERENCES

1. Ebel C (ed.). Understanding Herpes. Research Triangle Park, NC: American Social Health Association, 1991.
2. Johnson R, Lee F, Hadgu A, et al. U.S. genital herpes trends during the first decade of AIDS. Presented at the ISSTDR, Helsinki, August 1993, abstract 22.
3. Brookes JL, Haywood S, Green J. Adjustment to the psychological and social sequelae of recurrent genital herpes simplex infection. Genitourin Med 1993; 69:384–387.
4. Zorilla EP, McKay JR, Luborsky L, Schmidt K. Relation of stressors and depressive symptoms to clinical progression of viral illness. Am J Psychiatry 1996; 153:626–635.

7

The Dermatology Life Quality Index

Initial Experience of a Simple Practical Measure

Andrew Y. Finlay *University of Wales College of Medicine, Cardiff, United Kingdom*

INTRODUCTION

Many skin diseases can have a major impact on patients' quality of life. In the 1980s there was initial work on the development of disease-specific methods to measure this impact (1), and disability indices were described for use in psoriasis (2) and acne (3). The Psoriasis Disability Index (PDI) was also modified for use in eczema (4), but it became clear that patients' lives are affected in broadly similar ways, whatever the type of skin disease. There was therefore both a need for and the possibility of producing a single quality-of-life measure that could be used across a wide range of skin diseases. This chapter describes the first attempt at meeting this need: the creation, initial validation, and use of the Dermatology Life Quality Index (DLQI) (5) and the children's version, the CDLQI (6).

OBJECTIVE OF THE DLQI

The aim of creating the DLQI was to meet the need for a short, simple, and validated questionnaire to measure the impact of skin disease on patients' quality of life. The instrument was designed for use in a busy clinical setting, for clinical research, and for health service outcome research.

METHODS

The DLQI questionnaire was based on information directly received from patients with skin disease. One hundred and twenty consecutive patients attending a hospital outpatient department with a variety of different skin diseases were asked about the impact of their disease and its treatment on their lives. More than 32 different diagnoses were represented. Every patient who was asked cooperated with the study. Each answer was analyzed to identify every aspect of life quality affected. Forty-nine different aspects were recorded, sorted into overall categories, and ranked according to their frequency of mention. After the first 70 replies were analyzed, no additional information was gleaned from the subsequent 50 replies. This suggests that all of the most common ways in which skin disease affects patients lives were noted by the investigators.

The wording of the DLQI was designed to encompass as closely as possible all of the aspects mentioned, although because the questionnaire was specifically designed to be short and easy to use, there was some inevitable loss of specific information in this process of distillation. Each question was designed to refer to the experience of the previous week. The questionnaire was piloted twice on a series of patients with skin disease and minor changes made as a result. The question topics of the DLQI (5) are given in Table 1. The scoring system is simple, with each of the 10 questions having four alternative responses scored from 0 to 3. The maximum score is therefore 30, representing maximum handicap. It is suggested (5) that the results of the questionnaire could also be presented by grouping the

Table 1 DLQI Question Topics

1. Symptoms, including itchiness, soreness, pain
2. Feelings of embarrassment or self-consciousness
3. Interference with shopping or looking after home or garden
4. Clothes
5. Social or leisure activities
6. Sport
7. Effect on working or studying
8. Problems with partner or close friends or relatives
9. Sexual difficulties
10. Treatment effects

Source: Ref. 5. The DLQI is copyright by A. Y. Finlay and G. K. Khan, April 1992. It must not be copied without permission of the authors.

answers as follows: symptoms and feelings (questions 1 and 2); daily activities (questions 3 and 4); leisure (questions 5 and 6); work/school (question 7); personal relationships (questions 8 and 9); and treatment (question 10).

RESULTS

The DLQI was initially completed by 200 consecutive new patients attending a dermatology clinic. This initial study confirmed that atopic dermatitis (DLQI mean score = 12.5), psoriasis (8.9), and generalized pruritus (10.5) have a greater impact on quality of life than basal cell carcinomas (2.0) or seborrheic warts (1.8).

INITIAL VALIDATION OF THE DLQI

Validity testing of the DLQI has included test-retesting and comparison with a control "normal" population. In addition there has been demonstration of change following improvement of the clinical condition and demonstration of cross-validity with other measures of quality of life. In the group of 200 patients described above, 98% correctly completed all 10 questions, confirming the accuracy with which this instrument is completed and its ease of use.

Test-retest reliability assessment of the DLQI was checked (5) by giving it to 53 patients with relatively stable disease and then asking them to complete it again after an interval of 7–10 days. There were very high correlations between overall DLQI scores ($\gamma_s = 0.99$; $p < 0.0001$) and individual question scores ($\gamma_s = 0.95$–0.98; $p < 0.001$).

A control "normal" group of 100 healthy volunteers was asked to complete the DLQI: the mean score was 0.5 (5). Every individual question showed a highly significant difference between the mean of the scores of the controls and the patients.

Detailed analysis of the content and structure of the DLQI has been carried out following its use in atopic dermatitis (7). In a study of 614 patients with vitiligo who completed the DLQI (8), factor analysis indicated that the DLQI consists of three dimensions: questions 2–7 and 10 refer to the social and emotional aspects of vitiligo, questions 8 and 9 refer to the interpersonal aspects, and question 1 concerns the extent to which vitiligo causes physical discomfort.

DLQI: RESPONSE TO CHANGE

The ability of the DLQI to respond to changes in clinical condition or disease activity following treatment has been demonstrated in several studies, three of which have so far been published. These concern improvement with psoriasis and with atopic dermatitis after inpatient therapy (9), improvement in patients with acne after oral isotretinoin (10), and change after surgical therapy for basal cell carcinoma (11).

Over 6 months, 230 patients admitted to a teaching hospital dermatology ward were asked to complete the DLQI on admission and again 4 weeks after discharge (9). One hundred and eighty-one (83%) patients returned both questionnaires. The mean DLQI on admission was 13.2 (SD 7.6) and after discharge was 7.7 (SD 6.8; $p < 0.001$). Patients with psoriasis improved from 13.7 (SD 6.5) to 6.7 (SD 5.6; $n = 63$; $p < 0.001$). Patients with eczema improved from 16.2 (SD 6.3) to 9.6 (SD 7.6; $n = 56$; $p < 0.001$). "Control" groups of patients admitted for investigation of pruritus or for liver biopsy showed no change in the mean scores.

Patients with acne referred to a dermatology clinic completed the DLQI before being seen and again 4 and 12 months later (10). Forty-two patients completed all three questionnaires: the mean DLQI scores improved from 9.3 (baseline) to 2.6 (4 months) and finally to 1.5 (12 months). At the start of the study there was no relationship between the clinical score of the acne and the DLQI ($r = -0.17$; $p = 0.07$; $n = 109$). However, the improvement in the mean DLQI scores paralleled an improvement in the mean clinical score of acne severity. The mean DLQI scores showed a much greater percentage reduction following therapy than the General Health Questionnaire (GHQ) and the SF-36, which were used in parallel, demonstrating the greater responsiveness to change of the DLQI in this condition.

Although basal cell carcinomas cause very little impact on life quality at the time of presentation (mean score 5.3) (11), there was an elevation of the mean DLQI score to 8.7 one week after therapy, and the score returned to an even lower level (1.3; $p < 0.01$) 3 months after therapy. The DLQI can therefore detect the relatively subtle impact on quality of life of therapeutic procedures. Another study of 100 patients with facial nonmelanoma skin cancer showed a mean DLQI score of 2.3, compared to a mean score of 2.0 in 100 controls (Robinson JK, personal communication).

GENERAL HEALTH MEASURES AND THE DLQI

The use of general health measures is essential in order to draw any comparison between the impact of skin disease and other, nonskin diseases on patients' lives. General health measures used with the DLQI include the Sickness Impact Profile (SIP) (11), the Short-Form Health Survey Questionnaire (SF-36) (10,12), the GHQ (8,10), and the Patient Generated Index (PGI) (7). The problem with the use of any general health measure in patients with skin disease is that many of the questions are inevitably irrelevant. However, their number and the occasional positive response to questions caused by factors unrelated to the patient's skin disease will mean that there is likely to be a level of "background noise" in the score, possibly masking minor scores from the skin disease itself.

The United Kingdom version of the SIP (UKSIP) consists of 136 health-related statements grouped into 12 areas of daily living. This measure was used in parallel with the DLQI in patients before and after treatment for basal cell carcinoma (11). There was a significant correlation one week after treatment between the DLQI and the overall UKSIP score, and between some subcategories of the UKSIP and the overall DLQI. However, at baseline, when the level of quality-of-life impairment was very low, only the psychosocial dimension of the UKSIP correlated with the DLQI.

The SF-36 and the DLQI was self-administered to 668 adults with stable plaque psoriasis in a multicenter study in the United States (12). The mean DLQI score was 7.02; the SF-36 scores were within or slightly above U.S. population mean ranges for all scales. The DLQI had significant ($p < 0.001$) inverse relationships (ranging from -0.13 to -0.43) with all of the SF-36 scales. The DLQI was most highly correlated with the mental health subscale. The SF-36 was also used in parallel with the 28 question version of the GHQ and the DLQI in 111 patients in the acne study described above (10). In vitiligo (8), the DLQI correlated with the GHQ ($r = 0.39$; $p < 0.001$; $n = 599$) and with perceived stigma ($r = -0.65$; $p < 0.001$; $n = 418$).

The DLQI has been used in parallel with the PGI in a community-based study of 56 adults with atopic dermatitis (7). The PGI can be used in any medical condition and was designed to measure the effects on their lives that patients themselves consider the most important. There was a significant correlation between the two methods, but the use of the PGI did highlight some areas of concern to patients not directly addressed in the DLQI.

DISEASE-SPECIFIC QUESTIONNAIRES AND THE DLQI

The disease-specific PDI questionnaire was cross-validated with the DLQI in the study described above (12). There was a very strong correlation of 0.82 ($p < 0.001$). The original PDI (2) was modified; a 15-question version of the PDI (13) was used in a national structure of patients with severe psoriasis. Further studies of its structure (14,15), cross-validation with the UKSIP (16), and use in a community-based study (17) have been reported.

A study of acne (18) using the DLQI in parallel both with the short five-question version (Cardiff Acne Disability Index) (19) of the Acne Disability Index (14) and with the Assessment of the Psychological and Social Effects of Acne (APSEA) questionnaire has shown good correlation between the CDLQI and CADI ($r = 0.77$; $p < 0.001$) and between the DLQI and APSEA ($r = 0.65$; $p < 0.001$).

CROSS-SECTIONAL SURVEYS USING THE DLQI

As well as the psoriasis study described above, the DLQI has been used in several other cross-sectional surveys. The original study of patients in a general dermatology clinic (5) demonstrated the range of mean scores associated with different conditions. The finding of a high mean score for atopic dermatitis in this first study has been confirmed by a subsequent multicenter survey of 92 adult patients with severe atopic dermatitis (20), which revealed a mean DLQI of 18. This study also presented data from some utility measure questions. However, in contrast to this selected patient group, when all patients in a community who had atopic dermatitis were studied the median DLQI score was only 5.5 (7).

325 patients with Behçet's syndrome completed the DLQI, with a mean score of 5.7 (21). Patients who had suffered genital ulcers in the previous week had a mean score of 10.8 ($n = 95$), whereas those who had not had genital ulcers in the previous week had a score of 3.9 ($n = 230$, $p < 0.001$).

Table 2 DLQI Mean Scores Reported in Different Conditions

Diagnosis	DLQI score (SD)	n	Ref.
Acne	7.5 (5.5)	109	10
Alopecia	8.3 (5.6)	70	24
Atopic dermatitis (adults, severe)	18 (7.1)	92	20
Atopic dermatitis (community sample)	5.5 (median)	56	7
Basal cell carcinoma	5.3 (4.1)	44	11
Behçet's syndrome (with genital ulcers)	10.8 (7.7)	95	21
Behçet's syndrome (no genital ulcers)	3.9 (5.4)	230	21
Darier's disease	5.9 (5.7)	137	22
Hailey-Hailey disease	6.1 (5.5)	66	22
Nonmelanoma skin cancer	2.3	100	Robinson JK
Psoriasis (moderate)	7.0 (5.2)	644	12
Psoriasis (on admission)	8.9	52	9
Seborrheic keratoses	1.86	45	25
Vascular anomalies of face	5.6 (4.7)	24	23
Vitiligo (Caucasian)	4.6	567	8
Vitiligo (non-Caucasian)	7.8	46	8

In a survey of 137 patients with Darier's disease, the mean DLQI was 5.9, and in 66 patients with Hailey-Hailey disease, the mean was 6.06 (22). The DLQI scores did not correlate with the physician's assessment of clinical severity in both diseases, emphasizing the importance of remembering the potential for handicap even in patients with disease that appears to be mild.

Over 600 predominantly Caucasian patients with vitiligo completed the DLQI, with a mean score of 4.82 (8). The mean score of Caucasians (4.59; $n = 567$) was higher than the mean score of non-Caucasians (7.78; $n = 46$; $p < 0.001$). In a study (23) of 24 adult patients with congenital vascular anomalies of the face attending before laser therapy, the mean DLQI score was 5.6 (SD 4.7), and 70 patients with alopecia (24) had a mean score of 8.3. The very low to absent levels of impairment of life quality caused by seborrhoeic keratoses has been confirmed in a study of 45 patients; the mean DLQI was only 1.86 (25). A multicenter study is in progress in Wales of 10,000 patients referred to dermatologists to determine comparative ranges of DLQI scores. Mean scores of the DLQI in several conditions are summarized in Table 2.

CURRENT USE

Currently the DLQI is being used in the United States, Europe, and Australia in studies of patients with acne, alopecia, atopic dermatitis, congenital vascular malformations, hidradenitis suppurativa, ichthyosis, leg ulcers, pemphigus, photodamage, psoriasis, and urticaria, as well as being used to assess the effectiveness of a dermatology specialist nurse service. There are DLQI translations in Danish, Dutch, Finnish, French, German, Gujarati, Italian, Norwegian, Spanish, Swedish, and Turkish.

CHILDREN'S VERSION

Quality-of-life measures in dermatology are required not only for adults but also for children. The difficulties in creating appropriate and validated instruments for children are compounded by several additional factors, including questions of comprehension and requirements for different age groups. A Pediatric Symptom Checklist (26) has been used to screen for psychosocial dysfunction in children attending general and dermatological pediatric clinics, but this technique is not suitable for handicap comparison.

The Children's DLQI (CDLQI) was created in the same way as the adult DLQI from information gained from 169 children with skin disease attending a pediatric dermatology clinic (6). Ten questions were composed (Table 3) using a pattern based on the adult DLQI to cover the 111 different aspects identified. The CDLQI was piloted on two series of children and minor alterations were made. Validity testing has included test-

Table 3 CDLQI Question Topics

1. Itchiness, soreness, pain
2. Embarrassment, self-consciousness, being upset, sadness
3. Friendships
4. Clothes, shoes
5. Going out, playing, hobbies
6. Swimming, sports
7. Schoolwork or holiday enjoyment
8. Teasing, calling names, bullying, questions
9. Sleep
10. Treatment problems

Source: Ref. 6. The CDLQI is copyright by M. S. Lewis-Jones and A. Y. Finlay, May 1993. It must not be copied without permission of the authors.

retesting, confirming acceptable repeatability, and use in two control populations of normal children (mean score = 0.4; SD 0.7; $n = 47$) and of children with nondermatological disease (mean score = 0.7; SD 2.5; $n = 55$). Mean scores of several diagnostic groups are given in Table 4 (27): this information is taken from patients attending a hospital pediatric dermatology clinic after referral from their general practitioner.

There is evidence (27) of sensitivity of the scores of change following inpatient treatment of psoriasis and atopic dermatitis (mean CDLQI = 11.7 before, 3.5 after; $n = 15$; $p = 0.002$) and outpatient treatment of acne (9.2, 1.3, 15, p = 0.01). A printed color cartoon version of the CDLQI, using the same text, has been constructed and is undergoing cross-validation with the original CDLQI.

Table 4 CDLQI Mean Scores in Different Conditions

Diagnosis	CDLQI score (SD)	*n*
Acne	6.4 (5.2)	111
Atopic dermatitis	8.1 (5.6)	97
Moles	1.8 (2.5)	104
Molluscum contagiosum	5.2 (4.8)	31
Psoriasis	6.0 (4.9)	54
Viral warts	4.0 (4.1)	61

Source: Ref. 27.

CONCLUSIONS

The DLQI and the CDLQI are potentially of value for clinical purposes, for clinical research studies of new management methods, and for health service audit and research. The choice of their use in a wide range of current studies indicates the previously unmet need for such measures. In addition to the information provided in this volume, advice concerning decisions about which QOL measures may be most suitable for different purposes is given in a recent review (1).

REFERENCES

1. Finlay AY. Quality of life measurement in dermatology: a practical guide. Br J Dermatol 1997; 136: 305–314.
2. Finlay AY, Kelly SE. Psoriasis—an index of disability. Clin Exp Dermatol 1987; 12: 8–11.
3. Motley RJ, Finlay AY. How much disability is caused by acne? Clin Exp Dermatol 1989; 14: 194–198.
4. Salek MS, Finlay AY, Luscombe DK et al. Cyclosporin greatly improves the quality of life of adults with severe atopic dermatitis. Br J Dermatol 1993; 129: 422–430.
5. Finlay AY, Khan GK. Dermatology Life Quality Index (DLQI): a simple practical measure for routine clinical use: Clin Exp Dermatol 1994; 19: 210–216.
6. Lewis-Jones MS, Finlay AY. The Children's Dermatology Life Quality Index (CDLQI): initial validation and practical use. Br J Dermatol 1995; 132: 942–949.
7. Herd RM, Tidman MJ, Ruta DA, Hunter JAA. Measurement of quality of life in atopic dermatitis: correlation and validation of two different methods. Br J Dermatol 1997; 136: 502–507.
8. Kent G, Al-Abadie M. Factors affecting responses on Dermatology Life Quality Index items among vitiligo sufferers. Clin Exp Dermatol 1996; 21: 330–333.
9. Kurwa H, Finlay AY. Dermatology inpatient admission greatly improves life quality. Br J Dermatol 1995; 133: 575–578.
10. Mallon E, Newton JN, Klassen A, Ryan TJ, Finlay AY. Standard patient assessed quality of life instruments can be used to measure the benefits of acne treatment. Br J Dermatol 1995; 133 (suppl 45): 35.
11. Blackford S, Roberts DL, Salek MS, Finlay AY. Basal cell carcinomas and their treatment cause little handicap—the reason for delayed presentation? Qual Life Res 1996; 5: 131–138.
12. Nichol BM, Margolies JE, Lippa E, Rowe M, Quell J. The application of multiple quality of life instruments in individuals with mild-to-moderate psoriasis. Pharmacoeconomics 1996; 10: 644–653.
13. Finlay AY, Coles EC. The effect of severe psoriasis on the quality of life of 369 patients. Br J Dermatol 1995; 132: 236–244.

14. Kent G, Al-Abadie M. The Psoriasis Disability Index-further analyses. Clin Exp Dermatol 1993; 18:414–416.
15. Root S, Kent G, Al-Abadie MSK. The relationship between disease severity, disability and psychological distress in patients undergoing PUVA treatment of psoriasis. Dermatology 1994; 189:234–237.
16. Finlay AY, Khan GK, Luscombe DK, Salek MS. Validation of Sickness Impact Profile and Psoriasis Disability Index in psoriasis. Br J Dermatol 1990; 123:751–756.
17. O'Neill P, Kelly P. Postal questionnaire study of disability in the community associated with psoriasis. Br Med J 1996; 313:919–921.
18. Clark SM, Goulden V, Finlay AY, Cunliffe WJ. The psychological and social impact of acne: a comparison study using three acne disability questionnaires (abstr). Br J Dermatol 1997; 137(suppl 50):41.
19. Motley RJ, Finlay AY. Practical use of a disability index in the routine management of acne. Clin Exp Dermatol 1992; 17:1–3.
20. Finlay AY. Measures of the effect of adult severe atopic eczema on quality of life. J Eur Acad Dermatol Venereol 1996; 34:1016–1021.
21. Blackford S, Finlay AY, Roberts DL. Quality of life in Behçet's syndrome: 335 patients surveyed. Br J Dermatol 1997; 136:293.
22. Harris HA, Burge SM, Dykes PJ, Finlay AY. Handicap in Darier's disease and Hailey-Hailey disease. Br J Dermatol 1996; 135:959–963.
23. Al-Amri MSA. Quality of life studies in patients with vascular abnormalities. M.Sc. thesis, University of Wales, Cardiff, United Kingdom, 1995.
24. Williamson D, Gonzalez M, Finlay AY. Quality of life in patients with hair loss (abstr). Br J Dermatol 1997; 137(suppl 50):47.
25. Alam MZ. Seborrhoeic warts—an assessment of the disability they cause and their association with other medical disorders. M.Sc. thesis, University of Wales, Cardiff, United Kingdom, 1996.
26. Rauch PK, Jellinek MS, Murphy JM, Schachner L, Hansen R, Esterly NB, Prendiville J, Bishop SJ, Goshko M. Screening for psychosocial dysfunction in pediatric dermatology practice. Clin Pediatr 1991; 30:493–497.
27. Lewis-Jones MS, Lawson V, Hill G, Finlay AY. Monitoring childhood skin disease handicap. Br J Dermatol 1996; 135 (suppl 47):52.

8

Structural Validation of the DSQL

Confirmation of the Factor Structure and Justification of the Scoring Algorithm

Richard D. Lennox *Outcomes Research Associates, Hillsborough, North Carolina*

INTRODUCTION

The Dermatology-Specific Quality-of-Life (DSQL) questionnaire was designed to measure the individual differences in the quality of life (QOL) associated with dermatological diseases and changes in QOL due to their effective treatment. A report on the development and validation of the DSQL is provided in Anderson and Rajagopalan (1). As a disease-specific measure, the DSQL was designed to focus on the adverse impact of dermatological diseases without contamination by other diseases (e.g., heart conditions), adverse personal circumstances (unemployment), or sociological characteristics (e.g., social economic status). The disease focus is obtained by asking the patients to report impacts or effects upon QOL that they believe are caused by the dermatological disease. Although there are limits to the extent to which patients are able to make these attributions, targeting these measures is necessary in order to control the confounding effects of other medical and nonmedical factors that may also impact QOL but that cannot be treated or otherwise ameliorated by dermatological interventions. The conceptual framework underlying the instrument is multidimensional, based on the assumption that not all QOL domains are equally affected by all forms of dermatological diseases and that some forms of treatment may be more effective in changing some domains than others. The framework does, however, assert enough commonality among the domains to allow them to be subsumed under a superordinate construct that can be referred to as General Dermatology-Specific Quality of Life and should apply to several cutaneous diseases rather than a specific disease. The general QOL construct is considered to be the unifying focus of the instrument that permits all of the domains to be considered QOL-related.

The DSQL is a self-report measure intended to be used primarily as an outcome measure of dermatological diseases/conditions and/or treatment. The DSQL's five subscales are designed to evaluate three areas of functioning, a physical symptom construct, and a self-perception construct, each of which is likely to be adversely affected by dermatological diseases. The domains are also expected to improve with effective dermatological interventions. The total DSQL score evaluates the general QOL construct as an unweighted total of the individual subscales.

This report describes tests of the structural validity of the DSQL in terms of the correspondence between its empirical covariance structure and that expected based on the conceptual framework referred to above. The material includes data from two studies: a sample of patients with contact dermatitis (CD)(2) and a sample of patients with acne vulgaris (1). The latter DSQL version is identical to the CD version except that it has an additional physical symptom item. The item content of the acne version is presented in the Appendix.

The specific aims of the analysis are several fold. The first aim is to provide empirical tests of the structure of the DSQL that supports the calculation of five separate subscales: (1) physical symptoms, (2) activities of daily living, (3) social functioning, (4) work or school functioning, and (5) self-perception. A second aim is to provide justification for the calculation of a unit-weighted average score for each subscale. A third aim is to test the stability of the factor structure across time, after treatment for cutaneous diseases has occurred. A final aim is provide justification for the calculation of a single general QOL score.

THE DSQL

The DSQL contains five separate subscales, each directed at a particular facet of the patient's quality of life. Three of the facets refer to specific forms of functioning, one to self-perception, and one to physical symptoms. The scales are based on an effect-indicator measurement model (3, 4), in which the latent variable derived by the subscale average is thought to be the source of the covariance among the items. The subscales are theorized to represent distinct, yet related subconstructs of a general dermatology-related QOL construct. Therefore, the subscales are expected to form distinct empirical item sets that are at the same time positively correlated with one another.

The DSQL is administered as a multiscale inventory with the subscales clustered together using a common box-oriented response frame. These devices are thought to focus the respondent's attention on the construct at hand and are expected to reduce the cognitive effort of moving among different constructs and among differently structured items. According to this logic, allowing respondents to focus attention on one construct at a time keeps them from being confused or becoming fatigued by the measurement process.*

The subscales were all constructed using a rationally based scale-construction strategy (5). The domains of the construct were first defined, and then items were constructed that were logically linked to each of the domains. The items, therefore, all possess some degree of face validity in that their intuitive meaning is consistent with the apparent meaning of the construct. The subscales are described below.

Physical

The nine items of the physical symptoms subscale are designed to characterize patients' particular symptom profile as it relates to their specific types of dermatological disease. The items inquire about how frequently a patient's skin is accurately characterized by a set of symptoms commonly caused by dermatological disease (e.g., skin feels dry, tender, oily, painful, itchy, or is characterized as having burning sensations and/or other physical discomforts). Patients are also asked how often they experience intolerable physical discomfort or lose sleep because of the disease. The response format used is a five-point Likert scale (0 = never; 1 = rarely; 2 = sometimes; 3 = often; 4 = most of the time/constantly).

ADL

The activities-of-daily-living (ADL) subscale contains five measures of disability related to the disruption of normal activities caused by the disease.

---

* The logic of grouping items together and using box-oriented response options is almost certain to reduce cognitive strain and fatigue for the respond. Whether reducing strain increases the validity of the responses is open to question.

Patients are asked to report limitations they experience participating in normal daily activities, such as physical activities, shaving, wearing clothes, selecting hairstyles, and eating food or drinking beverages. The same response format is used as in the physical functioning subscale.

Social

The social functioning subscale contains 10 items designed to assess the degree to which the disease limits the patient's social activities, as in making friends, being comfortable in social situations, doing things that are enjoyable, being with friends, having dates, being satisfied with personal relationships, and going shopping. The same Likert format is used in the physical functioning and the ADL subscales, but with an additional "not applicable" option mainly to distinguish an absence of limitations in dating or other personal relationships due to skin disease from those not seeking such relationships.

Work

Items in the work functioning subscale are designed to measure limitations caused by disease on the job or at school, inquiring about the extent to which the disease inhibits the patient in getting ahead at the job or getting a good job, talking with co-workers, being effective in meetings, being effective at giving instructions, and being punctual. A Likert scale with the special "not applicable" option is used in this scale to distinguish not being affected in work functioning from not being exposed to work environments that involve substantial face-to-face interactions with others or not being employed.

Self-Perception

The self-perception subscale contains five items designed to assess the way the disease makes the patient feel about himself or herself. The items ask about the degree to which the patient lacks self-confidence, feels frustrated, feels embarrassed, feels angry, and worries about others' negative appraisals. The items are answered on a Likert scale of 0 = not at all, 1 = a little bit, 2 = sometimes, 3 = quite a bit, 4 = always.

DSQL Total Score

The total QOL score is used as a unifying mechanism for capturing all of the relevant domains in a single score. As such, this index score is thought to represent the combined adverse impact the disease has on the patient.

The measurement model of the general QOL score is based on classical psychometric theory, which assumes that each of the subscales is a fallible indicator of the general construct.*

ANALYTICAL RATIONALE

The design of the structural validation test is based on the assumption that the DSQL contains distinct yet related subscales, each of which is expected to have a unique measurement model that is empirically detectable with factor analysis. The scoring algorithm of each subscale is based on a simple unit-weighted sum. The sum is then divided by the number of items in the subscale to create an average that provides a theoretical range directly comparable to other subscales in the instrument and that permits the total subscale scores to be interpreted on the same scale as the original items. The average score is a commonly used device for maintaining comparability between and among subscale scores and between subscales and items.

Data from two distinct studies are used to confirm the factor structure of the DSQL. Subjects were 565 contact dermatitis patients and 392 acne patients who participated in separate dermatological clinical studies. Patients in both studies completed multi-inventory questionnaires simultaneously with clinical data collection; they were also retested at a subsequent follow-up. Both samples completed core DSQL items, the energy/fatigue subscales of the SF36, and several single-item general measures of the DSQL core constructs. The acne-specific instrument has an extra item for measuring physical symptoms.

CONFIRMATORY FACTOR ANALYSIS

The factor structure of the DSQL was tested using a structural equation approach to confirmatory factor analysis (CFA). It was assumed that the measurement models underlying subscales of the DSQL are based on classical psychometric theory and its corollary of internal consistency. In this model, the variance in the individual item is thought to be composed of a "true score" and a random error component, which for the sample (1) is normally distributed around zero, (2) has an expectation of zero, and (3)

* The use of the sum of the averages for the measure of general QOL produces a psychometrically superior measure because it removes the measurement error in the individual components before the average is created, thus giving a further refinement to the scale over the sum of simple single general items.

when included in the sum of a number of parallel items, has a sum of zero. Theoretically, the asymptotic sum of the random errors cancels out the errors in the items, and the "true score" emerges.

Confirmatory factor analysis formally estimates the random error component and removes it from the latent construct to permit formal examination of the relationship between the individual items and the "true score." The "true score" is estimated as the shared variance among multiple indicators of the latent construct as follows:

$$Y_i = \lambda_{i1}\eta_1 + \varepsilon_i \tag{1}$$

where Y_i is the ith indicator in the subscale, η_1 is the single latent construct assumed to underlie the subscale, λ_{i1} is the factor loading connecting the indicator to the latent construct, and ε_i is the random measurement in the ith indicator. Modeling the latent construct permits a testable hypothesis of the structural validity of the measurement model underlying the unit-weighted scoring algorithm used in practice.

In the study, maximum likelihood estimation (MLE) is used to test the measurement models of the DSQL. Models are evaluated based on the χ^2 test of differences between the observed and modeled covariance matrix and the average absolute residual covariance. Quantitative model fits were evaluated using Bentler-Bonnet normed and nonnormed fit indices (BB_N and BB_R, respectively)* and the Comparative Fit Index (CFI).†

RESULTS

Table 1 presents descriptive statistics for the DSQL for the two samples of patients at baseline and at follow-up. The responses for the acne sample show means for all DSQL variables clustered at the low end of the scale,

* To avoid confusion of the subscripts with Bentler-Bonnet fit indices (BBFI), we use the subscript "R" to signify nonnormed (to indicate the coefficient in raw form) and "N" to indicate normed.

† The BBFI are used to measure the fit of the modeled covariance to the observed covariance with a metric that goes beyond the χ^2 test of significance in much the same as a R^2 measures effect size. Like other measures of effect size, their interpretation relies more on convention than on hard rules. Conventional wisdom suggests that in general fit indices of 0.70–0.79 indicate an adequate fit, 0.80–0.89, indicate a good fit, and 0.90–0.99 indicate an excellent fit. The normed BBFI correct for number of variables in the covariance matrix, and the CFI is designed to test competing models.

Table 1 Means, Standard Deviations, and Standardized Coefficients for the DSQL at Baseline and Follow-Up

	Acne						Contact dermatitis					
	M_B	SD_B	l_B	M_F	SD_F	l_F	M_B	SD_B	l_B	M_F	SD_F	l_F
1	1.4	0.9	0.46	1.4	1.1	0.43	3.1	1.1	0.46	2.0	1.3	0.75
2	1.5	1.0	0.67	1.1	0.9	0.71	2.1	1.4	0.72	1.2	1.2	0.85
3	2.0	1.1	0.36	1.4	1.1	0.39	—	—	—	—	—	—
4	1.2	1.0	0.71	0.9	0.9	0.70	1.9	1.4	0.76	1.0	1.2	0.87
5	1.1	1.1	0.65	0.9	0.9	0.53	3.0	1.1	0.47	2.0	1.3	0.76
6	0.6	0.8	0.66	0.6	0.8	0.60	2.0	1.4	0.62	1.1	1.3	0.79
7	0.5	0.7	0.70	0.4	0.7	0.69	1.4	1.4	0.65	0.8	1.1	0.72
8	0.6	0.9	0.65	0.5	0.7	0.59	2.0	1.4	0.69	0.9	1.2	0.78
9	0.3	0.6	0.64	0.2	0.5	0.50	1.7	1.3	0.63	0.8	1.1	0.72
10	0.5	0.9	0.71	0.5	0.8	0.66	1.0	1.3	0.67	0.7	1.1	0.74
11	1.0	1.2	0.66	0.7	1.1	0.63	1.2	1.5	0.55	0.8	1.2	0.64
12	0.5	0.9	0.78	0.4	0.8	0.77	1.2	1.4	0.53	0.7	1.2	0.64
13	0.9	1.2	0.77	0.7	1.1	0.77	0.5	1.0	0.57	0.4	0.9	0.61
14	1.0	1.2	0.69	0.9	1.1	0.65	0.5	1.0	0.58	0.5	1.0	0.57
15	0.7	0.9	0.77	0.5	0.8	0.78	0.6	1.1	0.72	0.3	0.8	0.80
16	1.2	1.2	0.85	0.8	1.0	0.84	1.5	1.4	0.79	0.8	1.1	0.83
17	0.7	1.0	0.87	0.5	0.9	0.88	1.3	1.4	0.77	0.7	1.1	0.84
18	0.7	1.0	0.90	0.5	0.8	0.88	0.8	1.2	0.80	0.4	0.9	0.88
19	1.1	1.2	0.81	0.8	1.1	0.89	0.6	1.2	0.66	0.3	0.9	0.70
20	0.8	1.1	0.79	0.7	1.0	0.86	0.9	1.2	0.74	0.4	0.9	0.79
21	0.7	1.1	0.80	0.5	0.9	0.83	0.9	1.3	0.85	0.4	0.9	0.83
22	1.0	1.2	0.83	0.7	1.1	0.89	0.9	1.3	0.83	0.4	0.9	0.85
23	0.8	1.1	0.89	0.6	0.9	0.92	1.0	1.3	0.89	0.5	1.0	0.92
24	0.7	1.0	0.90	0.5	0.9	0.92	0.8	1.2	0.90	0.5	0.9	0.92
25	0.4	0.7	0.78	0.3	0.7	0.82	0.4	0.9	0.73	0.3	0.8	0.78
26	0.3	0.7	0.77	0.3	0.6	0.77	0.4	0.9	0.70	0.3	0.8	0.79
27	0.7	1.0	0.79	0.6	0.9	0.86	0.5	1.0	0.83	0.3	0.8	0.90
28	0.6	0.9	0.86	0.5	0.9	0.88	0.5	1.0	0.87	0.3	0.8	0.92
29	0.4	0.8	0.85	0.3	0.7	0.85	0.4	0.9	0.77	0.2	0.7	0.78
30	0.2	0.6	0.60	0.3	0.7	0.61	0.5	0.9	0.66	0.2	0.7	0.63
31	0.4	0.8	0.67	0.3	0.7	0.66	0.5	1.0	0.67	0.2	0.7	0.69
32	1.1	1.2	0.84	0.9	1.0	0.82	0.9	1.1	0.78	0.6	1.0	0.84
33	1.4	1.2	0.85	1.1	1.1	0.85	2.0	1.3	0.70	1.1	1.2	0.85
34	1.7	1.3	0.90	1.3	1.2	0.91	1.8	1.4	0.85	1.1	1.3	0.88
35	1.5	1.3	0.84	1.2	1.2	0.86	1.6	1.4	0.80	0.9	1.2	0.86
36	1.4	1.3	0.84	1.1	1.2	0.86	1.3	1.4	0.83	0.8	1.1	0.86

M = Mean; SD = standard deviation; 1 = standardized coefficient linking the items to their respective latent factor; $_B$ = baseline; $_F$ = follow-up.

suggesting that the patients on average did not experience substantial adverse impact on their QOL. There was, however, a substantial amount of heterogeneity as indicated by the large standard deviations, and there was a consistent pattern of skewness in the work items, with very few patients indicating that their disease affected the work environment at all. Though substantial, the skewness is probably not high enough to seriously threaten the assumptions of multinormality used in the robust MLE procedures.

The descriptive statistics for the contact dermatitis QOL study are also presented in Table 1. In general, the means on the contact dermatitis sample baseline visit were higher than they were in the acne baseline, particularly among the physical items. None of the physical items had means less than 1.0, and several had means greater than 2.0 and 3.0. This trend suggests a greater impairment of physical functioning than that produced by acne. The same pattern of high QOL was apparent on the work items as was seen in the acne sample, again indicating that the disease has very little adverse impact on the job. The work variables also show the same level of high variability and high skewness as was seen in the acne data.

The follow-up descriptive statistics for the acne sample are also presented in Table 1. As expected, the posttreatment scores decrease from baseline, despite the fact that the scores showed fairly high levels of QOL before treatment. The differences in the work items may have been attenuated somewhat by the ceiling effects and skewness at baseline. The follow-up data for the contact dermatitis sample also showed the same patterns of variability and skewness as in the baseline sample. In contrast to the baseline measurement, only one of the physical items had a mean greater than 2.0, and none of the items had a mean greater than 3.0. Several of the means dropped a full point. The standard deviations and skewness indices remained relatively constant across the intervention. These results suggest a general parallel shift of the distribution toward improved QOL.

Taken together, the descriptive statistics for the two samples suggest that the DSQL items possess sufficient distributional sensitivity, free of ceiling and floor effects, to permit reliable detection of the relevant individual differences in dermatology-specific QOL when they are present. The changes in scores on the individual items across treatment suggest that they have the potential to detect QOL change associated with clinical improvement as well.

CONFIRMATORY FACTOR ANALYSIS

Confirmatory Factor Analysis (CFA) moves beyond the univariate distributions to consider the bivariate and multivariate associations between and among the items as indications of the structural validity (6). The Basic

Model tests the DSQL's capacity to identify five distinct positively intercorrelated factors that correspond to the subscales. The factor loadings and the residual covariance address the justification of the scoring algorithm as an unit-weighted average. The Invariance Model tests the stability of the measurement model across treatment. This would provide assurance that mean differences are not confounded by a difference in meaning of the scores across time. The General DSQL Model tests a superordinate factor model that addresses the scale's capacity to support a single unit-weighted sum of the subscale scores as a measure of general disease-related QOL across the functional domains.

The Basic Model

The basic confirmatory factor model for the DSQL is depicted in Figure 1. The figure shows that the five latent factors are each defined by the subscales and their relevant indicators. Accordingly, the five latent factors that parallel the subscales are considered to represent the source of the covariance among the subscale indicators. The small arrows under each indicator represent the measurement error in each item, which is, in the confirmatory factor model, the unique variance in each item representing random measurement error. The arrows connecting the latent factors to their indicators represent factor loadings. Finally, the curved lines between each pair of latent factors represents the interfactor correlations. In the DSQL the latter is assumed to be positive and significantly different from zero.

The MLE of the model depicted in Figure 1 provides a reasonable approximation of the covariance matrix of the DSQL indicators. Although the χ^2 of 2006 with 584 degrees of freedom suggested a significant difference between the observed and model covariance matrix, the fit indices suggested that the difference was not substantial.* However, the average of the residuals was only 0.04 and the residuals were normally distributed around zero, indicating that there was little systematic variance left to be explained by other factors not included in the model. The fit indices were in the 0.85 range ($BB_N = 0.826$; $BB_R = 0.859$; $CFI = 0.869$) and are all consistent with a respectable fit to the data. The contact dermatitis sample yielded virtually the same fit ($\chi^2 = 2262$ (550), $p < 0.001$; $BB_N = 0.818$; $BB_R = 0.844$;

* The fact that χ^2 increases with sample size limits its utility as a statistical test of goodness-of-fit when the sample size is large (3), and most analysts agree that it is best to rely on multiple measures to avoid concluding that a model fit is nonsignificant, and to instead focus attention on the goodness-of-fit, size of the residuals, and shape of the distribution of residuals as a basis for determining if there is any systematic covariance left to be explained in the covariance matrix.

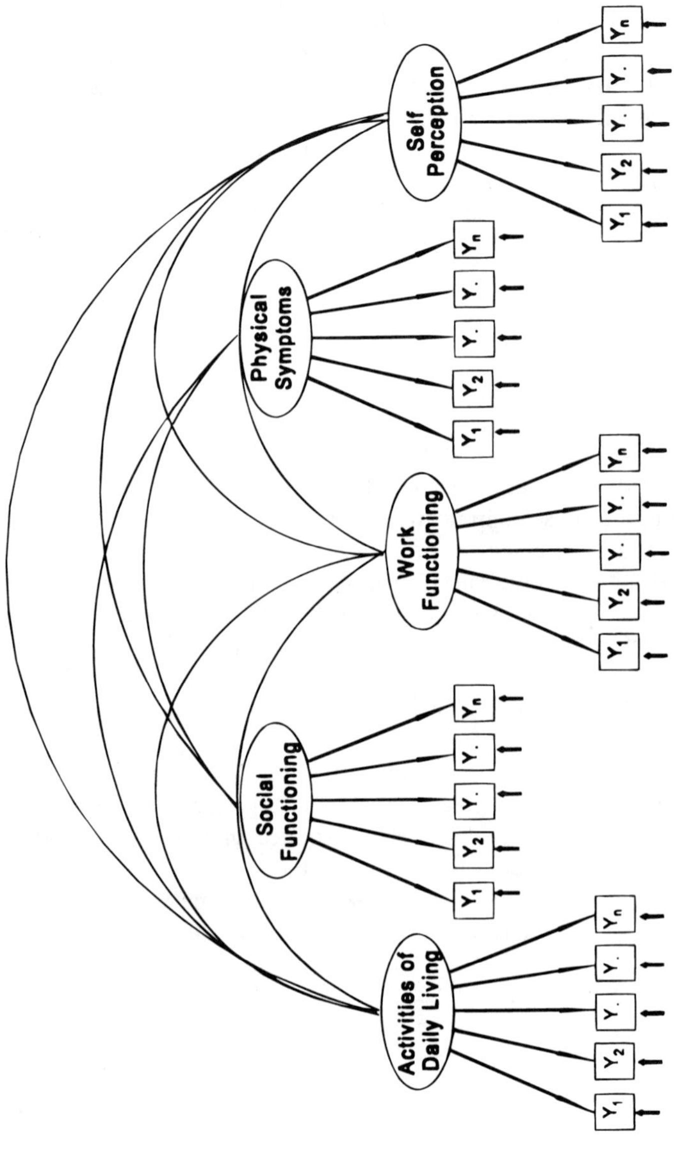

Figure 1 Basic confirmatory factor model.

CFI = 0.856). From a model perspective, the five-correlated-factor model seems consistent with the data.

Table 1 also contains the factor loadings for the DSQL items on their five respective latent factors. All coefficients were significantly different from zero and substantial, with the lowest factor loading in the entire two columns being for the PHY3 (0.358) in the acne instrument. All of the other DSQL items appeared to be strong indicators of their latent constructs. With the exception of the single physical symptom item in the acne instrument, the factor loadings of all DSQL items were sufficiently high and similar to one another to support the unit-weighted scoring algorithm.

Table 2 contains the interfactor correlations among the five latent constructs. The correlations were all significantly different from zero and high enough to provide convincing evidence that the five constructs are relevant to a single QOL construct.

Follow-Up

CFA also showed that the follow-up data provide a relatively good fit to the model presented in Figure 1. Here again, in the acne data the χ^2 of 1968 with 584 degrees of freedom suggests a significant difference between the observed and model covariance matrix, but the fit indices suggest that the difference was trivial. The average residual was only 0.04, and the residuals were normally distributed around zero. The fit indices again clustered

Table 2 Intercorrelations Among Latent Factors of the DSQL

	Factor combinations			
	CD_B	CD_F	$Acne_B$	$Acne_F$
ADL—physical	0.58	0.64	0.74	0.53
Social—physical	0.51	0.62	0.67	0.49
Work—physical	0.47	0.47	0.63	0.50
Personal—physical	0.55	0.69	0.66	0.53
Social—ADL	0.69	0.80	0.87	0.77
Work—ADL	0.53	0.49	0.83	0.77
Personal—ADL	0.62	0.70	0.75	0.71
Work—social	0.69	0.70	0.81	0.79
Personal—social	0.73	0.76	0.82	0.76
Personal—work	0.73	0.62	0.65	0.67

ADL = Activities of daily living; physical = physical symptoms; social = social functioning; work = work functioning; personal = self-perceptions.

around the 0.85 range ($BB_N = 0.834$; $BB_R = 0.867$; CFI = 0.877). The contact dermatitis sample produced a fit very similar to the acne sample ($\chi^2 = 2589$ (550), $p < 0.001$; $BB_N = 0.814$; $BB_R = 0.834$; CFI = 0.847).

Table 1 presents the standardized factor loadings for the DSQL items no the latent factors. All coefficients were significantly different from zero and substantial. The low loading for the acne sample PHY3 item appeared again in the follow-up sample (0.389), suggesting that this item may not be contributing much to the DSQL, and the current version of the DSQL does not obtain this item. As in the baseline data, the large and generally equivalent factor loadings support the unit-weighted scoring algorithm.

The CFA on the baseline and follow-up data provide convincing evidence in support of the structural validity of the scale. In both trials, the empirical tests of the factors show close correspondence to the subscales. The high factor loadings, the low average residual covariances, and the normal distribution of the model errors all support the unit-weighted scoring algorithms in both measurements trials. Taken together, these analyses show the DSQL to possess adequate psychometric characteristics.

Test of Invariance

Figure 2 models the invariance in the factor structures across treatment. This analysis tests a fully constrained model in which the factor loadings and the factor intercorrelations are assumed to be equal to one another across treatment. As discussed above, this technique formally tests whether the pattern found in the baseline data can be considered identical to that found in the follow-up data. The fully constrained model produced a respectable fit to the covariance matrix in the acne sample. Although the χ^2 of 4080 with 1214 degrees of freedom was statistically significant, the fit indices suggested a fairly good fit to the data. All indices were again in the 0.85 range ($BB_N = 0.825$; $BB_R = 0.866$; CFI = 0.870). A cumulative La Grange multiplier test showed that the bulk of the error in the model was explained by constraining the factor loadings item 2 (feel sore/tender) on factor 1 (physical symptoms) and item 39 (talking to coworkers) on factor 4 (work functioning) across the treatment measurements. The two modifications produced a decrease in the χ^2 of 34.426, a reduction that still does not indicate a nonsignificant difference between the observed and modeled covariance matrices.

The contact dermatitis sample yielded a slightly weaker fit to the data ($\chi^2 = 5129$ (1145), $p < 0.001$; $BB_N = 0.805$; $BB_R = 0.835$; CFI = 0.842). In this model there were six constraints that accounted for most of the lack of fit to the observed covariance matrices: item 1 (feel drier than nonaffected areas) on factor 1; item 4 (feel painful) on factor 1 (physical symptoms);

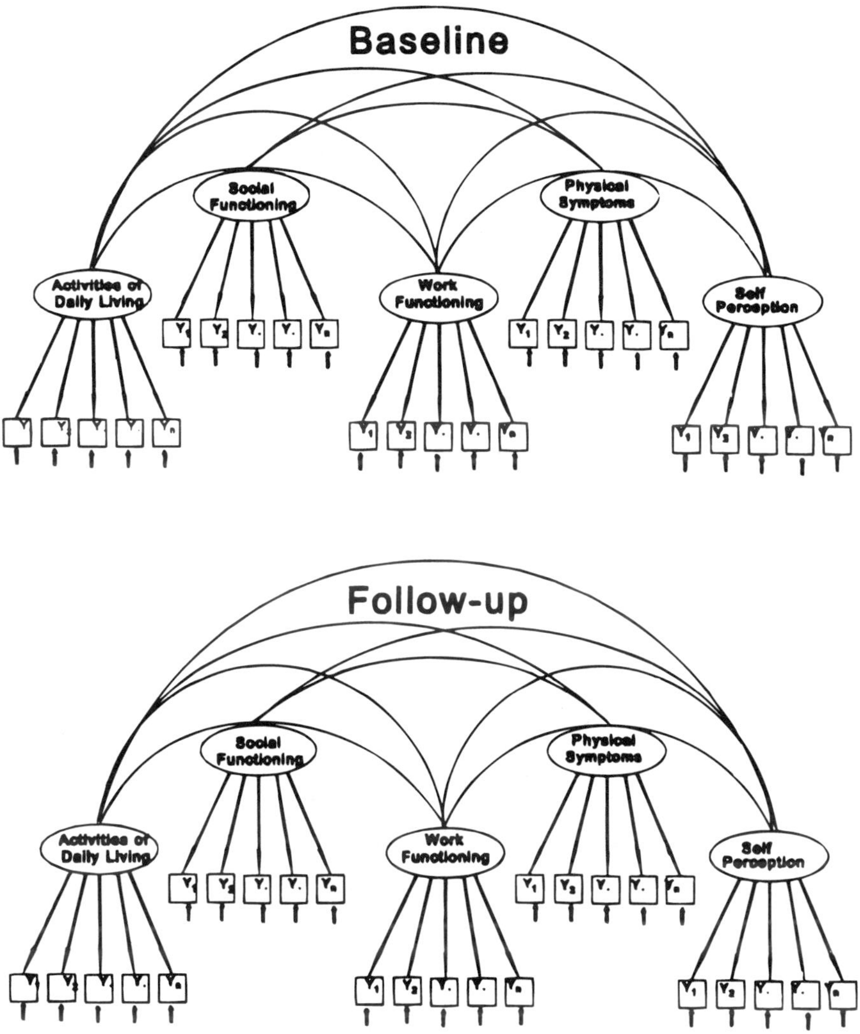

Figure 2 Test of invariance.

item 20 (desire to be with friends) on factor 3 (social functioning); item 41 (being effective in giving directions) on factor 5 (work functioning); item 21 (desire to date) on factor 3 (social functioning); and the correlations between factors 1 and 3 (physical symptoms and work functioning, respectively). Although the reduction on the χ^2 of 164.012 is substantial, it is

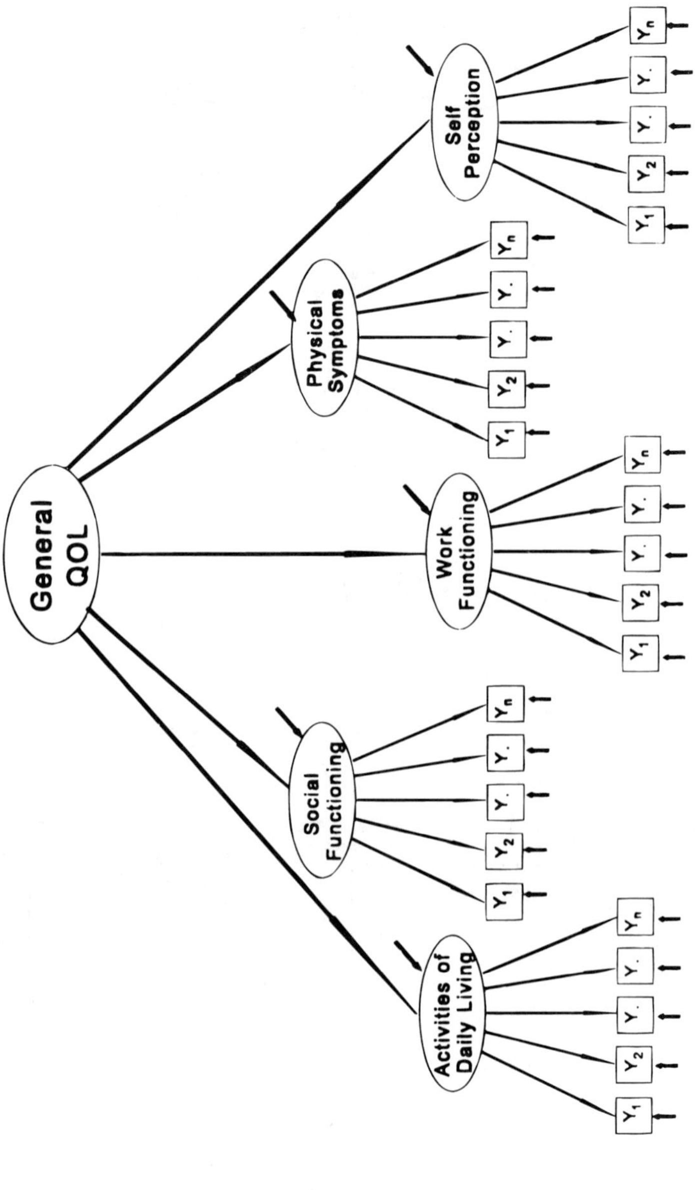

Figure 3 Test of second-order model.

minor compared to the overall model fit. This suggests that the invariance is minor and poses no serious threat to the interpretation of the changes in scores across treatment.

Test of the Total Score

The size of the intercorrelations seen in the basic model analysis suggests that the correlations among the subscales of the DSQL are high enough to permit the calculation of a single total scale score. The total score captures the commonality among the subscales and permits a straightforward test of QOL hypotheses in which a given treatment is expected to improve health status in all functional areas. Figure 3 depicts a second-order factor that tests the ability of the five latent factors to emerge from a single underlying superordinate construct global QOL. Here the first-order factors are modeled in the same way as the measured indicators, with their own error terms indicated by the small diagonal arrow next to each first-order factor. The larger arrows connecting the global QOL latent factor to the first-order latent factors represent standardize loadings on the second-order factor. The invariance found in the previous test suggests that separate analyses of the baseline and follow-up data are not needed in this model. We therefore present only the results for the baseline data.

Estimation of the factor model suggests a respectable fit to the data in both samples. For the acne data, the χ^2 of 1983 with 589 degrees of freedom was statistically significant, but the fit indices suggested that the difference was small, and in the acceptable range ($BB_N = 0.833$; $BB_R = 0.867$; $CFI = 0.876$). Table 3 shows that standardized loadings on the second-order factor were also extremely high, with all but one being above 0.80. The contact dermatitis sample yielded a similar fit to the data ($\chi^2 = 2281$

Table 3 Factor Loadings on the Second-order factor

	First-order factors	
Subscale	Acne	CD
Physical symptoms	0.59	0.62
Activities of daily living	0.87	0.76
Social functioning	0.90	0.88
Work functioning	0.86	0.76
Self-perception	0.83	0.83

All coefficients are significantly different from zero at the 0.01 level.

(555), $p < 0.001$; $BB_N = 0.817$; $BB_R = 0.844$; CFI = 0.854). All first-order factors produced loadings greater than 0.60 on the general QOL second-order factor.

SUMMARY

The structural validation of the DSQL showed it to be comprised of a set of internally consistent items capable of defining its intended disease-specific content. The univariate analysis showed the scale to contain sufficiently broad distributions, which although somewhat skewed appear to possess enough sensitivity to detect individual differences in both tails of the distributions without excessive concern for ceiling or floor effects. The confirmatory factor analysis supported the earlier exploratory factor analysis by showing that the five correlated factors identified in the obliquely rotated exploratory analysis did in fact account for the majority of the covariances among the indicators, and that these factors are themselves highly correlated with one another.

The factor loadings supported the proposed unit-weighted scoring algorithm by producing significant and substantial loadings on the relevant factors with little evidence of cross-loadings on the other factors. Because the averaging of the subscale scores is obtained by simply dividing by a constant, there is no further need to validate the averaging part of the algorithm. The averaging approach is widely used in psychological research using self-reported measures, offering a form of standardization that facilitates cross-subscale interpretation.

The second-order factor analysis provided support for the interpretation of a unit-weighted sum of the subscale scores as a total. This empirical support for the combination of the scale is valuable in understanding the total impact of disease and has great benefit in pharmacoeconomic research, in which QOL is used as an outcome parameter. In utility analysis, for example, the total score can be used as an unweighted sum of the subscales for a unitary outcome. The coefficients in the factor analysis may also be used to create different weights for this purpose.

The test of the stability of the factor structure across treatment suggests that difference scores can be used without concern for confounding as a result of a changed structure due to treatment. This finding justifies the use of traditional General Linear Model (GLM) change procedures such as analysis of covariance, raw change scores, residualized change score, and simple postreatment differences as a method for testing effectiveness of treatments.

The data support the basic psychometric properties of the individual subscales, and the high intercorrelations among the subscales are consistent with a superordinate QOL model. An additional inquiry into the DSQL, as well as other QOL instruments, should focus on the extent that the intercorrelations observed among subscales reflect the true underlying structure of QOL, with highly interdependent domains, vs. correlated errors from a common set of instructions or methods, thus inflating the interscale correlations (7).

REFERENCES

1. Anderson RT, Rajagopalan R. Development and validation of a quality of life instrument for cutaneous diseases. J Am Acad Dermatol 1997. In press.
2. Rajagopalan R, Anderson RT. The profile of a patient with contact dermatitis and a suspicion of contact allergy: history, physical characteristics and dermatology-specific quality of life. Am J Contact Dermatitis 1997; 8(1): 26–31.
3. Bollen KA. Structural Equations with Latent Variables. New York: Wiley, 1989.
4. Bollen KA, Lennox RD. Conventional wisdom on measurement: a structural equations perspective. Psychol Bull 1991; 110(2): 305–314.
5. Nunnally JC, Bernstein IH. Psychometric Theory. 3rd ed. New York: McGraw-Hill, 1995.
6. Lennox RD, Dennis ML. Measurement error issues in substance abuse services research: lessons from structural equation modeling and psychometric theory. Eval Prog Plan 1994; 17(4): 399–407.
7. Lennox RD. Correlated errors among items linked to a common set of instructions. Annual Meeting of the American Statistical Association, Chicago, Aug 4–8, 1996.

APPENDIX

I. Abbreviated DSQL scale items (item number in parentheses)
   A. Symptoms. How often did the affected area(s) of your skin: (1) feel dryer than nonaffected areas, (2) feel sore/tender, (3) feel more oily, (4) feel painful, (5) feel itchy (6) cause a burning sensation, (7) cause other symptoms? How often did you (8) experience intervals of discomfort? How often did your discomfort cause you (9) to lose sleep or sleep badly?
   B. ADL. Because of your *skin condition*, how often did you limit yourself in: (11) participating in vigorous physical activity, (12) shaving or wearing makeup, (13) choice of clothes worn, (14) choice of hairstyle, (15) choice of food or beverage?
   C. Social functioning. How often did you feel that your *skin condition* limited your: (17) chances for making friends, (18) being comfortable in group activities, (19) freedom to do things you enjoy, (20) desire to be with friends, (21) desire to date, (22) extent of satisfac-

tion with personal relationships, (23) readiness to go shopping or browsing, (24) dating habits or plans, (25) planned social activities, (26) time spent in the community?

D. Work or school performance. To what extent has your *skin condition* interfered with: (37) getting ahead at work or school, (38) getting a better job, (39) talking to co-workers or classmates, (40) being effective in meetings, (41) being effective in giving directions, (42) being punctual because of doctor's appointments; (43) being punctual due to physical or emotional discomfort?

E. Personal perceptions. To what extent has your *skin condition* caused you to: (45) lack self-confidence, (46) feel frustrated, (47) feel embarrassed about appearance, (48) feel angry, (49) worry about what others think of you?

II. Abbreviated DSQL global items (item number in parentheses). On scale of 1 to 10:

(10) How bothered were you by any physical symptoms due to your *skin condition*?

(16) How much did your *skin condition* interfere with grooming or styling?

(27) How much did your *skin condition* interfere with your social activities?

(44) How satisfied have you been with how others respond to you at work or school?

(40) How satisfied have you been with your social life?

(51) How satisfied have you been with your skin appearance?

(50) How severe is your *skin condition* today?

(53) How severe has your *skin condition* been in the last month?

9

Impact of Acne on Quality of Life in Adolescents

Jeffrey A. Smith and Daniel P. Krowchuk *Bowman Gray School of Medicine of Wake Forest University, Winston-Salem, North Carolina*

INTRODUCTION

Acne vulgaris affects an estimated 17 million people in the United States, including 85% of adolescents and young adults (1). It is the most common skin condition treated by physicians (2). The etiology of acne is multifactorial, involving the interaction of sebum, bacteria, and androgenic hormones (3). The observation that severe acne is common in some families suggests that genetic factors also may be important (2). A number of factors may worsen acne. Certain cosmetics, emollients, and sunscreens may physically obstruct follicles, thereby creating more lesions. Medications with hormonal effects, including progestins and corticosteroids, may exacerbate acne, as can certain nonhormonal therapeutic agents.

The lesions of acne occur on the face, chest, and back, areas in which pilosebaceous follicles are concentrated. Beginning in late childhood, coincident with increased secretion of androgenic hormones characteristic of early puberty, acne first appears. Initially the lesions often are obstructive in nature, so-called "blackheads" and "whiteheads," and are concentrated in the midportion of the face (3). Later, inflammatory lesions (papules and pustules) are seen that upon resolution may leave pigmentary changes, cysts, or scars. The peak incidence of acne occurs at age 17 years (1); in most individuals the disease undergoes complete involution, usually by late adolescence or early adulthood (2).

A cutaneous condition such as acne that has a predilection for the face might be anticipated to have considerable impact on quality of life. This chapter reviews published studies that address quality-of-life issues in adolescents and young adults with this disorder. To identify relevant publications, a search employing Medline and Psychological Abstracts was conducted. Empirical studies appearing in English-language journals were then reviewed. This chapter will provide an overview of health-related quality-of-life assessment and will then review studies that have examined quality of life in young adults and adolescents with acne. The concluding section will discuss possible future directions for research in this area.

HEALTH-RELATED QUALITY-OF-LIFE ASSESSMENT

As an increasing number of successful medical treatments have been developed, there is growing evidence that nondisease factors, such as the intrusiveness of the treatment and the frequency of hospital admissions, affect patient adjustment (4). Therefore, recent years have witnessed a growing recognition among medical investigators of the importance of supplementing traditional morbidity and mortality indices of disease severity and treatment efficacy with measures of health-related quality of life (HRQL) (5). Frequently, HRQL assessments are aimed at identifying psychological dysfunction among patients with a primary physical illness. HRQL assessments are also particularly valuable in clinical trials in which improved functioning serves as an indicator of benefit, the study population is of mild to moderate disease status and the intervention may have undesirable effects, or a new treatment is being compared with standard therapy to determine both its clinical and functional benefits. Much of the research on acne involves at least one of these factors and suggests an important role for HRQL assessment.

Most definitions of HRQL are multidimensional (6,7) and include elements from the following four domains: physical symptoms, functional status, psychological functioning, and social functioning. Although much progress has been made in recent years in the definition and assessment of HRQL in adults, this has not been the case in research on children. To date, HRQL is rarely assessed in a systematic and integrated manner in studies involving children (8). A modified battery approach to HRQL is the norm, where investigators use a number of instruments to assess each of the core HRQL domains (9).

The issues that make the assessment of HRQL important in the study of adults' responses to both disease and its treatment are also relevant to children and adolescents. Yet as difficult as it may be to assess and interpret HRQL in adults, children and adolescents present an even greater challenge. Specifically, child and adolescent researchers must take into consideration the relatively rapid developmental shifts that occur within the time frame of most longitudinal assessment and clinical trials research and their subjects' self-report limitations, especially at the younger age ranges. Therefore, the ideal HRQL assessment for youths would include instruments that are reliable, brief, easy to administer, and have age-adjusted norms available.

HRQL AND ACNE

Although usually a self-limited disorder, acne has traditionally been perceived as having significant adverse effects on the acne sufferer's HRQL. Nearly 50 years ago, Sulzberger and Zaidens (10) commented: "There is no single disease which causes more psychic trauma . . . than does acne vulgaris." Over the years, that sentiment has been echoed by many other clinicians and researchers. Hurwitz (11), for example, stated that acne "should never be dismissed as being of no consequence . . . for the psychosocial scars and trauma are often deeper and more disastrous than the blemishes . . . ." Unfortunately, empirical support for the association between acne and diminished quality of life has lagged far behind the clinician's belief that such a relationship exists.

Young Adult Studies

Single Assessment Design

Most attempts to examine acne's influence on HRQL have focused on the assessment of psychopathology among its sufferers. Due to the paucity of research that has focused solely on the impact of acne on the HRQL in adolescents, a critical review of studies that used either a combination of adolescents and young adults or only young adults will follow.

In a published abstract, Shuster et al. (12) observed that dissatisfaction with facial appearance was common and correlated with disease severity. They concluded, therefore, that acne had a negative impact on self-image. However, no information was provided on the sample's characteristics, the methodological soundness of the assessment tool, or the statistical analyses utilized (12).

Medansky et al. (13) investigated the relationship between acne severity and anxiety in a sample of older adolescents and young adults. Using the Speilberger State-Trait Anxiety Inventory (STAI), they found anxiety levels among their subjects that were comparable to those found in the general population, despite intuitively expecting "acne to be a devastating psychological event for some individuals" (13). Furthermore, neither the patient's age nor the duration or severity of their acne was found to be correlated with their self-reported trait anxiety (13). No mention was made about any analyses performed on the relationship of severity and duration of acne with trait anxiety, the dimension of anxiety most likely to be affected by situational as opposed to constitutional factors. In contrast, van der Meeren et al. (14) found higher levels of social anxiety among their acne patients using the Social Anxiety Scale, an instrument the authors claimed was comparable to the STAI.

In an effort to expand our knowledge of the impact of acne on HRQL, Jowett and Ryan (15) collected detailed information about the effect that a variety of skin diseases, including acne, had on several domains of patients' lives. Using a structured interview format, nearly half of the acne sufferers reported experiencing interpersonal difficulties due to their skin condition, and two thirds reported experiencing acne-related shame and anxiety (15). Few acne sufferers reported that their condition had much of an impact on their relationship with family. The results of this study, however, are difficult to interpret given the absence of a control group, the wide age range of subjects (16–79 years), and the use of a nonstandardized assessment instrument.

In an attempt to improve upon some of the methodological shortcomings of earlier studies, Wu et al. (16) used previously standardized instruments to evaluate the relationship between a variety of psychological constructs and both an objective as well as a patient's subjective rating of acne severity. A control group of individuals who had never experienced any type of skin disorder was also incorporated into the study. The sample was comprised primarily of young adults. The findings revealed a positive correlation between both self- and physician-rated acne severity and anxiety. A similar relationship was found between physician-rated severity and anger (16). Although this study improved upon the methodology of prior research in this area, the results are confounded by the statistically significant age differences between the most severely affected group of acne patients and the less affected patients and the control group. Without having statistically controlled for patient age and perhaps duration of condition, it is impossible to determine if the reported group differences in anger and anxiety were solely a function of acne severity.

In a relatively recent attempt to understand the impact of acne on HRQL, Motley and Finlay (17) constructed a 10-item Acne Disability Index (ADI) containing questions that were highly correlated with acne severity and administered it to a sample of teenagers and young adults.

Patients with facial acne rated themselves as aggressive, unhappy with their physical appearance, inhibited in their ability to meet individuals of the opposite sex, and reluctant to go out socially. Patients were also asked the amount of money they would be willing to pay for a cure for their acne. Interestingly, ADI scores and not objective acne severity ratings were found to be correlated with the amount patients would pay for a cure for their acne (17).

As part of a larger study, Al'Abadie et al. (18) examined the relationship between stress and acne in adults. Sixteen percent of a mixed-diagnosis group, some of whom had acne, reported that stress contributed to the onset of their condition, whereas 36% reported that stress exacerbated their symptoms. Both of these percentages were considerably lower than those reported by a group of psoriasis patients (70% and 67%, respectively) and were equivalent to another mixed-diagnosis group comprised primarily of patients with malignant melanomas and basal cell carcinomas. However, the authors acknowledge limitations to this study. First, the mixed-diagnosis groups were created based on the untested assumption that stress functioned similarly for each of the diagnostic entities included. Thus, the possibility exists that a weak relationship between stress and a particular skin condition (e.g., eczema) may have masked the presence of a strong relationship between stress and another skin condition (e.g., acne) in the same group (18).

An important advance in the study of the impact of skin disease was the development of the Dermatology Life Quality Index (DLQI), a 10-item questionnaire that provides a global assessment of quality of life (19). Scores on the DLQI range from 0 to 30; higher scores reflect greater perceived effect of the disease. In initial studies, Finlay and Khan (19) administered the DLQI to 200 new patients with various inflammatory dermatoses attending a dermatology clinic and to 100 healthy controls. DLQI scores for the 18 patients with acne (mean 4.3, range 0–11) were significantly greater than for controls (mean 0.5; range 0–6).

In sum, the preponderance of data suggests that acne negatively affects the HRQL of young adults. However, future studies will need to improve upon the methodological limitations of the existing literature if the association between acne and HRQL is to be understood more fully.

Effects of Treatment of HRQL

An additional method used to examine the impact of acne on HRQL has been to assess psychopathological variables both before and after medical treatment. In the earliest study of this kind, van der Meeren et al. (14) examined the psychological response of a small group of patients ($n = 12$) to successful treatment of their acne. Results revealed a nonsignificant trend toward reduced anxiety levels. The importance of this study lies in its pioneering use of pre- and posttreatment assessments of HRQL variables to evaluate the therapeutic efficacy of an acne treatment, rather than in the reliability of its findings. Given the small sample size and absence of a control condition, the results of the study must be interpreted cautiously.

Rubinow et al. (20) evaluated the psychiatric morbidity of 72 young adults with cystic acne enrolled in a National Institutes of Health treatment efficacy study. The assessment battery included the Profile of Mood States Scale (POMS), the Hopkins Symptoms Checklist (HSCL), the Rosenberg Self-Esteem Questionnaire, the NIMH Mood Scale, as well as a semi-structured psychiatric interview. The results revealed significantly elevated scores on all scales of the HSCL prior to treatment, but on none of the other instruments. Posttreatment, patients showed a significant reduction in anxiety as reflected by both the HSCL and the NIMH Mood Scale. Extracting and focusing solely on the data from individuals with predominantly facial as opposed to truncal acne, significant reductions in both anxiety and depression as a function of treatment were demonstrated. The authors suggest that the results of their study be interpreted with caution due to the enhanced risk, given the number of analyses performed, that a Type I error was committed (20). Additional reasons for caution include the absence of a control group and the lack of information provided on the particular semi-structured psychiatric interview utilized.

Gupta et al. (21) assessed depression, anxiety, body dissatisfaction, and general emotional well-being in 10 consecutive acne patients prior to and following treatment using a variety of well-validated psychological instruments. Despite recruiting only patients with mild to moderate levels of acne, significantly higher pretreatment rates of clinical depression (three subjects at the time of assessment, four additional subjects with a positive history), anxiety, and body dissatisfaction were observed than would be found in the general population. The authors reported that improvements in acne were associated with declines to the average range in each of these psychological characteristics. Thus, the authors concluded that even patients with only mild to moderate acne can experience significant psychological distress and that improved psychological functioning can be achieved via successful medical treatment (21). However, given the small sample size, the possibility of an ascertainment bias resulting in inflated levels of pretreatment psychopathology, and the lack of a control group, additional research is needed to confirm the study's findings.

Taken together, these studies indicate that positive responders to acne treatment experience a reduction in their levels of psychological distress. However, due to the absence of control groups, this conclusion must remain tentative.

Adolescent Studies

As mentioned earlier, surprisingly little is known about the impact of acne on the HRQL of adolescents. It might be hypothesized that the psychosocial impact of this disorder would be greater in teenagers than in adults for two reasons. First, adolescence is the phase of life during which acne occurs, thus creating the need for many persons to develop new coping skills in order to accept their changes in physical appearance. Second, the teenage years are widely regarded as critical to the development of one's self-identity, a portion of which is determined by an individual's physical self-image. Therefore, despite the temptation to assume that the relationship between acne severity and HRQL among adolescents mirrors that found in the adult literature, the developmental uniqueness of adolescence requires that this relationship be examined in studies that restrict themselves to teenage subjects and employ age-appropriate assessment instruments.

Our review of the literature through both Medline and Psychological Abstracts uncovered only three studies that limited their investigation of the impact of acne on HRQL to teenagers. In the first study, Schachter et al. (22) assessed the psychological effects of acne in a sample of 1254 high school students. The subjects ranged in age from 14 to 18 years, with the majority being either 15 or 16 years of age. Subjects were asked 46 questions about various aspects of their quality of life. Significant differences between subjects with and without acne were revealed on several items. Specifically, individuals with acne reported feeling more socially isolated and self-conscious than did their unaffected peers. The strengths of this study were its exclusive focus on teenagers and its attempt to examine the impact of acne on several domains of adolescent life (e.g., social acceptance, academic achievement, familial cohesion) (22). Unfortunately, its strengths are overshadowed by its methodological shortcomings. First, HRQL was assessed with a nonstandardized interview format. Second, the authors failed to describe the type of statistical analyses they employed. Third, the considerable number of statistical tests performed likely increased the chance that a Type I error was committed.

A second study to provide information on the relationship between acne and HRQL in teenagers was performed by Lewis-Jones and Finlay (23). In an effort to develop and validate the Children's Dermatology Life Quality Index (CDLQI), data were collected from 233 pediatric dermatology patients, 47 normal controls, and 55 pediatric patients attending nondermatological clinics. The CDLQI contains 10 questions, which provide information on the impact of pediatric skin diseases on emotions, leisure activities, school performance, friendships, and sleep, as well as data on the inconvenience of symptoms and treatment. Scores on the CDLQI can range from 0 to 30; higher scores reflect greater perceived effect of skin disease on quality of life. Results of the study demonstrated that pediatric dermatology patients reported a significantly higher CDLQI mean score (5.1) than either of the two control groups (0.4, 0.7). The diagnostic groups with the highest mean CDLQI scores were patients with eczema (7.7), acne (5.7), and psoriasis (5.4). Across dermatological conditions, the questions most frequently endorsed pertained to symptoms and feelings (23). However, data on the responses to individual items for each diagnostic condition were not provided, thus making it impossible to determine which domains addressed by the CDLQI are most affected among acne patients. Overall, the development of the first reliable instrument to assess the HRQL of children with various skin diseases is a clear strength of this study. In addition, the CDLQI is easy to complete and score. However, it remains unclear how useful the CDLQI would be at assessing HRQL in clinical research studies involving teenage acne patients. The brevity of the measure, though clinically useful, might not lend itself to providing comprehensive information on the physical, social, psychological, and general role (i.e., school and home) functioning of an adolescent. In addition, the CDLQI was validated on a sample of 3- to 16-year-olds, and, therefore, it is unclear how older adolescents with acne would respond to the instrument. Finally, substantial age differences existed between acne patients (mean age = 14.4 years) and the remainder of the pediatric dermatology sample (mean age ≅ 10.5 years), the normal control group (mean age = 9.0 years), and the nondermatological control condition (mean age = 7.8 years). This is of concern because a group of adolescent control subjects might have provided significantly different responses than did the young subjects used in this study.

In the third study, Krowchuk et al. (24) evaluated teenagers presenting for care to a community-based dermatologist in order to assess the psychological impact of acne on adolescents and, in particular, to evaluate whether self-concept was affected by medical treatment. Subjects were 39 consecutive healthy adolescents presenting for initial care of their facial acne who ranged in age from 13 to 19 years (mean age 15.6 years). At the initial visit, subjects completed a series of instruments. A nonstandardized self-assessment questionnaire was employed to elicit the subject's self-perception of the severity and social consequences of their acne. With regard to social consequences, subjects were asked about their levels of dissatisfaction with their facial appearance, levels of peer disapproval of their facial appearance, embarrassment due to acne, and acne-related social inhibition. Subjects also completed the Piers-Harris Self-Concept Scale, a standardized instrument designed to assess self-concept in children and adolescents. The severity of acne was then assessed using a validated grading scale, revealing that acne was mild in 28% of subjects, moderate in 41%, severe in 28%, and very severe in 3% (24).

Analysis of the data revealed that acne negatively impacted upon self-reported satisfaction with facial appearance. Similar to the findings of Motley and Finlay (17) with adults, the most important predictor of personal dissatisfaction with facial appearance was the adolescent's subjective perception of acne severity, rather than the clinician's objective evaluation. This dissatisfaction, in turn, was significantly related to embarrassment and social inhibition. Furthermore, subjects' perceived dissatisfaction with facial appearance and embarrassment and social inhibition stemming from acne were positively correlated with feelings of unhappiness and anxiety. Surprisingly, however, subjects' pretreatment self-concept scores were still within the statistically normal range. Treatment-related improvement in acne severity was found to be associated with significant reductions in many of its perceived adverse consequences, such as peer disapproval of facial appearance and embarrassment and social inhibition stemming from acne. In addition, statistically significant increases in subjects' self-concept scores were also observed from pre- to posttreatment (24). These treatment effects are consistent with the results of Rubinow et al. (20) and Gupta et al. (21).

Specific limitations of this study were discussed by its authors. First, the use of an uncontrolled design limited interpretation of the increases in self-concept scores that accompanied treatment. Second, the finding of baseline self-concept scores within the normal range raised the question of whether self-concept was unaffected by acne or whether a global instrument such as the Piers-Harris Self-Concept Scale was insufficiently sensitive to detect the possibly subtle self-esteem concerns that might exist among adolescents with acne. It is possible, for example, that an instrument that is more sensitive to the influences of physical appearance would have detected changes in self-concept.

The results of these three studies mirror the general findings of the adult literature. That is, HRQL among teenagers is negatively affected by acne, and improvements in acne are associated with significant elevations in individuals' self-appraisals. However, these adolescent studies suffer from methodological limitations similar to those found in the adult literature—specifically, the absence of appropriate control conditions and the lack of a comprehensive assessment of multiple HRQL domains.

SUMMARY AND FUTURE DIRECTIONS

The majority of studies that have examined the impact of acne suggest that various components of HRQL are negatively affected. Unfortunately, this body of research is fraught with methodological problems, such as the use of nonstandardized assessment tools, the lack of clarity regarding statistical models used, and the absence of control groups. On an optimistic note, research performed in the recent past has made efforts to address these methodological concerns. Regardless, further research is needed in the area of acne's impact upon the HRQL of its teenage sufferers.

The following is offered as a possible model for future research on adolescent acne and its impact on HRQL. The sample would consist of teenagers, ages 13–19 years. Acne severity would be determined by a dermatologist using a validated grading system, but subjects would also be asked to self-rate their acne severity. Subjects would be assigned to either a treatment or wait-list control condition, matched for age, sex, and dermatologist-rated acne severity. HRQL would be operationally defined as comprising the dimensions of psychological functioning, social functioning, and physical symptomatology. As functional status is unlikely to be affected in acne patients, we would recommend excluding this dimension from the investigation. The remaining domains should be evaluated with instruments designed for adolescents and appropriate proxies (e.g., parents and teachers). When available, the instruments selected for inclusion in the study should have demonstrated reliability and validity, be age-adjusted and normalized, and allow for a broad range of performance from below to above average. Although we propose a comprehensive assessment of the critical indices of HRQL for this patient population, instruments would need to be selected for brevity as well as their psychometric properties in order to minimize patient and family burden. These might include the multidimensional CDLQI as well as specific measures like the Child Behavior Checklist (25), the Beck Depression Inventory (26), the Children's Manifest Anxiety Scale–Revised (27), and the Perceived Competence Scale for Children (28). Each of these measures is standardized and would provide valuable information on acne's effects on general psychological health, including levels of anxiety and depression and self-perception. Using this type of research design would provide important, reliable information regarding the impact of acne on quality of life in adolescents.

REFERENCES

1. Leydon JJ, Shalita AR. Rational therapy for acne vulgaris: an update on topical treatment. J Am Acad Dermatol 1986; 15:907–915.
2. Pochi PE. The pathogenesis and treatment of acne. Annu Rev Med 1990; 41:187–198.
3. Rothman KF, Lucky AW. Acne vulgaris, Adv Dermatol 1993; 8:347–375.
4. Barbarin OA. Adjustment to serious illness. Adv Clin Child Psychol 1990; 13:377–403.

5. Pantell RH, Lewis CC. Measuring the impact of medical care on children. J Chron Dis 1987; 40(suppl 1): 99S–108S.
6. Aaronson NK, Meyerowitz BE, Bard M, et al. Quality of life research in oncology. Past achievements and future priorities. Cancer 1991; 67: 839–843.
7. Eisen M, Ware JE, Donald CA, Brook RH. Measuring components of children's health status. Med Care 1979; 17: 902–921.
8. Speith LE, Harris CV. Assessment of health-related quality of life in children and adolescents: an integrative review. J Pediatr Psychol 1996; 21: 175–193.
9. Shumaker SA, Anderson RT, Czajkowski SM. Psychological tests and scales. In: Spilker B, ed. Quality of Life Assessment in Clinical Trials. New York: Raven, 1990: 95–113.
10. Sulzberger MB, Zaidens SH. Psychogenic factors in dermatologic disorders. Med Clin North Am 1948; 32: 669–685.
11. Hurwitz S. Clinical Pediatric Dermatology. Philadelphia: WB Saunders, 1981.
12. Shuster S, Fisher GH, Harris E, Binnell D. The effect of skin disease on self image. Br J Dermatol 1978; 99(suppl 16): 18–19.
13. Medansky RS, Handler RM, Medansky DL. Self-evaluation of acne and emotion: a pilot study. Psychosomatics 1981; 22: 379–383.
14. van der Meeren HLM, van der Schaar WW, van den Hurk CMAM. The psychological impact of severe acne. Cutis 1985; 36: 84–86.
15. Jowett S, Ryan T. Skin disease and handicap: an analysis of the impact of skin conditions. Soc Sci Med 1985; 20: 425–429.
16. Wu SF, Kinder BN, Trunnell TN, Fulton JE. Role of anxiety and anger in acne patients: a relationship with the severity of the disorder. J Am Acad Dermatol 1988; 18: 325–333.
17. Motley RJ, Finlay AY. How much disability is caused by acne? Clin Exper Dermatol 1989; 14: 194–198.
18. Al'Abadie MS, Kent GG, Gawkrodger DJ. The relationship between stress and the onset and exacerbation of psoriasis and other skin conditions. Br J Dermatol 1994; 130: 199–203.
19. Finlay AY, Khan GK. Dermatology Life Quality Index (DLQI)—a simple practical measure for routine clinical use. Clin Exper Dermatol 1994; 19: 210–216.
20. Rubinow DR, Peck GL, Squillace KM, Gantt GG. Reduced anxiety and depression in cystic acne patients after successful treatment with oral isotretinoin. J Am Acad Dermatol 1987; 17: 25–32.
21. Gupta MA, Gupta AK, Schork NJ, Ellis CN, Voorhees JJ. Psychiatric aspects of the treatment of mild to moderate facial acne. Some preliminary observations. Int J Dermatol 1990; 29: 719–721.
22. Schachter RJ, Pantel ES, Glassman GM, Zweibelson I. Acne vulgaris and psychologic impact on high school students. NY State J Med 1971; 24: 2886–2890.
23. Lewis-Jones MS, Finlay AY. The Children's Dermatology Life Quality Index (CDLQI): initial validation and practical use. Br J Dermatol 1995; 132: 942–949.

24. Krowchuk DP, Stancin T, Keskinen R, Walker R, Bass J, Anglin TM. The psychosocial effects of acne in adolescents. Pediatr Dermatol 1991; 4: 332–338.
25. Achenbach TM. Integrative Guide for the 1991 CBCL/4–18, YSR, and TRF Profiles. Burlington, VT: University of Vermont Department of Psychiatry, 1991.
26. Beck A, Ward C, Mendelson M, Mock J, Erbaugh J. An inventory for measuring depression. Arch Gen Psychiatry 1961; 4: 53–63.
27. Reynolds C, Richmond B. What I think and feel: a revised measure of children's manifest anxiety. J Abnorm Psychol 1978; 6: 271–280.
28. Harter S. Manual for the Self-Perception Profile for Adolescents. Denver, CO: University of Denver, 1988.

10

Health-Related Quality of Life in Psoriasis

A Biopsychosocial Model and Measures

Stephen R. Rapp, Steven R. Feldman, Alan B. Fleischer, Jr., David M. Reboussin, and M. Lyn Exum *Bowman Gray School of Medicine of Wake Forest University, Winston-Salem, North Carolina*

While not life threatening, psoriasis poses a severe threat to its victims' quality of life. By interfering with a wide range of everyday activities, disrupting social relations, and undermining a sense of psychological well-being, psoriasis tears indiscriminately at the fabric of patients' lives.

To better understand and ultimately reduce the negative impact of psoriasis, therefore, we must consider a very broad range of factors that conspire to produce their deleterious effects. Moreover, we need also to explain why some, but not all, patients suffer negative effects by examining the influences of modifying variables that moderate the influence of psoriasis on physical, psychological, social, and vocational outcomes. If interventions are to be developed that reduce psoriasis' negative impact, then we must understand not only how patients' quality of life is affected, but also why. To do so we need conceptual models that begin to incorporate biological, psychological, and social variables that are testable. Despite recent calls for such models (1), none has been developed to date.

The present chapter has four aims. First, we describe a multifactorial theoretical model developed to study the negative impact of psoriasis. It incorporates many factors identified in prior research and several new ones. Next, we describe the development and evaluation of key measures needed to test our model: disease severity, functional impairment, and psoriasis-related stressors. Then we describe the types and prevalence of functional impairment and psoriasis-related stressors reported to us by a group of 317 psoriasis patients. Finally, we describe several studies in which predictions of the model are tested. It is hoped that other investigators interested in the impact of psoriasis will find this information helpful in developing and testing their own models and that eventually research will lead us to discover ways to prevent or reduce patients' suffering.

A MULTIFACTORAL MODEL OF THE IMPACT OF PSORIASIS

The existing literature on the impact of psoriasis reveals that it can disrupt daily personal care activities (2–5), interfere with work performance (2,5,6), and disturb social relationships (2,4,5,7–9). Disfigurement caused by the disease leads to heightened self-consciousness (4,7), shame, and embarrassment (6,10) leading to social stigmatization (7,11). Not surprisingly then, psoriasis patients are at high risk for developing significant psychological morbidity like depression and anxiety (6,12–18) and suicidal intent (19–21).

Presumably, these adverse outcomes result primarily from the disease but covary with severity. However, factors like stress (17,22–27), personality (28), and coping strategies can play a role in moderating the impact of psoriasis. Other potential modifiers of importance include age, educational level, economic resources, and social resources. The disease itself can create stressors that can exacerbate the severity of the disease and increase functional impairment. As with exogenous stressors, modifying variables may affect disease-related stressors. Figure 1 shows a diagram of the model incorporating these and other factors. Biological factors including genetic abnormalities, neuroendocrine abnormalities, and immunological abnormalities have been identified as possibly important factors in psoriasis (26, 29–32) and are considered primary causes of disease onset and severity in our model. Disease severity, measured in terms of the acute condition of the skin (erythema, induration, scaliness, and body surface area involved), must be assessed independently from disease impact if we are to study how disease severity affects functional outcomes.

The impact of psoriasis on physical function is described in terms of the level of interference with activities like dressing, bathing, gripping, reaching, and so on. The impact on social functioning involves disruptions in casual and intimate social relations as well as increased social sensitivity, social avoidance, and ultimately feelings of stigmatization. The psychological impact is reflected in higher self-consciousness, perceptions of no control

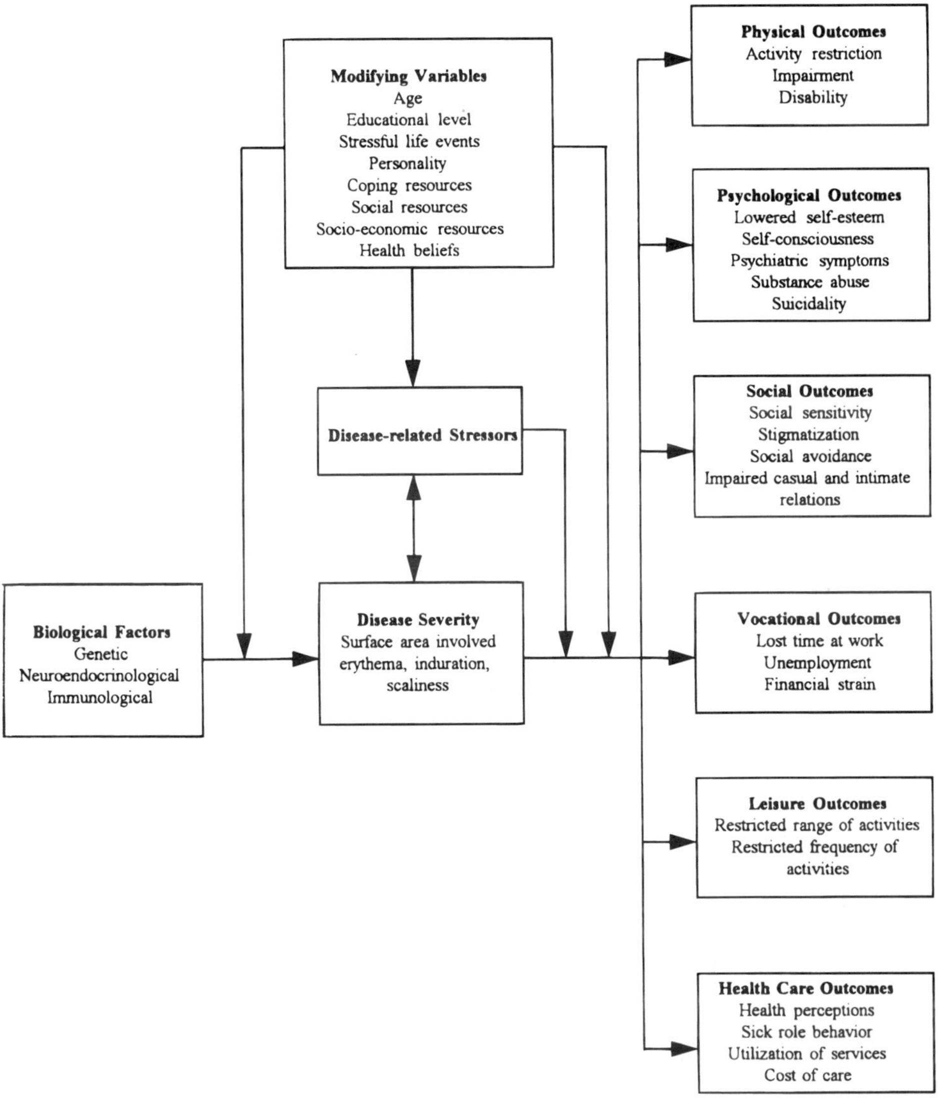

Figure 1 Biopsychosocial model of the impact of psoriasis.

over the disease and its impact, psychological distress such as depression and anxiety, substance abuse, and suicidality. Psoriasis can impact vocational functioning by increasing absenteeism, by interfering with finding or keeping a job or job advancement, and by creating financial strain. Finally, leisure activities can be disrupted or prevented because of psoriasis. For example, patients might avoid some leisure activities requiring public skin exposure like swimming or sunbathing or engage in certain hobbies less often because of physical discomfort or disability.

In addition to these primary functional outcomes, psoriasis severity also influences health care behavior such as the amount of time spent caring for the skin, the use of conventional and unconventional treatments, and the use of inpatient and outpatient dermatological services. Health perceptions are also influenced by disease severity and modified by personality and coping style. These health care functions presumably not only affect the other functions but also can influence disease severity.

Another component of the model is disease-related stressors. Disease-related stressors are aspects of psoriasis that force the individual to make behavioral or psychological adjustments and are perceived as bothersome. Aspects like pain, itching, burning, the relative uncontrollability of the disease, people staring, time lost from work, the cost of caring for one's skin, and doctors' attitudes are just some of the aspects identified by patients as bothersome. The importance of disease-related stressors is just that—they are stressors born of the disease that can contribute to the global negative impact of psoriasis. Psoriasis-related stressors are distinct from exogenous stressful life events (e.g., death of a loved one) although they are presumed to exert similar effect on the individual. Stressors may also reciprocally influence disease severity, too.

Modifying factors in the model are those variables presumed to alter the influence of one factor on another. For example, several studies have suggested that stressful life events may play a role in the onset and exacerbation of psoriasis (17,22,33,34) and that high-stress reactors have more severe disease (33). Thus life stresses may modify the influence of biological factors on disease severity as well as modify the influence severity has on functional impairment. Similarly, specific personality characteristics could be important, such as introversion-extroversion or the dispositional tendency to fear negative evaluation from others (35), which is related to self-consciousness, social anxiety, and embarassability (35,36–38). Personal coping resources (e.g., social assertiveness) used to deal with unpleasant social interactions or pain might also buffer patients from negative impact. Likewise, patients who enjoy greater social support from family and friends might be better protected from the negative reaction of others or develop more benign self-images than persons with low social support. Finally, eco-

Table 1 Primary Variables and Measures Used for Biopsychosocial Model

Variable	Measure	Description
Disease severity	Self-Administered Psoriasis Area and Severity Index (SAPASI)	Self-shaded silhouette of surface area affected multiplied by overall ratings of redness, thickness and scaliness of "average spot"
Functional impairment	Psoriasis Disability Scale (PDS)	35 physical, social, vocational, and leisure activities rated on 3-point Likert scale from 1 ("has not interfered") to 3 ("has interfered a lot")
Psoriasis-related stressors	Psoriasis Stressor Scale (PSS)	20 physical, social, economic vocational, medical, and psychological aspects of psoriasis self-rated for how bothersome it is from 1 ("not at all") to 4 ("a lot")
Psychological distress	Brief Symptom Inventory (BSI)	53 psychological distress symptoms self-rated for severity from 1 ("not at all") to 5 ("extremely"); three global indexes and 9 clinical subscales
Fear of negative evaluation by others	Fear of Negative Evaluation (12-item short form) (FNE-12)	12 statements reflecting a propensity toward heightened social sensitivity; items are self-rated for how descriptive each is from 1 ("not at all like me") to 5 ("extremely like me")
Non–disease-specific health-related quality of life	Short-Form-36 (SF-36)	36 self-ratings of physical, social, and mental functioning, and ratings of pain, perceived health and health beliefs; composite summary scores are calculated for physical and mental health
Coping	Modified (COPE)	22 coping strategies used when "people react negatively to my psoriasis"; items are self-rated from 1 ("I usually don't do this at all") to 4 ("I usually do this a lot")
Social support	Modified Social Support Scale (SOCSUP)	9 types of social support self-rated for frequency from 1 ("none of the time") to 5 ("all of the time")

nomic resources might influence the amount and type of health care a patient receives or the access to other resources that enhance quality of life like education and leisure activities. The next sections describe the methods we used to develop measures of disease severity, functional impairment, and psoriasis-related stressors. We also describe the type and prevalence of each functional impairment and each psoriasis-related stressor.

THE GENERAL METHODOLOGY

A multidiscipline research team representing psychology, dermatology, epidemiology, and biostatistics was assembled and a list of relevant variables was generated. A patient focus group (5 women, 3 men) was then convened to validate and to further develop the list. A series of structured and open-ended questions was discussed with participants. The proceedings were transcribed and reviewed by the research team before the final list of variables for the model was selected.

The next step was to locate good measures of the variables in the model. Preference was given to measures with documented reliability and validity. Table 1 gives a partial listing of the primary constructs in the model and a brief description of the instruments used to measure them. Preexisting measures selected included the Brief Symptom Inventory (BSI; 39); the Short-Form-36 (SF-36; 40), the short form of the Fear of Negative Evaluation Scale (FNE; 41), an abbreviated version of the Medical Outcome Study Social Support Scale (SSS; 42), and the COPE scale (43). We decided to develop novel measures for several variables. For disease severity, we found no self-report measure with adequate reliability and validity (44). Existing measures either require a clinician to make ratings of skin condition (e.g., Psoriasis Area and Severity Index; 45) or confounded severity with impact with items such as "rate how severe your psoriasis is." Therefore, we needed a measure of skin condition that could be completed by patients themselves and that did not confound severity and outcomes.

Most studies of disability include similar items covering physical, social, and vocational functioning. With some exceptions, however, very few studies documented the reliability and validity of their disability scales. One exception is the 15-item Psoriasis Disability Index (2,3), which appears to have good psychometric properties but is very brief. We, however, needed a measure that provided a more detailed picture of disability across each activity domain, so we were required to develop one ourselves. Because we needed a measure of disease-related stressors and found none, we set out to develop a self-report psoriasis-related stressor scale. Before describing each instrument in detail, we will describe the sample of psoriasis patients recruited to test the measures and to test our model.

THE STUDY SAMPLE

A roster of psoriasis patients treated for psoriasis between July 1, 1992, and June 30, 1993, at the Bowman Gray School of Medicine (BGSM) of Wake Forest University was obtained. After removing the names of persons under the age of 18 years, a total of 571 patients remained. A packet containing the questionnaires described in this chapter was sent to each person. Packets were also made available to patients seen in the BGSM dermatology clinic and in a local, private dermatology practice. If packets were not returned within 3 weeks, follow-up phone contacts and repeat mailings were made. Of the 571 packets, 11 were returned unopened, 10 persons denied having psoriasis, and 5 persons were deceased. Thus, of the 545 eligible respondents, 309 returned completed surveys. Twelve surveys were removed due to excessive missing data, resulting in a completion rate of 297/545 or 54.5%. Twelve of the 25 surveys distributed through the BGSM dermatology clinic were returned (48%), while 8 of 9 surveys from the community clinic were returned (88.9%). Since there were no statistically significant differences on clinical or demographic variables between respondents by location of recruitment, surveys were combined for all analyses. The overall return rate for the three groups was 317/579 (54.7%).

The medical records of 25 survey respondents were compared to records of 25 nonrespondents for potential differences. Nonrespondents were randomly selected from among persons sent the survey packet who did not return it. Eight of the nonresponders did not have psoriasis, indicating that our original list of 571 psoriasis patients was somewhat inflated, so the actual response rate was about 55%. After removing these 8 patients from the subsample of 25, responders and nonresponders did not differ significantly in age, race, gender, psoriatic severity, or treatment intensity, suggesting that responders were representative of the entire list of patients.

The entire sample of patients who responded to the survey ($n = 317$) had an average age of 49 years, were predominantly Caucasian (92%), and were only slightly more likely to be female (57%). Seventy-four percent were married and 44% had competed high-school. Sixty-eight percent of respondents had household incomes of less than $50,000. Regarding psoriatic severity, 1% was in remission, 23% had mild, 67% moderate, and 9% severe psoriasis at the time of the survey. Patients had psoriasis for an average of 14 years. For additional information about the sample, see Fleischer et al. (46).

In the sections that follow, three measures we developed 1 of disease severity, functional impairment, and psoriasis-specific stressors—are described in detail and the psychometric properties are presented. Together with other measures, these three are then used to test our conceptual model.

THE SELF-ADMINISTERED PSORIASIS AREA AND SEVERITY INDEX

A common, standardized way to measure psoriasis disease severity is the Psoriasis Area and Severity Index (PASI; 45). The PASI has been used in a variety of clinical studies (47–50). A major limitation of the PASI is that it requires a clinician to make 16 different measurements of each patient, which is impractical in nonclinic samples or in large-scale studies. We felt that a self-administered psoriasis severity measure was needed for studying the relationships between disease severity, host factors, and disability.

To respond to this need, we developed a structured PASI-like instrument that allows patients to accurately report the severity of psoriasis called the Self-Administered Psoriasis Area and Severity Index (SAPASI; 51). The instrument, printed on a single page, consists of two parts: (1) front and back silhouettes, on which respondents shade in the body surface areas affected, and (2) three 100-mm visual analog scales (VAS), on which they rate the average redness, thickness, and scaliness of their lesions. Based on the silhouette shading, a technician assigns a numerical value of 0–6 corresponding to 0–100% involvement for each of four areas—head, upper extremities, trunk, and lower extremities—as in the PASI scoring system. Each VAS is normalized to a continuous equivalent of a 5-point scale (0–4). The SAPASI score is then calculated from the following formula:

$$\text{SAPASI} = [(0.1{*}A_H) + (0.2{*}A_U) + (0.3{*}A_T) + (0.4{*}A_L)]{*} \\ \times [0.0333{*}(\text{VAS}_E + \text{VAS}_I + \text{VAS}_S)$$

where A_H is the head area score, A_U is the upper extremity score, A_T is the trunk area score, A_L is the lower extremities score, VAS_E is the VAS erythema score, VAS_E is the VAS induration score, and VAS_S is the VAS scale score.

We assessed the criterion validity, reliability, and responsiveness of the SAPASI in subjects who received no training in the measurement of psoriasis or in the use of the instrument beyond the simple one-page instructions. The criterion validity of the SAPASI was determined by comparison with the clinician-rated PASI scores (51,52). In the Fleischer et al. study, SAPASI scores predicted 71% of the variance in the clinician-rated PASI scores, while in the Feldman et al. study (52) it predicted 59%, both highly significant. Feldman et al. further reported that when individual subcomponents of the SAPASI were analyzed, significant correlations were found between clinician-rated and patient-rated body surface area (BSA) scores ($0.62 < r < 0.75$) and scores for redness, thickness, and scaling ($0.24 < r < 0.39$).

The test-retest reliability of the SAPASI scores was determined in a sample of patients presenting to the Bowman Gray School of Medicine Psoriasis and Skin Treatment Center for treatment of psoriasis vulgaris.

New and returning patients were recruited when they arrived for their appointments. Of 80 patients who completed the SAPASI instrument and had independent PASI ratings made by clinic specialists, 19 agreed to repeat the assessments 2 days later (see Ref. 52 for details of this study). We compared changes of the SAPASI score over the 2 days with changes in the PASI score. Strong correlations were found between SAPASI scores ($r = 0.82$; $p = 0.0001$). The changes in the PASI and SAPASI between administrations were also strongly correlated ($r = 0.63$; $p = 0.0002$).

The interrater reliability of technician's scoring of the SAPASI was tested by having five raters (three dermatology specialists and two nonspecialists) independently score the BSA shadings on 40 body silhouettes. There was excellent agreement among the raters with an intraclass correlation coefficient of 0.95.

The responsiveness of the instrument to change over an average of 18 days was evaluated in 15 patients (9 women, 6 men) receiving treatment at our center (51). Patients completed the SAPASI twice and were evaluated twice by clinicians who completed PASI ratings and were blinded to the SAPASI data. One way t-tests for paired samples showed significant pre- and postimprovements in the SAPASI ratings ($p < 0.003$) as well as in PASI scores ($p < 0.05$), indicating that the SAPASI is sensitive to clinically measurable changes in severity.

The construct validity of the SAPASI was demonstrated further in a study using the present sample of 317 psoriasis patients (53). The SAPASI was significantly and positively correlated with the severity of pruritus, burning, joint pain, and psoriatic arthritis. SAPASI scores were also significantly correlated with the time spent caring for the skin ($r = 0.32$).

We expected the SAPASI to be unrelated to age, gender, and race. A correlation between the SAPASI and age revealed no association ($r = -0.02$; $p = 0.77$). T-tests on the differences between Caucasians ($n = 289$) and non-Caucasians ($n = 26$) in our sample were also nonsignificant ($t = 0.95$; $p = 0.35$), and there was no significant difference between men ($n = 135$) and women ($n = 180$) ($t = 1.12$; $p = 0.23$).

In addition to being valid and reliable, we have found the SAPASI to be a practical instrument for the study of psoriasis. We have incorporated the instrument into a variety of studies requiring measurement of psoriasis disease severity, including clinical studies of topical therapy, evaluation of ultraviolet light therapy, and studies of the efficacy of psychological interventions for psoriasis. The instrument is easy for patients to complete and can be easily scored by technicians.

PSORIASIS DISABILITY SCALE

The Psoriasis Disability Scale (PDS; 2) is a 15-item, disease-specific scale with items covering daily activities including work (8 items), personal relationships (2 items), leisure activities (4 items), and treatment (1 item). The PDS is brief and easy to complete and has been validated with patients (3). However, one limitation of the PDS is its rather narrow range of functional activities. Our review of the literature and focus groups suggested that a larger number of items and a broader range of disabilities would be needed to study the many effects of psoriasis on functional status.

After reviewing the literature and convening the focus group, items were generated by the research team that assessed physical functioning, social functioning, self-care, leisure activities, vocational activities, and being around the public. For each item respondents are asked to judge how much their psoriasis has interfered with the activity during the past 4 weeks and rate their judgments: "Has not interfered at all" (1), "Has interfered a little" (2), or "Has interfered a lot" (3). Two blank "Other" items were included to allow respondents to identify impairments not listed. These items are not include in the overall scoring of the PDS, however. After pilot testing items on patients and eliminating redundant and irrelevant items, we had a final list of 34 activities, plus two "Other" items.

The PDS was administered as part of our survey of 317 psoriasis patients. Table 2 shows the percentage of respondents reporting some disability. All item scores ranged from 1 to 3, and item frequencies ranged from 18% for "reaching" to 54% for "choice of clothes." Between one fifth and one quarter of respondents described difficulties with getting out of a chair, reaching, gripping objects, preparing food, shaking hands, engaging in hobbies, choosing where to sleep, exercising, planning for the future, being with family, dating, kissing or hugging, making friends, relating to coworkers, getting or maintaining a job, or being promoted. A third of our sample reported interference with activities like cleaning their home, sleeping, shopping, intimate sex, going out socially, traveling or vacationing, being around others in public, being at work, or visiting a barber. Over 40% of the sample reported problems with house/yard work, using public facilities, recreational and sports activities, how often they change clothes, their choice of clothes, and swimming in public. The mean item frequency was 31.2%, and none of the frequencies was so high as to be universally present for patients (e.g., >90%) nor so low as to be considered rare (e.g., <10%). Twenty-three of 34 item frequencies were between 25 and 75%, suggesting a fairly broad distribution.

A principal-components factor analysis with varimax rotation was performed on the PDS items to assess the factor structure. Four factors had eigenvalues greater than 1 and accounted for a total of 62% of the variance in scores. All items loaded rather heavily on the first unrotated factor suggesting a common underlying construct. After rotation, the four factors primarily represented disability in daily activities, in social activities, in

Table 2 Item Frequencies and Factor Loadings for Psoriasis Disability Scale

Item	Percentage reporting interference	Factor loadings (rotated) 1	2	3	4
Gripping	24	*0.76*	0.05	0.28	0.07
Getting out of chair	19	*0.73*	0.14	0.04	0.13
Reaching	18	*0.64*	0.21	0.05	0.34
Cleaning home	35	*0.63*	0.13	0.42	0.11
Sleep adequacy	39	*0.63*	0.17	0.21	0.29
House/yard work	41	*0.62*	0.22	0.40	−0.04
Preparing food	28	*0.61*	0.10	0.38	0.02
Shaking hands	29	*0.60*	0.18	0.40	0.11
Doing hobbies	27	*0.56*	0.35	0.26	0.07
Being with family	19	*0.56*	0.43	0.14	0.20
Sleep location	21	*0.55*	0.34	0.16	0.28
Exercise	29	*0.55*	0.33	0.30	0.18
Planning for future	29	*0.52*	0.52	0.21	0.21
Shopping	35	*0.47*	0.37	0.30	0.26
Kissing/hugging	23	0.22	*0.77*	0.14	0.15
Intimate sex	36	0.07	*0.75*	0.19	0.13
Dating	19	0.11	*0.74*	0.15	0.03
Making friends	26	0.48	*0.66*	0.23	0.14
Using public facilities	47	0.17	*0.65*	0.16	0.40
Going out socially	38	0.47	*0.64*	0.10	0.29
Going to parties	32	0.48	*0.60*	0.16	0.34
Travel/vacation	35	0.48	*0.57*	0.28	0.27
Going out in public	39	0.52	*0.53*	0.14	0.33
Recreation/sports	43	0.46	*0.51*	0.24	0.27
Getting new job	20	0.23	0.20	*0.82*	0.09
Maintaining job	21	0.31	0.14	*0.78*	0.09
Being promoted	16	0.27	0.21	*0.77*	0.20
Relating to coworkers	19	0.29	0.34	*0.62*	0.27
Being at work	39	0.32	0.27	*0.55*	0.30
Visiting barber	39	0.09	0.14	0.00	*0.78*
Frequency of bathing	30	0.31	0.14	0.18	*0.71*
Frequency of clothes change	41	0.34	0.14	0.18	*0.65*
Choice of clothes	54	0.06	0.34	0.18	*0.59*
Swimming in public	51	0.00	0.49	0.22	*0.51*

Italics indicate heaviest loadings on each factor.

Table 3 Comparison of Patients with Low and High Psoriasis Severity

Scale	Low severity ($n = 68$–72) Mean	SD	High severity ($n = 222$–239) Mean	SD	p-value
PDS (total)	39.25	7.75	50.59	15.94	0.0001
PDS (overall item mean)	1.21	0.27	1.53	0.47	0.0001
PDS—Physical Function	1.21	0.32	1.44	0.49	0.0001
PDS—Social Function	1.14	0.27	1.58	0.59	0.0001
PDS—Vocational Function	1.12	0.29	1.38	0.57	0.0001
PDS—Public Skin Exposure	1.35	0.42	1.82	0.58	0.0001
PSS (total)	37.43	12.14	49.23	11.75	0.0001
PSS (overall item mean)	2.04	0.63	2.65	0.61	0.0001
PSS—General	2.65	0.88	3.36	0.68	0.0001
PSS—Inconvenience	1.74	0.65	2.37	0.72	0.0001
PSS—Aches/Pains	2.12	0.84	2.53	0.84	0.0002
PSS—Negative Social Reaction	1.39	0.58	2.02	0.94	0.0001

PDS = Psoriasis Disability Scale, PSS = Psoriasis Stressor Scale. Low-severity group had Self-Administered Psoriasis Area and Severity Index scores of less than or equal to 3. High-severity group had scores greater than 3. Group *ns* varied because of missing values for some items.

vocational activities, and in avoidance of public skin exposure, respectively. Table 2 also shows the factor loadings for each rotated factor. The first factor, Personal Care Activities, has 14 items with loadings of 0.47 or greater. The internal consistency of this scale is 0.92, indicating very high interrelatedness among items. The Personal Care Activities factor correlated significantly with the SAPASI ($r = 0.51$; $p = 0.0001$) and with the BSI ($r = 0.34$; $p = 0.0001$) indicating that as severity increased, so did impairment and psychological distress symptoms. Ten items loaded most heavily on the Social Activities factor, which has a coefficient alpha of 0.93. This factor also correlated significantly with SAPASI scores ($r = 0.53$; $p = 0.0001$) and with the BSI ($r = 0.40$; $p = 0.0001$). Five items loaded most heavily on the Vocational Activities factor, including finding new employment, maintaining one's current job, being promoted, relations with coworkers, and being at work or school. This factor also correlated with both SAPASI ($r = 0.44$; $p = 0.0001$) and the BSI ($r = 0.29$; $p = 0.0001$) and had an internal consistency of 0.89. Going to the barber, frequency of bathing, frequency of clothes changes, choice of clothes, and swimming in public all loaded not heavily on the Avoidance of Public Exposure factor. It correlated with the SAPASI ($r = 0.51$; $p = 0.0001$) and with the BSI ($r = 0.33$; $p = 0.0001$) and had an alpha coefficient of 0.77.

When all 34 items were combined, the PDS had an alpha of 0.96, indicating excellent internal consistency. Total scores ranged from 23 to 102, with a mean score of 47.7 (SD = 15.17), and all items had ranged from 1 to 3. The total PDS correlated significantly with the SAPASI ($r = 0.58$; $p = 0.0001$) and with the BSI ($r = 0.40$; $p = 0.0001$), supporting its construct validity. To further assess its construct validity, the PDS was correlated with the SF-36 summary scale scores. Significant negative correlations were found for the Physical Health summary score ($r = -0.33$; $p = 0.0001$) and for the Mental Health summary score ($r = -0.38$; $p = 0.0001$), indicating that the PDS is associated with global physical and mental functioning as well as with psychiatric symptoms and psoriasis severity. Next, PDS scores were compared for patients with low severity (i.e., SAPASI < or = 3.0) and with high severity (SAPASI > 3.0) (Table 3). The low-severity group ($n = 72$) had significantly lower total PDS scores (mean = 39.25; SD = 7.75) than the high-severity group ($n = 239$; mean = 50.59; SD = 15.94; $p < 0.0001$). All four factors scores were also significantly greater in the high-severity group ($p < 0.0002$).

We did not expect the PDS to be significantly associated with race, gender, or age. *T*-tests revealed no differences for gender ($t = -0.29$; $p = 0.77$) or for race ($t = 0.95$; $p = 0.35$), but age was negatively correlated with the PDS ($r = -0.13$; $p = 0.02$), indicating that younger patients experienced more disability from their psoriasis in this sample.

PSORIASIS STRESSOR SCALE

In addition to interfering with a wide range of daily activities, psoriasis can create secondary stressors, which further strain patients and increase distress and dysfunction. It is important to identify specific stressful aspects of the disease if disease-specific, stress reduction interventions are to be developed to help patients cope with this chronic condition.

We identified 19 bothersome aspects of the illness from the literature and from our focus groups. Items were written describing each aspect and pilot tested. The resulting Psoriasis Stressor Scale (PSS) requires respondents to rate how much they are bothered by each aspect of the disease on a scale from 1 ("not at all") to 4 ("a lot"). An overall PSS sum score and an overall item mean can be calculated.

Table 4 presents the percentage of respondents in our survey who rated each item "moderately" or "a lot" bothersome. The percentage of patients reporting substantial strain varied across stressors; for each PSS item the range of ratings was from 1 to 4. Between one fifth and one third of the

Table 4 Item Frequencies and Factor Loadings for Psoriasis Stressor Scale

Item	Percentage reporting "Mod./A lot"	Factor loadings (rotated)			
		1	2	3	4
Scales	75	*0.80*	0.09	0.24	0.15
Appearance	83	*0.77*	0.25	0.10	0.19
No control	80	*0.73*	0.29	0.08	0.17
Self-consciousness	37	*0.65*	0.25	0.15	0.47
Itching	75	*0.64*	0.06	0.40	0.02
Medication side effects	34	0.15	*0.68*	0.21	0.05
Time lost from work	16	−0.06	*0.64*	0.32	0.19
Cost of care	68	0.38	*0.64*	−0.11	0.09
Odors	37	0.26	*0.64*	0.17	0.22
Time spent on care	57	0.52	*0.58*	0.12	0.17
Stains	48	0.38	*0.57*	0.09	0.29
Hair loss	30	0.00	*0.49*	0.30	0.20
Joint pain	49	0.04	0.25	*0.77*	0.06
Burning	56	0.43	0.03	*0.68*	0.09
Skin soreness	61	0.42	0.13	*0.67*	0.16
How joints/bones look	30	0.11	0.30	*0.54*	0.19
Being avoided by others	22	0.15	0.16	0.17	*0.88*
People staring	36	0.27	0.20	0.10	*0.86*
Doctors' attitudes	27	0.12	0.31	0.08	*0.44*

respondents were bothered by time lost from work, being avoided by others, people staring at them, how their joints or bones look, hair loss, odors, medication side effects, self-consciousness, and doctors' attitudes. Between 40 and 70% of patients reported the cost of care, stains, joint pain, skin soreness, and burning as quite bothersome. For the remaining items—scales, the appearance of the skin, not being able to control the illness, and itching—more than 70% of respondents reported aggravation. While a few of the frequencies are relatively high (i.e., appearance of the skin, no control over the psoriasis), none is so high as to be a universal stressor (>90%) and none is rare (<10%). Fifteen of 19 frequencies are between 25 and 75%, and the mean frequency is 48.5%, indicating a fairly normal distribution.

A principal-components factor analysis was performed with a varimax rotation. Four factors had eigenvalues greater than unity and together explained 62% of the overall variance. All PSS items loaded on the first unrotated factor with loadings between 0.49 and 0.79, indicating that a common factor underlies the PSS. Table 4 shows the rotated factor loadings for each factor. The first factor, accounting for 39% of the total variance and labeled a General factor, is composed of a broad range of stressors: scales, appearance of skin, no control over psoriasis, self-consciousness, itching, time spent caring for skin, and, to a lesser extent, burning and soreness. The second factor, labeled Inconvenience, accounted for an additional 8% of the variance. Items loading most heavily were medication side effects, time lost from work, the cost of psoriasis care, unpleasant odors, time spent caring for skin, stains on clothing and furniture, and hair loss. The third factor accounted for 7% of the variance and was labeled Aches and Pains. Items loading most heavily on this factor included itching, joint pain, burning, soreness and appearance of joints and bones. The fourth factor, called Reaction to Others, accounted for an additional 6% of variance and weighted items such as being avoided by others, people staring in a negative way, feeling self-conscious, and doctors' attitude. The coefficient for internal consistency for the total PSS was 0.90, and the coefficients for the four factors were 0.85, 0.81, 0.74, and 0.75, respectively, indicating adequate reliability.

To evaluate the construct validity of the PSS, scores were compared for patients with low and high psoriasis severity (see Table 4). The overall sum score, the overall mean item rating, and each of the factor scores were significantly greater in the high-severity group. Also, as seen in Table 5, the PSS total score was also significantly correlated with the SAPASI score ($r = 0.47$; $p = 0.0001$), the PDS score ($r = 0.63$; $p = 0.0001$), the BSI ($r = 0.46$; $p = 0.0001$), the SF-36 Physical Health composite score ($r = -0.29$; $p = 0.0001$), and the SF-36 Mental Health composite score ($r = -0.45$; $p = 0.0001$). Finally, all of the PSS items correlated significantly with SAPASI scores with a range from 0.11 (Doctor's attitude) to 0.38 (Time spent caring for psoriasis) and a mean correlation of 0.28.

Table 5 Correlations Between Measures and Independent Measures of Quality of Life

	1	2	3	4	5	6
1. SAPASI	—					
2. PDS	0.58	—				
3. PSS	0.47	0.63	—			
4. BSI	0.19	0.40	0.46	—		
5. SF-36 Physical	−0.23	−0.33	−0.29	−0.30	—	
6. SF-36 Mental	−0.20	−0.38	−0.45	−0.68	0.20	—

SAPASI = Self-Administered Psoriasis Area and Severity Index; PDS = Psoriasis Disability Scale; PSS = Psoriasis Stressor Scale; BSI = Brief Symptom Inventory; SF-36 Physical = Short-Form-36 Physical Function Composite Score; SF-36 Physical = Short-Form-36 Mental Function Composite Score. All correlations are significant at the 0.0006 level or less.

Finally, we did not expect the PSS to be associated with either age, gender, or race. *T*-tests revealed that it was not associated with gender ($t = -0.19$; $p = 0.85$) or race ($t = 0.26$; $p = 0.80$), but was weakly correlated with age ($r = -0.19$; $p = 0.0005$), indicating that as age increases overall stress levels decline. Taken together, these correlations strongly support the validity of the PSS as a measure of stressors associated with psoriasis.

SUPPORT FOR THE MODEL

The results described thus far provide support for the theoretical model of the impact of psoriasis presented earlier. Patients reported a broad range of functional disabilities and a broad range of disease-related stressors associated with psoriasis. Moreover, as predicted by the model, both functional impairment and stressors increase as severity increases. We also confirmed that these two variables are strongly associated with psychological distress, global physical functioning, and global mental functioning.

The findings on functional impairment are quite consistent with previous research, demonstrating that psoriasis interferes with everyday personal care activities, social relations, job-related activities, leisure activities, and merely being in public (2–4). By assessing a wide variety of specific functions we were able to see important inter- and intradomain variability in the disability reported by patients across and within functional domains, which can help in the selection of treatment aims. For example, the mean item rating for the Public Skin Exposure factor was greater than any of the other factors, indicating that helping patients to feel more comfortable in public places may be a very good goal of adjunctive counseling. Similarly, if we look at social functioning, we see that there is less impact on dating (19%) or kissing/hugging (23%) than on using public facilities (47%), suggesting that the latter might be a better target for counseling programs.

Our data on psoriasis-related stressors replicate and extend previous research. They support the impression that a disease like psoriasis produces disease-specific stress on patients. This has important implications for the study of stress and psoriasis. We found, as others have, that psoriasis and its treatment produces a wide array of stressors, some physical, some vocational, some interpersonal, and some associated with treatments. While physical aspects of psoriasis are among the most stressful, we also see that negative reactions from others like staring at or avoiding the individual can lead to self-consciousness, shame, and embarrassment (6), and perceptions of stigmatization (11) are troublesome for many patients.

Other analyses of our data set have provided additional insights into the impact of psoriasis. Rapp et al. (54) studied suicidal ideation among patients. They found that 27% of survey respondents had wished they were dead because of their psoriasis and/or tried to kill themselves, a finding observed by others (19–21). There were a number of differences between these "high-strain" patients and nonsuicidal patients, including higher SAPASI scores, greater functional impairment, greater psychological distress, and higher levels of psoriasis-related stress. These differences were not attributable to comorbid psychiatric or medical problems. When the SAPASI, PDS, PSS, and BSI were used together to predict suicidality in a logistic regression analysis, all were significant predictors except the SAPASI, suggesting that each of these variables contributes independently to suicidality associated with psoriasis and that the effect that psoriasis has on strain is through functional impairment, psoriasis-related stress, and the psychological distress it generates, as predicted by the model.

We also looked at health care outcomes, specifically the use of unconventional treatments like herbal remedies, dietary manipulations, vitamin treatments, homeopathy, nonprescription tanning, and other nontraditional treatments (53). Sixty-two percent of the sample had used alternative treatments. Use was positively correlated with severity, but uncorrelated with education or income.

Leary et al. (55) found that personality can affect the impact of psoriasis. Respondents who are characteristically concerned about how they are perceived and evaluated by others reported more negative effects of the disease than those who showed less of this tendency. The fear of negative evaluation (FNE; 35) correlated with perceptions of being stigmatized, interpersonal discomfort, stress over others' reactions, distress regarding the observable symptoms of psoriasis, and the degree to which psoriasis interfered with aspect of the patients' social lives. Respondents who scored higher in FNE worked harder to conceal their disease than low scorers. Not only did people with high FNE report greater difficulties overall, but individual differences in FNE moderated the effects of disease severity on several outcomes. At low levels of disease severity, FNE had no apparent effect on outcomes, but for patients who reported both high disease severity and high fear of negative evaluation, the consequences were particularly negative. It appears then that when one's psoriasis symptoms are not severe enough to evoke negative reactions from others, one's tendency to worry about what others are thinking is relatively unimportant. However, as symptoms become more observable and generate negative reactions, persons with a greater interpersonal fear will become increasingly distressed and dysfunctional.

CONCLUSION

The first aim of this chapter was to describe a biopsychosocial conceptual model for the impact of psoriasis. We tried to include many variables identified in prior research and by patients themselves. The result is an incomplete picture, to be sure. Many factors that could have been included were not. We hope that the model stimulates further refinements and ultimately helps researchers to isolate the most important contributors to distress and dysfunction. The second aim of the chapter was to present data on three measurement tools developed to assess key variables in the model—disease severity, functional impairment, and psoriasis-related stressors. We demonstrated that the SAPASI, the PDS, and the PSS have adequate to excellent reliability and correlated in expected ways to each other and to other variables in the predicted direction. Despite these encouraging results, the test-retest reliability, responsiveness to change, and the criterion validity of the SAPASI, and PDS, and the PSS will have to be demonstrated in large samples to be generalizable. Measurement of these constructs is necessary if we are to disentangle disease severity from its impact and look at the role of modifying variables like personality, coping skills, social resources, and the like. They are also useful as outcome measures in treatment studies. For example, if two medications have equivalent effects on disease severity, but one reduces functional disability or stress more, it is preferable. The third aim of this chapter was to present data on the prevalence of functional impairments and on the stressors associated with the disease. We noted that, on average, approximately one third of the survey respondents reported significant functional impairment caused by their psoriasis, indicating clearly that psoriasis can have profound effects on the quality of life. This point is further emphasized when we consider the accumulation of stress it causes. Half of the survey respondents reported significant aggravation from stressors specific to psoriasis.

The high incidence of negative physical, social, and psychological effects underlines the need to develop treatments that reduce distress and disability, not just disease severity. These findings reiterate the complexity of psoriasis' impact and the wide range of variables that conspire to produce the negative effects. We hope that this chapter stimulates other researchers to develop and test models like the one presented here, models that will lead to the development of biopsychosocial interventions to reduce the multifaceted negative impact of psoriasis.

ACKNOWLEDGMENTS

This work was supported by the National Institute of Mental Health (grant MH-51552). We express our gratitude to Adele Clark, PA-C, for her assistance in collecting these data.

REFERENCES

1. Ginsburg IH. Psychological and psychophysiological aspects of psoriasis. Dermatol Clin 1995; 13:793–804.

2. Finlay AY, Kelly S. Psoriasis—an index of disability. Clin Exp Dermatol 1987; 12:8–11.
3. Finlay AY, Khan GK, Luscombe DK, Salek MS. Validation of Sickness Impact Profile and Psoriasis Disability Index in psoriasis. Br J Dermatol 1990; 123:751–756.
4. Ramsey B, O'Reagan M. A survey of social and psychological effects of psoriasis. Br J Dermatol 1988; 118:195–201.
5. Finlay AY, Coles EC. The effect of severe psoriasis on the quality of life of 369 patients. Br J Dermatol 1995; 132:236–244.
6. Jowett S, Ryan T. Skin disease and handicap: an analysis of the impact of skin conditions. Soc Sci Med 1985; 20:425–429.
7. Savin JA. Patients' beliefs about psoriasis. Trans St. John's Hosp Dermatol Soc 1970; 56:139–147.
8. Jobling R. Psoriasis—a preliminary questionnaire study of suffer's subjective experience. Clin Exp Dermatol 1979; 1:233–236.
9. Roenigk RK, Roenigk HH Jr. Sex differences in the psychological effects of psoriasis. Cutis 1978; 21:529–533.
10. Stankler L. The effect of psoriasis on the sufferer. Clin Exp Dermatol 1981; 6:303–306.
11. Ginsburg IH, Link BG. Feelings of stigmatization in patients with psoriasis. J Am Acad Dermatol 1989; 20:53–6.
12. Bennett P, Thomas B, Gawkrodger D. Anxiety and psoriasis. Practitioner 1993; 237:539–543.
13. Gilbert AR, Rodgers DA, Roenigk HH Jr. Personality evaluation in psoriasis. Cleveland Clin Q 1973; 40:147–152.
14. Goldsmith LA, Fisher M, Wacks J. Psychological characteristics of psoriatics. Arch Dermatol 1969; 100:674–676.
15. Hardy GE, Cotterill JA. A study of depression and obessionality in dysmorpho-phobic and psoriatic patients. Br J Psychiatry 1982; 140:19–22.
16. Lyketsos GC, Stratigos J, Tawil G, Psaras M, Lyketsos CG. Hostile personality characteristics, dysthymic states and neurotic symptoms in urticaria, psoriasis and alopecia. Psychother Psychosom 1985; 44:122–131.
17. Fava GA, Perini GI, Santonastaso P, Formasa CV. Life events and psychological distress in dermatologic disorders: psoriasis, chronic urticaria and fungal infections. Br J Med Psychol 1980; 53:277–282.
18. Hughes JE, Barraclough BM, Hamblin LG, White JE. Psychiatric symptoms in dermatology patients. Br J Psychiatry 1983; 143:51–54.
19. Ginsburg IH, Link BG. Psychological consequences of rejection and stigma feelings in psoriasis patients. Int J Dermatol 1993; 32:587–591.
20. Gupta MA, Schork NJ, Gupta AK, Kirkby S, Ellis CN. Suicidal ideation in psoriasis. Int J Dermatol 1993; 32:188–190.
21. Sandborn PE, Sandborn CJ, Cimbolic P, Niswander GP. Suicide and stress-related dermatoses. Dis Nerv System 1972; 33:391–394.
22. Seville RH. Psoriasis and stress. Br J Dermatol 1977; 97:297–302.
23. Baughman R, Sobel R. Psoriasis, stress, and strain. Arch Dermatol 1971; 101:599–605.

24. Farber EM, Nall ML. The natural history of psoriasis in 5600 patients. Dermatologica 1974; 148:1–18.
25. Farber EM, Bright RD, Nall ML. Psoriasis: a questionnaire survey of 2144 patients. Arch Dermatol 1968; 98:248–259.
26. Farber EM, Nall ML. Psoriasis: a stress-related disease. Cutis 1993; 5:322–326.
27. Gaston L, Crombez J, Lassonde M, Bernier-Buzzanga J, Hodgins S. Psychological stress and psoriasis: experimental and prospective correlational studies. Acta Dermato-Venereol 1991; 156:37–43.
28. Matussek P, Agerer D, Seibt G. Aggression in depressives and psoriatics. Psychother Psychosom 1985; 43:120–125.
29. Arnetz BB, Fjellnet B, Eneroth P, Kallner A. Stress and psoriasis: psychoedocrine and metabolic reactions in psoriatic patients during standardized stressor exposure. Psychosom Med 1985; 47:528–541.
30. Farber EM, Lanigan SW, Baer J. The role of cutaneous sensory nerves in the maintenance of psoriasis. Int J Dermatol 1990; 9:418–420.
31. Farber EM, Rein G, Lanigan SW. Stress and psoriasis, psychoneuroimmunologic mechanisms. Int J Dermatol 1991; 30:8–12.
32. Matis WI, Lauker RM, Murphy GF. Substance P induces the expression of an endothelial leukocyte adhesion molecule by microvascular endothelium. J Invest Derm 1990; 94:492–495.
33. Gupta MA, Gupta AK, Kirkby S, Schork NJ, Gorr SK, Ellis CN, Voorhees JJ. A psychocutaneous profile of psoriasis patients who are stress reactors: a study of 127 patients. Gen Hosp Psychiatry 1989; 11:166–173.
34. Susskind W, McGuire RJ. The emotional factor in psoriasis. Scottish Med J 1959; 4:503–507.
35. Watson D, Friend R. Measurement of social-evaluative anxiety. J Consult Clin Psychol 1969; 33:448–457.
36. Heimberg RG, Hope DA, Rapee RM, Bruch MA. The validity of the Social Avoidance and Distress Scale and the Fear of Negative Evaluation Scale with social phobic patients. Behav Res Ther 1988; 26:407–410.
37. Leary MR, Kowalski RM. The Interaction Anxiousness Scale: construct and criterion-related validity. J Personality Assess 1993; 61:136–146.
38. Miller RS. On the nature of embarassibility: Shyness, social evaluation, and social skill. J Personality 1995; 63:315–339.
39. Derogatis LR, Spencer PM. The Brief Symptom Inventory (BSI): Administration, Scoring and Procedures Manual. Baltimore: Johns Hopkins University Press, 1982.
40. Ware JE Sherbourne CD. The MOS 36-item Short-Form Health Survey (SF-36): I. Conceptual framework and item selection. Med Care 1992; 30:473–483.
41. Leary MR. A brief version of the Fear of Negative Evaluation Scale. Personality Soc Psychol Bull 1983; 9:371–376.
42. Sherbourne CD, Stewart AL. The MOS Social Support Survey. Soc Sci Med 1991; 32:705–714.
43. Carver CS, Scheier MF, Weintraub JK. Assessing coping strategies: a theoretically based approach. J Personality Soc Psychol 1989; 56:267–283.

44. Exum ML, Rapp SR, Feldman SR, Fleischer AB, Reboussin DM, Clark AR. Measuring severity of psoriasis: methodological issues. J Derm Treat 1996; 7:119–124.
45. Fredriksson T, Pettersson U. Severe psoriasis—oral therapy with a new retinoid. Dermatologica 1978; 157:238–244.
46. Fleischer AB, Feldman SR, Rapp SR, Reboussin DM, Exum ML, Clarke AR, Rajashekhar V. Disease severity measures in a population of psoriasis patients: the symptoms of psoriasis correlate with the Self-Administered Psoriasis Area and Severity Index scores. J Invest Dermatol 1996; 107:26–29.
47. Cecchi R, Seghieri G, Gironi A, Tuci F, Giomi A. Relationship between urinary albumin excretion and skin involvement in patients with psoriasis. Dermatology 1992; 185:93–95.
48. Collins P, Rogers S. Bath-water compared with oral delivery of 8-methoxypsoralen PUVA therapy for chronic plaque psoriasis. Br J Dermatol 1992; 127:392–395.
49. Harland CC, Whitaker RP, Barron JL, Holden CA. Increased urine neopterin levels in psoriasis. Br J Dermatol 1992; 127:453–457.
50. Lauharanta J, Geiger JM. A double-blind comparison of acitretin and etretinate in combination with bath PUVA in the treatment of extensive psoriasis. Br J Dermatol 1989; 121:107–112.
51. Fleischer AB Jr, Rapp SR, Reboussin DM, Vanarthos JC, Feldman SR. Patient measurement of psoriasis disease severity with a structured instrument. J Invest Dermatol 1994; 102:967–969.
52. Feldman SR, Fleischer AB Jr., Reboussin DM, Rapp SR, Exum ML, Clark AR. The Self-Administered Psoriasis Area and Severity Index is valid and reliable. J Invest Dermatol 1996; 106:183–186.
53. Fleischer AB Jr., Feldman SR, Rapp SR, Reboussin DM, Exum ML, Clark AR. Alternative therapies commonly used within a population of patients with psoriasis. Cutis 1996; 58:216–220.
54. Rapp SR, Exum ML, Reboussin DM, Feldman SR, Fleischer A, Clark A. The physical, psychological and social impact of psoriasis. J Health Psychol. In press.
55. Leary MR, Rapp SR, Berbst K, Exum ML, Feldman SR. Interpersonal concerns and psychological difficulties of psoriasis patients: effects of disease severity and fear of negative evaluation. Health Psychol. In press.

11

Psoriasis Life Stress Inventory

An Index of the Stress Associated with the Impact of Psoriasis on the Quality of Life

Madhulika A. Gupta *University of Western Ontario, London, Ontario, Canada*

INTRODUCTION

The impact of psoriasis on the quality of life, which arises largely as a result of the cosmetic disfigurement and social stigma (1–5) associated with psoriasis, can result in significant stress for the patient. It is well recognized that psychosocial stress can exacerbate psoriasis (6,7). The psoriasis-related stress, therefore, can adversely affect the course of psoriasis (1,5) (Fig. 1).

OBJECTIVE

The Psoriasis Life Stress Inventory (PLSI; 1) (see Appendix), which is an instrument developed to measure the stress resulting from the impact of psoriasis upon the quality of life, is described in this chapter.

METHODS

Development of the Psoriasis Life Stress Inventory

The 15-item PLSI (1) was developed using 217 psoriasis patients (139 inpatients and 78 outpatients; 113 males and 104 females) representing a wide

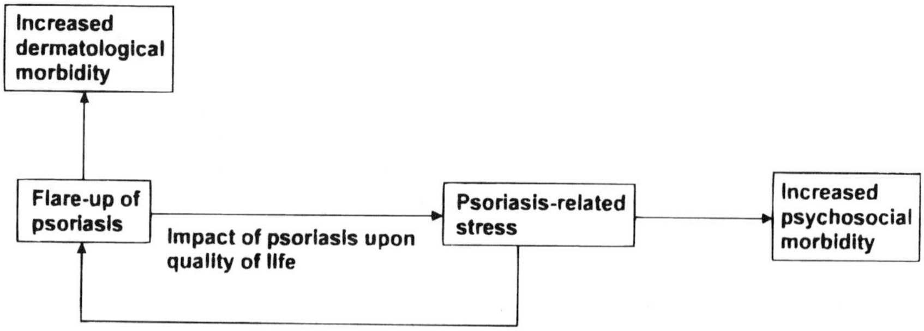

Figure 1 Proposed model for the role of psoriasis-related stress on the course of psoriasis.

range of psoriasis severity who were attending the Department of Dermatology at the University of Michigan, Ann Arbor, Michigan. The original inventory consisted of 41 psoriasis-related items based on the results of a field test with 50 psoriasis patients. Fifteen of the original 41 items, each of which had been endorsed by at least 15% of the 217 patients, were included in the final version of the PLSI. In the final version, the events related to the impact of psoriasis upon the quality of life could be classified into two general categories: those resulting from the cosmetic disfigurement and social stigma associated with having psoriasis, for example, feeling self-conscious among strangers, and those associated with the physical aspects of psoriasis and its treatments, for example, being inconvenienced by shedding of the skin or having to set aside a large portion of time to take care of the psoriasis. The patients endorsed the events that they had experienced over the previous month by checking a "Yes" or "No" to the question "Did this happen in the past 1 month? Second, when an event was reported as having occurred, the patient rated the degree of stress associated with the event using a 4-point scale, where a rating of 0 denoted "not at all," 1 denoted "slight degree," 2 denoted "moderate degree," and 3 denoted a "a great deal" of stress.

The overall psoriasis-related stress score was derived from the sum of all stress ratings. If a patient did not experience a particular event, a stress score of 0 was assigned to that event (in this instance the patient is asked to leave the stress rating blank on the PLSI instrument). Alternately, a stress score of 0 was also assigned if an event occurred but no stress was experienced as a result of it. The total stress score could therefore theoretically range from 0 to 45. The total PLSI score from the 15-item instrument was cut at a value of 10, and patients with scores of <10 (representing 52% of the 217 patients) were classified as having "low" PLSI scores, whereas patients with scores of ≥ 10 (representing 48% of patients) were classified as having "high" PLSI scores. The cutoff value of 10 was chosen because this value discriminated between the "high" and "low" stress reactor groups in a manner consistent with an earlier study (5), where the high stress reactors had more cosmetically disfiguring psoriasis and reported a greater number of flare-ups of their psoriasis, supporting the model in Fig. 1.

Validation of the PLSI

We examined the relation between the PLSI scores and patient rated measures of psoriasis severity (rated on a 10-point scale). There was a direct correlation between the PLSI score and patient self-ratings of "overall redness of skin rash" (Pearson $r = 0.15$, $p = 0.04$), "overall scaling or shedding of skin" (Pearson $r = 0.20$, $p = 0.008$), "overall thickness of psoriasis plaques" (Pearson $r = 0.17$, $p = 0.02$), "itching due to psoriasis" (Pearson $r = 0.24$, $p = 0.001$), and "overall severity of psoriasis" (Pearson $r = 0.19$, $p = 0.01$). Second, examination of the correlation between the PLSI scores and psoriasis severity affecting individual body regions revealed that most of the body regions that correlated significantly with the PLSI scores (Pearson $r \geq 0.20$, $p < 0.05$) also tended to be associated with greater cosmetic disfigurement. Comparison of the groups with a low (< 10) PLSI score vs. a high (i.e., ≥ 10) PLSI score revealed that a PLSI score of ≥ 10 delineated a subgroup of patients with greater overall psoriasis severity ($p = 0.007$) and greater psoriasis severity ($p < 0.05$) affecting body regions that led to the greatest cosmetic disfigurement. These findings are consistent with the model described in Fig. 1.

Cronbach's alpha for all 15 items of the PLSI was 0.90, indicating a high degree of internal consistency within the items (1).

SUMMARY

The PLSI provides an index of the impact of psoriasis upon the quality of life and may be used to monitor the course of psoriasis and/or measure the efficacies of dermatological therapies for psoriasis. Furthermore, in addition to being an overall measure of the psychosocial morbidity associated with psoriasis, which is also measured by the generic and psoriasis-specific quality of life instruments, our initial studies (1,5) suggest that a PLSI score of ≥ 10 delineates a subgroup of patients who are likely to be most adversely affected, from both a psychosocial and dermatological perspective, by the impact of psoriasis upon their quality of life.

REFERENCES

1. Gupta MA, Gupta AK. The Psoriasis Life Stress Inventory: a preliminary index of psoriasis-related stress. Acta Dermato-venereol (Stockh) 1995; 75:240–243.
2. Ginsburg IH, Link BG. Feelings of stigmatization in patients with psoriasis. J Am Acad Dermatol 1989; 20:53–63.
3. Ramsay B, O'Reagan M. A survey of the social and psychological effects of psoriasis. Br J Dermatol 1988; 118:195–201.
4. Gupta MA, Gupta AK, Haberman HF. Psoriasis and psychiatry: an update. Gen Hosp Psychiatry 1987; 9:157–166.
5. Gupta MA, Gupta AK, Kirkby S, Schork NJ, Gorr SK, Ellis CN, Voorhees JJ. A psychocutaneous profile of psoriasis patients who are stress reactors. Gen Hosp Psychiatry 1989; 11:166–173.
6. Farber EM, Bright RD, Nall ML. Psoriasis, a questionnaire survey of 2,144 patients. Arch Dermatol 1968; 98:248–259.
7. Al'Abadie MS, Kent GG, Gawkrodger DJ. The relationship between stress and the onset and exacerbation of psoriasis and other skin conditions. Br J Dermatol 1994; 130(2):190–203.

APPENDIX: THE PSORIASIS LIFE STRESS INVENTORY (PLSI) (1)

Please indicate if you have experienced the following life situations over the past 1 month by marking the appropriate box with an X. If an item is not applicable to you, mark *no*. If an event occurred, then using the following ratings, write down the most appropriate number that describes how much stress the experience caused you.

Stress rating scale: 0 = "not at all"; 1 = "slight"; 2 = "moderate"; 3 = "a great deal."

Psoriasis-related event	Did this happen in the past 1 month? Check *one* box. Yes	No	If yes, how much stress did it cause you? (Write number from 0 to 3 using stress rating scale; leave blank if event did not occur.)
1. Inconvenienced by the shedding of your skin	☐	☐	—
2. Feeling self-conscious among strangers	☐	☐	—
3. Feeling that you have to set aside a large part of your time to take care	☐	☐	—

of your psoriasis			
4. Not going to a public place (e.g., swimming pool, health club, restaurant) when you would have liked to	☐	☐	—
5. Wearing unattractive or uncomfortable clothes in order to cover certain regions of the body	☐	☐	—
6. Having to avoid sunbathing in the company of others	☐	☐	—
7. Fear of having serious side effects from medical treatments	☐	☐	—
8. People treating you as if your skin condition is contagious	☐	☐	—
9. Avoiding social situations	☐	☐	—
10. Strangers (children or adults) making rude or insensitive remarks about your appearance	☐	☐	—
11. Not enough money to pay medical bills	☐	☐	—
12. Feeling like an "outcast" or "social misfit" a great deal of the time	☐	☐	—
13. People making a conscious effort not to touch you	☐	☐	—
14. Hairdresser or barber appearing reluctant to cut your hair	☐	☐	—
15. People implying that your skin condition may be due to AIDS, leprosy, or a venereal disease	☐	☐	—

12

Skindex, a Dermatological Outcomes Measure of the Effects of Skin Disease on Patients' Quality of Life

Mary-Margaret Chren* and Rebecca J. Lasek *Cleveland Veterans Affairs Medical Center, University Hospitals of Cleveland, and Case Western Reserve University, Cleveland, Ohio*

To study and improve the quality of care for our patients, we need accurate measures of the outcomes of skin diseases and their treatment. But health outcomes are especially problematic for dermatology. Traditional patient-based outcomes, such as mortality, length of hospital stay, surgical complications, or tumor recurrence rates, are not relevant to many dermatological diseases. The vast majority of our patients are ambulatory, and most of them have chronic diseases that do not impair survival.

The measurement of outcomes of skin diseases has included quantitative measures of disease extent and severity—for example, acne lesion counts or the Psoriasis Area Severity Index (PASI) (1). These are useful measures, although they must be demonstrated to be reliable and valid. In fact, this important testing is often lacking for the instruments we use (2): for example, a review of physicians' assessments of the area of psoriatic skin involvement discovered wide disagreement among physicians for the same

***Current affiliation**: University of California at San Francisco, and San Franciso Veterans Affairs Medical Center, San Franciso, California.

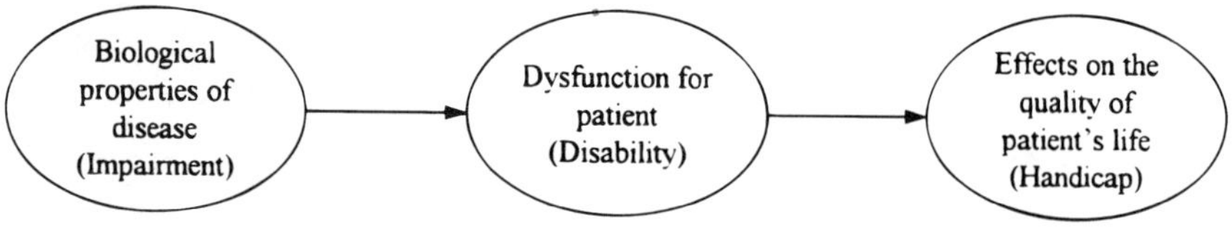

Figure 1 Framework for understanding the relationships between a disease and a patient's experience of it.

patients (3).

Moreover, these measures often do not comprehensively assess severity as perceived by the patient. In this regard, dermatological diseases illustrate well a fundamental but complex relationship among health outcomes from all diseases (Fig. 1): the biological properties of a disease (the impairment it causes) result in different degrees of dysfunction for patients (disability), which in turn result in different effects on their quality of life (their perceived handicap). Dermatologists, perhaps because they are accustomed to dealing with diseases whose biological properties can cause disfigurement and thus affect patients emotionally as well as physically, intuitively grasp that patients differ greatly in the dysfunction they experience from a given skin eruption and also differ greatly in how much that dysfunction bothers them. In fact, if the goal of health care is to make patients better, then their perceptions of the effects of skin disease on their well-being are paramount, especially for skin disease, where much of the severity of disease may not be visible to the physician. Thus, there is a compelling need for scientifically validated measures of the effect of skin disease and their treatment on patients' quality of life.

In this chapter, we will describe the sequential development and testing of an instrument called Skindex to measure the quality of life of patients with skin disease. We will begin with a description of our goals for the instrument and a brief overview of the measurement properties we intended it to demonstrate. We will then describe how we composed Skindex and its cross-sectional and longitudinal testing in a random sample of patients with skin disease. We will end with a discussion of future directions for the instrument and its use to improve the quality of care of skin diseases.

GOALS FOR SKINDEX

In developing Skindex, we were informed by much scholarly work regarding health status measurement in general and in other specialties (4–9). In particular, we explicitly intended the instrument to be used not only to distinguish the burden of skin disease in different populations at one point in time (its discriminative function), but also to be used as an outcomes measure, to gauge how patients' quality of life changes as their skin changes over time (its evaluative function) (5). These dual purposes affected the choice and phrasing of items in the instrument; for example, more common perceptions such as annoyance from skin disease may change as the skin disease changes but may not distinguish well between clinical groups. We specifically used these two functions as goals for the instrument in its development and testing.

MEASUREMENT PROPERTIES TO BE ASSESSED

Investigators (and clinicians) ask of quality-of-life measures what they ask of all scientific assays: that they have a high signal-to-noise ratio (reliability) and that they measure what they are supposed to measure, not measure what they are not supposed to measure (validity). The science of using standardized tests or scales to measure attributes of an individual is called psychometrics, and Skindex was designed using standard psychometric principles and techniques. In this description, *item* refers to a question in a survey instrument, *construct* refers to the theoretically derived notion of the concept being measured, and *scale* refers to an aggregation of one or more items to measure a construct.

By reliability is meant that the variability in scores between patients who truly vary is greater than the variability between patients who do not vary or within a stable of patients taking the test repeatedly. Reliability of a psychometric tool is measured in two ways. First, internal consistency reliability describes whether items inquiring about a similar construct (i.e., items in the same scale) vary appropriately with each other; this is reported as Cronbach's alpha coefficient, which is the average of all possible (split-half) correlations of items in a scale. Second, reproducibility, or test-retest reliability, describes the ability of the instrument to yield the same results on repeated trials and is often reported with Pearson's correlation coefficient. (For a more detailed discussion of psychometric properties, see Chapter 3.)

Validity of psychometric instruments is multidimensional (Table 1); because there is no criterion measure for the effects of skin disease on a patient's quality of life, we have examined the validity of Skindex by an incremental process, which tests many of the other types of validity. For example, in testing its construct validity, we quantitatively examined the logical relations that we hypothesized should exist between what the instrument is measuring and what we want it to measure. We expected that

Table 1 Types of Validity of Health Assessments

Type of Validity	Meaning
Face	Makes sense
Content	Covers the topic adequately
Criterion	Agrees with a gold standard
Construct	Correlates with other variables as hypothesized
Discriminant	Correlates more with concepts intended to measure than with other concepts
Predictive	Forecasts another event as hypothesized
Concurrent	Relates to another instrument administered simultaneously
Convergent	Strength of association between two measures of the same construct

patients with certain types of skin diseases might have greater effect on their quality of life than patients with other types. Similarly, we hypothesized that there are certain underlying themes that explain the way that skin disease affect people's quality of life—skin diseases may have annoying symptoms, cause physical limitations, affect one's ability to socialize, or affect one emotionally. One measure of construct validity is to examine quantitatively whether these underlying themes indeed hang together statistically—i.e., that the logical relations exist. To measure this aspect of construct validity, we used a form of multivariable analysis called factor analysis, in which the variance in a set of measured variables (e.g., the responses to questions in a questionnaire) are explained in term of underlying factors, assuming that the observed variables, or items, are linear combinations of the factors. In particular, factor analysis can be used to validate an instrument if the statistically derived factors correlate qualitatively and quantitatively with an a priori hypothesis of what the measured variables should be. In addition to its construct validity, we also measured the convergent and discriminant validities of Skindex compared to a commonly used, validated measure of general health status, the Short Form-36 (SF-36) of the Medical Outcomes Study (10–12). For this validity testing, we compared correlations between Skindex scores and SF-36 scores measuring constructs that we hypothesized each would measure better or worse. For example, for measuring the convergent validity of Skindex with the SF-36, we predicted that the correlations between Skindex scores and SF-36 scores for scales measuring related constructs would be moderately high, but not redundant.

Finally, because we intended Skindex for evaluative purposes as well, we also assessed its responsiveness, which is the extent to which it is able to measure clinical change.

COMPOSITION OF SKINDEX

We used a modification of the stepwise instrument development method described by Kirshner and Guyatt (5). First, we developed a comprehensive hypothesis—a conceptual framework—for the impact of skin disease on patients' quality of life. We reviewed the medical, psychological, sociological, and lay literature regarding quality of life in patients with skin diseases, ways in which skin diseases affect patients, and stigma associated with disfigurement (13–34). We also conducted structured interviews with patients with a wide variety of skin problems, and directed focus sessions with dermatologists, generalist physicians, and nurses who care for patients with skin disease. Based on this information, we hypothesized that the effects of skin disease on patients' quality of life are either psychosocial or physical. Psychosocial effects could be either cognitive, social, or emotional. Cognitive effects are beliefs about self or others related to skin disease (e.g., "People talk about my skin condition behind my back"). Social effects are those of avoidance of social situations that the patient ascribed to skin disease (e.g., "I do more things by myself because of my skin condition [watching TV, studying, reading]"). Emotional effects could be those of depression, fear, embarrassment, or anger. Depression refers to the experience of despondent feelings ascribed to skin disease (e.g., "This skin condition makes me feel hopeless"), fear refers to worry (e.g., "I am concerned that my skin condition has a bad effect on my family"), embarrassment refers to feelings of social anxiety ascribed to skin disease ("I am ashamed of my skin condition"), and anger refers to hostility ("My skin condition makes me irritable"). Physical effects of skin disease could be either discomfort or physical limitations. Discomfort refers to symptoms ascribed to skin disease (e.g., "My skin itches") and limitations to impaired physical functioning ascribed to skin disease (e.g., "My skin condition makes moving around difficult"). Using this conceptual framework (Fig. 2) and established guidelines for item construction (35), we composed 65 items to address the eight constructs. This draft instrument was pretested by 22 patients in the general dermatology clinics at a Veterans Affairs hospital and 24 patients at a suburban private dermatology practice. We interviewed these patients about items they found confusing and revised or deleted those items accordingly.

The resulting instrument was the version of Skindex that we pilot-tested. The instrument was a 61-item self-administered questionnaire (see

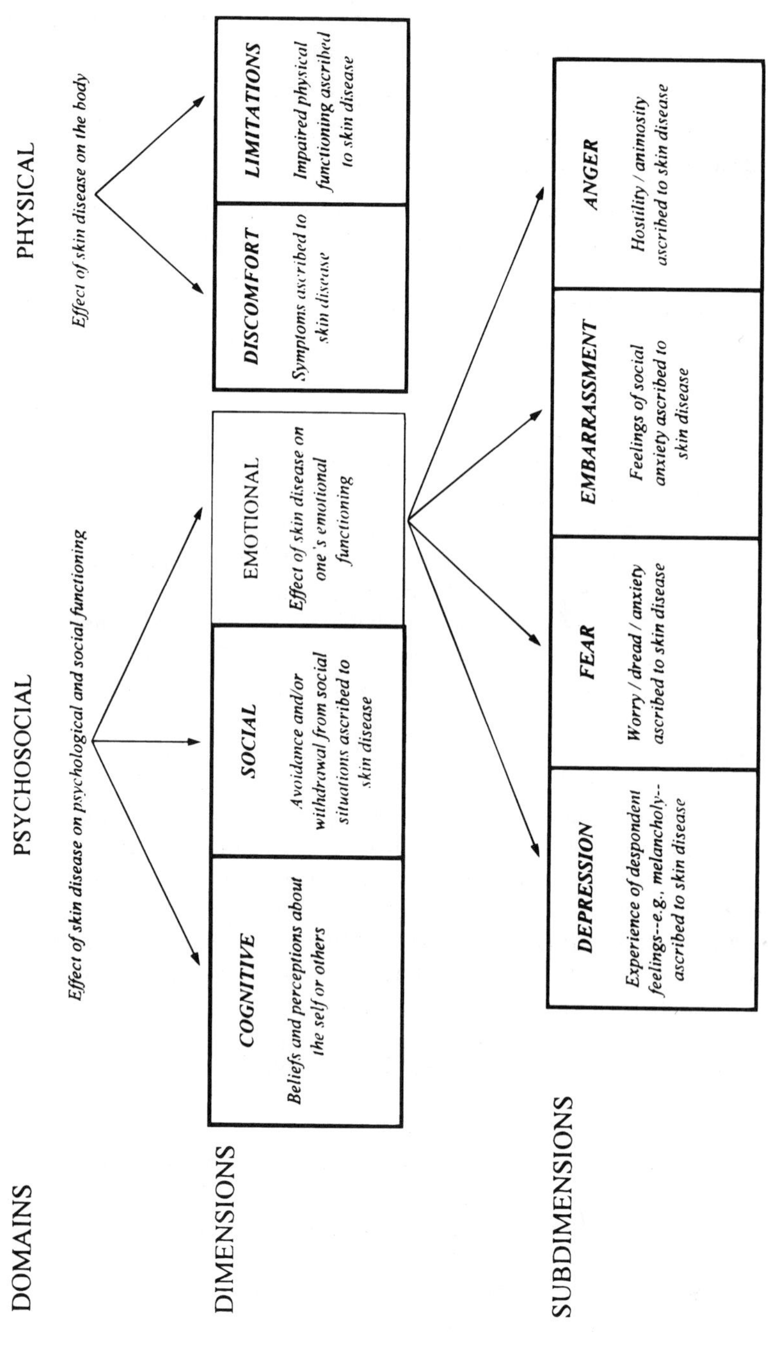

Figure 2 Conceptual framework for the effects of skin disease on a patient's quality of life.

Appendix). All items inquired about the patient's perceptions during the previous 4 weeks. The response categories had either five or six choices relating to frequency ("Never" to "All the time") or agreement ("Strongly disagree" to "Strongly agree"). Thirty-eight of the items were positively phrased, so that a patient experiencing this impact of skin disease responded with a higher response choice; the remaining 23 items were negatively phrased, so that this patient would choose a lower response choice (35).

TESTING OF SKINDEX

Data Collection

Patients were randomly selected from all adults receiving dermatology care in four private suburban practices of dermatologists on the faculty at Case Western Reserve University and the resident-staffed general dermatology clinics at the Cleveland Veterans Affairs Medical Center. To obtain a random sample, we consecutively numbered all scheduled patients during a data-collection session and used a computer-generated random number list of 50% of the total number of patients scheduled. We chose this arrangement to permit us adequate time to explain the study to all potential enrollees and to obtain consent. One of us approached and offered participation to all eligible patients in the reception room of the office while they were waiting for their appointments.

In addition to Skindex, enrolled patients also answered other questions about clinical and sociodemographic information, and some patients completed the generic health status measure, the SF-36 (10–12).

Samples

We assessed the measurement properties of Skindex in four groups or subgroups of patients. First, to test internal consistency reliability and construct validity, a cross-sectional sample of 266 patients was approached to participate in the study. Of these patients, 13 refused to participate, and 19 were deemed mentally or physically unable to complete the instrument, leaving 234 enrolled patients (88%). Next, to test responsiveness, a random sample of 100 of these patients was mailed a second copy of Skindex approximately 6 months after first completing the instrument. At that time, each patient also responded to a global question about change in their skin condition since they last completed the instrument. The response rate from this mailing was 67%. Third, to test convergent and discriminant validity, 132 of the 234 patients in the cross-sectional sample completed both Skindex and the SF-36. Finally, to test reproducibility, an additional sample of 40 patients responded to Skindex twice in 72 hours.

Analyses

To determine the analytic dataset, we eliminated questionnaires if an entire page of the four-page Skindex, or more than 25% of the 61 items, was left blank. We also eliminated questionnaires if responses indicated an obviously contradictory response pattern (i.e., if responses were the same for an entire page, except for "Sometimes," "Slightly agree," or "Slightly disagree"). All responses were standardized to a linear scale of 100, and responses to the negatively phrased items were reverse-scored so that for all items a higher score indicated a greater effect on quality of life. For scoring, a scale score was the mean of a patient's responses to items in that scale. For factor analyses, answers to missing items were imputed as the mean of the patient's responses to other items in the same scale. For comparing scales from the SF-36 and Skindex, we generated comparative scales measuring related constructs and composed of existing scales from each instrument (36). Analyses are summarized in Table 2.

Results

Of the 234 enrolled patients in the main cross-sectional sample, 28 were eliminated because they had completed less than 75% of the instrument and 5 because they had responded in a contradictory manner. Thus, the final size of this sample was 201 patients. The mean age was 51(± 17) years,

Table 2 Analyses Used in Initial Psychometric Testing of Skindex

Scale Scores	Mean of patient's responses to items in a scale
Reproducibility	Pearson's correlation coefficient
Internal Consistency Reliability	Cronbach's alpha coefficient
Construct Validity	Differences in scale scores in different diagnostic groups Principal axes factor analyses
Responsiveness	Change in scale score in patients who reported that their skin condition had changed
Convergent Validity Compared with SF-36	Correlations between comparative scales
Discriminant Validity Compared with SF-36	Correlations of scores from each instrument with responses to questions about general health and skin

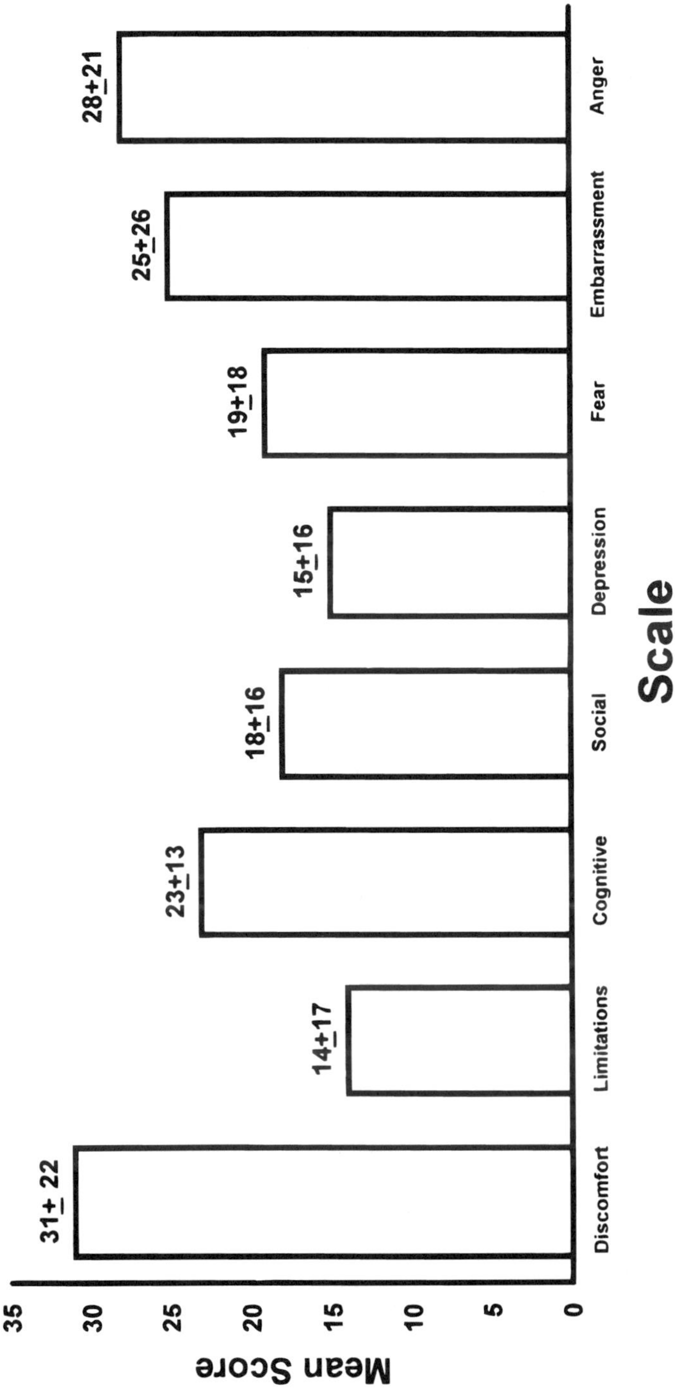

Figure 3 Mean Skindex scale scores of 201 dermatology patients. Higher scores indicate greater effect on quality of life.

60% were female, and 91% were white. Dermatological diagnoses were nonmelanoma skin cancer or actinic keratosis in 18%, isolated benign lesion in 17%, acne vulgaris or rosacea in 17%, eczematous dermatitis in 13%, and a variety of other skin problems in the remaining 36%. Most skin problems (58%) had been present at least a year.

Mean scores on the eight Skindex scales varied from 14 for physical limitations to 31 for physical discomfort (Fig. 3). The standard deviations were quite high, indicating that there were widely varying responses. For example, 10% of patients responded with physical discomfort, embarrassment, and anger scores of greater than 60 (i.e., they often or all the time experienced those symptoms or feelings).

Skindex scales were reproducible ($r = 0.68$–0.90) and internally reliable ($\alpha = 0.76$–0.86). Similarly, Skindex appeared to have evidence of construct validity both clinically and psychometrically. As we had hypothesized, patients with inflammatory skin diseases such as psoriasis or eczematous dermatitis had significantly higher scores than patients with isolated skin lesions for all scales except physical limitations. Also, factor analysis supported the conceptual framework. Of the common variance in patients' responses, 78% was accounted for by seven factors, which correlated with the constructs in the conceptual framework (Table 3). For example, the dominant factor, which we named embarrassment, was loaded on most heavily by items inquiring about embarrassment or shame. The second factor, which we labeled self-esteem, was loaded on most heavily by items inquiring about ability to make friends. Factor scores calculated using the regression coefficients of each item for a factor correlated most highly with

Table 3 Factors Extracted in Factor Analysis of Responses of 201 Dermatology Patients to Skindex

Factor	Name	Items with strong load	Scale with highest correlation (R)
I	Embarrassment	Embarrassed, ashamed	Embarrassment (0.91)
II	Self-esteem	Make friends	Depression (0.79)
III	Anxiety	Accomplish as much	Fear (0.79)
IV	Discomfort	Skin irritated	Discomfort (0.89)
V	Limits	Shake hands	Limitations (0.80)
VI	Self-consciousness	People talk behind back	Cognitive (0.73)
VII	Intimacy	Sex life	Social (0.76)

the appropriate scales from the conceptual framework, giving quantitative evidence for construct validity of the instrument.

Skindex also appeared to have both convergent and discriminant validity when compared to the SF-36. Correlations between scales of the two instruments measuring the same constructs were moderate, as hypothesized ($r = 0.44–0.56$), and patients with low, medium, or high responses to Skindex differed similarly in SF-36 scores. On the other hand, patients' responses to questions about their skin correlated more highly with their Skindex scores than their SF-36 scores, and, conversely, their scores about their general health correlated more highly with their SF-36 scores.

Finally, Skindex scores were responsive to clinical change. In the group of 34 patients who had reported that their skin condition overall was better than when they had taken Skindex originally (6 months before), the mean scores of seven Skindex scales decreased, three of which decreased significantly ($p \leq 0.05$). Similarly, in 27 patients who said their skin was unchanged, only one scale score (fear) changed significantly. In the six patients who reported that their skin was worse, all eight scale scores increased, four of them significantly ($p \leq 0.05$).

These studies document that Skindex has many features that make it likely to be an accurate outcomes measure of the effects of skin disease on patients' quality of life. It is reproducible and has internal reliability, and it has evidence of many types of validity. As we intended, it has both discriminative and evaluative capabilities, in that it is able to distinguish between different groups of patients and also appears to be able to measure change as patients' clinical conditions change.

FUTURE DIRECTIONS

Instrument development is an incremental process (5). These data showed that Skindex has promising psychometric properties (36,37), but also that it could be refined. For example, patients required 15 minutes to complete the instrument, which is not ideal for busy clinical or research settings. Likewise, in the small groups of patients we studied, not all scales were responsive to clinical change, and the evaluative capability of the instrument may be improved by eliminating items that seem more likely to be measuring stable traits rather than clinical states. We are presently refining the instrument and testing the newer version (38).

Our long-range goal for Skindex is that it be used as an outcomes measure to improve the quality of dermatological care. Many of our therapies that appear to give relatively equivalent clinical outcomes—PUVA and topical nitrogen mustard for early cutaneous T-cell lymphoma, or topical steroids, calcipotriene, UVB, and PUVA for moderate plaque-type psoriasis—may, in fact, vary significantly if patients' perceptions are included as outcomes. We plan to use Skindex in studies to examine these types of clinical questions.

Finally, we believe that skin diseases provide an interesting model to examine the relationship between biology and the patient's health. The World Health Organization has defined health as not only the absence of disease but also a person's perceived well-being, yet traditional medical investigation and clinical research has focused on biophysical measures of disease. Because skin diseases can be visible and disfiguring, they provide an intriguing setting in which to examine—and understand—the relationship between the physical characteristics of disease (Impairment, Fig. 1) and the patients' perceptions of illness.

ACKNOWLEDGMENTS

We thank the faculty, residents, and nurses of the Department of Dermatology, University Hospitals of Cleveland and the Cleveland Veterans Affairs Medical Center, for their cooperation. We also gratefully acknowledge the advice of Stephen J. Zyzanski, Ph.D., of the Department of Family Medicine, Case Western Reserve University, and the members of the Program in Health Care Research, Cleveland Veterans Affairs Medical Center.

This material is based upon work supported by the Office of Research and Development, Health Services Research and Development, Department of Veterans Affairs. Dr. Chren is Assistant Chief, Dermatology Service, Veterans Affairs Medical Center, Cleveland, OH. This work was also supported by a Mentored Clinical Scientist Development Award to Dr. Chren from the National Institute of Arthritis, Musculoskeletal and Skin Diseases (K08AR01962-01), National Institutes of Health, and United States Public Health Service.

APPENDIX: SKINDEX

Items 1–48: Never, Rarely, Sometimes, Often, All the Time.
Items 49–62: Strongly Disagree, Disagree, Slightly Disagree, Slightly Agree, Agree, Strongly Agree.

Item	Scale
1. My skin hurts.	discomfort
2. I think about my skin condition.	cognitive
3. My skin is in bad condition.	cognitive
4. I have control over my skin condition.	cognitive
5. I am humiliated by my skin condition.	embarrassment
6. My skin condition affects what I choose to wear (clothes, hats, wigs).	embarrassment
7. I go out as much as usual even though I have this skin condition.	social
8. I am angered by my skin condition.	anger
9. I am embarrassed by my skin condition.	embarrassment
10. Other people ignore my skin condition.	cognitive
11. My skin condition makes it difficult for me to accomplish as much as usual.	limitations
12. My skin condition makes me feel like an outsider	depression
13. I blame someone else for my skin condition.	cognitive
14. I am comfortable in situations where people can see my skin condition (swimming, exercising).	social
15. I worry about how old my skin looks.	fear
16. My skin itches.	discomfort
17. People make fun of me because of my skin condition.	cognitive
18. I feel good about myself even though I have this skin condition.	depression
19. My skin condition affects how close or intimate I can be with people I love.	social
20. Bathing is as easy as usual even though I have this skin condition.	limitations
21. I worry that therapy for my skin will harm my general health.	fear
22. I am concerned that my skin condition has a bad effect on my family.	fear
23. I am able to keep by home as clean as usual even though I have this skin condition.	limitations
24. People see my skin condition and think I am dirty.	cognitive
25. The physical symptoms from my skin condition have a bad effect on my sex life.	limitations
26. I am willing to shake hands with others even with this skin condition.	social

Item	Scale
27. I worry my skin condition will affect my general health.	fear
28. My skin is in bad condition.*	
29. I can put my hands in water as much as usual even with this skin condition.	limitations
30. I worry about scarring or disfigurement from this skin condition.	fear
31. My skin condition makes me feel depressed (down in the dumps).	depression
32. My skin condition makes me irritable.	anger
33. My skin condition bleeds.	discomfort
34. I am comfortable showing affection to others even though I have this skin condition.	social
35. I am frustrated by this skin condition.	anger
36. Other people understand my skin condition.	cognitive
37. I worry my skin condition will spread to other places on my body.	fear
38. I sleep as well as usual even though I have this skin condition.	limitations
39. People talk about my skin condition behind my back.	cognitive
40. I do more things by myself because of my skin condition (watching TV, studying, reading).	social
41. I blame myself for this skin condition.	cognitive
42. Using my hands (typing, cleaning, using tools) is as easy as usual even with this skin condition.	limitations
43. I am ashamed of my skin condition.	embarrassment
44. My skin condition makes moving around difficult.	limitations
45. My skin is irritated.	discomfort
46. My skin is in good condition.	cognitive
47. My skin condition makes me look disfigured.	cognitive
48. I worry my skin condition will spread to others.	fear
49. Life is fair even though I have this skin condition.	cognitive
50. My skin problem is the major thing people notice about me.	cognitive
51. Life is worthwhile even though I have this skin condition.	depression
52. I can still make new friends even with this skin condition.	social
53. In general, I am a confident person even though I have this skin condition.	depression
54. Even a compliment about the condition of my skin would bother me.	anger

Item	Scale
55. I visit the hairdresser/barber as much as usual even though I have this skin condition.	social
56. This skin condition makes me feel hopeless.	depression
57. I feel like myself even though I have this skin condition.	depression
58. Compared to others, I am fortunate to have the skin I have.	anger
59. My sex life is the same as usual even though I have this skin condition.	social
60. People who see my skin condition are as friendly as usual.	cognitive
61. My skin condition makes me tired more than usual.	limitations
62. I socialize less than usual because I have this skin condition.	social

* Item 28, a repeated item, was deleted before any analysis.

REFERENCES

1. Fredriksson T, Pettersson U. Severe psoriasis—oral therapy with a new retinoid. Dermatologica 1978; 157:238–244.
2. Chren MM. Dermatologic health services research. Dermatol Clin 1995; 13:689–695.
3. Marks R, Barton SP, Shuttleworth D, Finlay AY. Assessment of disease progress in psoriasis. Arch Dermatol 1989; 125:235–240.
4. Spitzer WO. State of science 1986: quality of life and functional status as target variables for research. J Chron Dis 1987; 40:465–471.
5. Kirshner B, Guyatt G. A methodological framework for assessing health indices. J Chron Dis 1985; 38:27–36.
6. Gill TM, Feinstein AR. A critical appraisal of the quality of quality-of-life measurements. JAMA 1994; 272:619–626.
7. Guyatt GH, Cook DJ. Health status, quality of life, and the individual. JAMA 1994; 272:630–631.
8. Guyatt GH, Feeny DH, Patrick DL. Measuring health-related quality of life. Ann Intern Med 1993; 118:622–629.
9. Wright JG, Feinstein AR. A comparative contrast of clinimetric and psychometric methods for constructing indexes and rating scales. J Clin Epidemiol 1992; 45:1201–1218.
10. Ware JE, Sherbourne CD. The MOS 36-item short-form health survey (SF-36): I. Conceptual framework and item selection. Med Care 1992; 30:473–483.
11. McHorney CA, Ware JE, Raczek AE. The MOS 36-item short-form health survey (SF-36): II. Psychometric and clinical tests of validity in measuring physical and mental health constructs. Med Care 1993; 31:247–263.

12. McHorney CA, Ware JE, Lu JFR, Sherbourne CD. The MOS 36-item short-form health survey (SF-36): III. Tests of data quality, scaling assumptions, and reliability across diverse patient groups. Med Care 1994; 32:40–66.
13. Jowett S, Ryan T. Skin disease and handicap: an analysis of the impact of skin conditions. Soc Sci Med 1985; 20:425–429.
14. Finlay AY, Khan GK, Luscombe DK, Salek MS. Validation of Sickness Impact Profile and Psoriasis Disability Index in psoriasis. Br J Dermatol 1990; 123:751–756.
15. Salek MS, Finlay AY, Luscombe DK, Allen BR, Berth-Jones J, Camp RDR, Graham-Brown RAC, Khan GK, Marks R, Motley RJ, Ross JS, Sowden JM. Cyclosporin greatly improves the quality of life of adults with severe atopic dermatitis. a randomized, double-blind, placebo-controlled trial. Br J Dermatol 1993; 129:422–430.
16. Shuster S, Fisher GH, Harris E, Binnell D. The effect of skin disease on self image. Br J Dermatol 1978; 99:18–19.
17. Porter JR, Beuf AH. Racial variation in reaction to physical stigma: a study of degree of disturbance by vitiligo among black and white patients. J Health Soc Behav 1991; 32:192–204.
18. Medansky RS, Handler RM, Medansky DL. Self-evaluation of acne and emotion: a pilot study. Psychosomatics 1981; 22:379–383.
19. Finlay AY, Kelly SE. Psoriasis—an index of disability. Clin Exper Dermatol 1987; 12:8–11.
20. Motley RJ, Finlay AY. How much disability is caused by acne? Clin Exper Dermatol 1989; 14:194–198.
21. Wessely SC, Lewis GH. The classification of psychiatric morbidity in attenders at a dermatology clinic. Br J Psych 1989; 155:686–691.
22. Dooley G, Finlay AY. Personal construct systems of psoriatic patients. Clin Exper Dermatol 1990; 15:401–405.
23. Motley RJ, Finlay AY. Practical use of a disability index in the routine management of acne. Clin Exper Dermatol 1992; 17:1–3.
24. Savin JA. Patients' beliefs about psoriasis. Trans St Johns Hosp Derm Soc 1970; 56:139–142.
25. McHenry PM, Doherty VR. Psoriasis: an audit of patients' views on the disease and its treatment. Br J Dermatol 1992; 127:13–17.
26. Lindholm C, Bjellerup M, Christensen OB, Zederfeldt B. Quality of life in chronic leg ulcer patients. An assessment according to the Nottingham Health Profile. Acta Derm Venereol (Stockh) 1993; 73:440–443.
27. Sonino N, Fava GA, Mani E, Belluardo P, Boscaro M. Quality of life in hirsute women. Postgrad Med J 1993; 69:186–189.
28. Kent G, Al-Abadie M. The psoriasis disability index—further analyses. Clin Exper Dermatol 1993; 18:414–416.
29. Lubeck DP, Patrick DL, McNulty P, Fifer SK, Birnbaum J. Quality of life of persons with onychomycosis. Qual Life Res 1993; 2:341–348.
30. Nadelson T. A person's boundaries: a meaning of skin disease. Cutis 1978; 21:90–94.

31. Whitlock FA. Psychophysiological aspects of skin disease. In: Rook A, ed. Major Problems in Dermatology. Philadelphia: W.B. Saunders Company, Ltd., 1976: 58–68.
32. Updike J. Personal history. At war with my skin. New Yorker 1985; (Sept. 2).
33. Bukowski C. Ham on Rye. Santa Rosa: Black Sparrow Press, 1993.
34. Updike J. Personal history. At war with my skin. New Yorker 1985; (Sept 2):39–57.
35. Comrey AL. Factor-analytic methods of scale development in personality and clinical psychology. J Consult Clin Psychol 1988; 56: 754–761.
36. Chren MM, Lasek RJ, Quinn LM, Covinsky KE. Convergent and discriminant validity of a generic and a disease-specific instrument to measure quality of life in patients with skin disease. J Invest Dermatol 1997; 108: 103–107.
37. Chren MM, Lasek RJ, Quinn LM, Mostow EN, Zyzanski SJ. Skindex, a quality-of-life measure for patients with skin disease: reliability, validity, and responsiveness. J Invest Dermatol 1996; 107: 707–713.
38. Chren MM, Lasek RJ. Skindex1.1. Reliability, validity, and responsiveness of a refined instrument to measure the effects of skin disease on quality of life (abstr). Invest Dermatol 1997; 108:366.

13

Profile of a Patient with Contact Dermatitis with a Suspicion of Contact Allergy

History, Physical Characteristics, and Dermatology-Specific Quality of Life

Rukmini Rajagopalan *Glaxo Wellcome Inc., Research Triangle Park, North Carolina*

Roger T. Anderson *Bowman Gray School of Medicine of Wake Forest University, Winston-Salem, North Carolina*

BACKGROUND

According to the National Center of Health Statistics survey, more than 717 million physician visits were recorded in 1994, approximately 31.5 million (4.39%) of which were dermatology-related. Among visits classified as for dermatitis, approximately 40% were to dermatologists (1) (Table 1).

It has been estimated that 70% of contact dermatitis is irritant and 30% allergic (2). Thus, treatment patterns depend upon differential diagnosis of the dermatitis. The North American Contact Dermatitis Group (NACDG) reports the results of their multicenter patch testing so that dermatologists, industry, and others may become aware of contact sensitivity to

Reprinted with permission from the American Journal of Contact Dermatitis 1997; 8(1): 26–31.

Table 1 Dermatology-Related Visits to Physicians, 1994

	Total	Visits to dermatologist	Visits to other specialties
Atopic dermatitis and other conditions	922,359 (100.00%)	378,082 (40.99%)	544,297 (59.01%)
Contact dermatitis and other eczema	6,918,548 (100.00%)	2,717,794 (39.28%)	4,200,754 (60.72%)

Source: Ref. 1.

chemicals used for patch testing and included in formulations. A total of 3541 subjects were patch-tested during a 2-year period (1992–94) by the 12 members of the NACDG. Of the subjects patch tested, 1788 (50%) showed a positive response to at lease one allergen from the first tray (a screening series of 20 allergens). If the positive findings were below 30% in the first tray, the testing would appear to have been overused, and a positive finding of over 75% would demonstrate underuse (3).

The entire health care industry in the United States as well as in the rest of the westernized world continues to undergo a steady transformation due to political, social, and economic pressures. These pressures are driven by increasing costs, an aging population, more expensive, high-technology medical solutions, and increasing patient expectations about the quality and quantity of health care. Both the public and private sectors continue to seek ways to reduce costs and control access. As a result, managed care is realizing steady growth. As the managed care system develops, its control over the access and use of medical care becomes stronger. In essence, more and more individuals seeking medical care will be channeled through the system before they access the appropriate care.

Thus, as one scenario, a larger proportion of patients seeking dermatological care within managed care organizations will be seen by primary care physicians (PCPs) initially, who will decide whether or not a patient should be referred to a dermatologist. Therefore it is imperative that all PCPs, or in some instances primary care nurse practitioners, have proper guidelines available for prompt referrals. Beyond educating PCPs about *which* patients to refer is the issue of *when* to refer. Too guick a referral may mar the cost-effectiveness of the therapeutic outcome, and too late a referral may jeopardize the clinical, economic, and dermatology-specific quality of life (DSQL) effectiveness of the treatment. Because many PCPs might not have sufficient experience treating skin diseases, a first step in developing practice guidelines for cost-effective treatment for dermatitis will be to review a profile of a patient with contact dermatitis. Data on characteristics such as duration and severity of dermatitis, number of office visits for dermatitis, multiple diagnoses, patient demographics, and DSQL can provide key information about the past and present economic and non-economic costs of the condition, as well as potential benefits from future therapy. Currently, there are few such reports in the literature which describe the general clinical and DSQL profile of patients with dermatitis.

STUDY OBJECTIVES

The objective of this study was to provide a profile of demographics and disease characteristics and quality-of-life aspects of patients who present themselves with signs and symptoms of allergic contact dermatitis (ACD) to the physician. These data were collected as an initial step for an observational study conducted prospectively to study the cost-effectiveness of patch-testing in patients with contact dermatitis.

MATERIALS AND METHODS

This was an observational study designed to be conducted in 10 study centers with 600 subjects presenting with signs and symptoms of ACD to evaluate the cost-effectiveness of patch-testing. The study results below describe the demographic and life-quality characteristics of these subjects.

The disease severity was classified as "moderate" (at least one characteristic from category 2 in Table 2) or "severe" (at least one characteristic from category 3 or two from category 2 as shown in Table 2). The disease was classified as "mild" if both of the following statements were true: (1) the dermatitis occurred only once, was easily tolerated, and has never recurred; (2) the dermatitis responded to mid- to low-potency corticosteroids (i.e., if all three category 1 findings (Table 2) are true).

Table 2 Disease-Severity Categories

Category	Duration of disease	Frequency of episodes	Severity of symptoms
1	Less than one year	Once in a while	Tolerable
2	1–5 years	1–5 per month	Frequently bothersome
3	More than 5 years	More than 5 per month or constant	Constantly unbearable

Those with multiple diagnosis were also included in the study as long as there was a suspicion of allergic component. Subjects were included in the study with one or more of the following conditions:

1. Subject has a suspected contact dermatitis (recurrent, chronic or acute) with undetermined etiology.
2. Subject has dermatitis in which contact dermatitis is a possible contributing secondary factor, e.g., atopic dermatitis that worsens despite previously effective therapy, stasis dermatitis, and vesicular hand dermatitis.
3. Subject has contact dermatitis that does not improve with avoidance of the suspected allergen or "obvious" allergen.
4. Subject has any "dermatitis" of unknown cause that prompts hospitalization for management or that limits a subject's ability to work or participate in usual activities of daily living.
5. Subject has any "dermatitis" that is recurrent after treatment courses of topical or systemic corticosterioids.
6. Subject's eczema/dermatitis is not controlled, even if patch tests were negative at some point in the past.
7. Subject with one or more contact allergies experiences new episodes of dermatitis.
8. Subject has other primary skin disease that worsens with topical therapy.

Percent disease activity is defined as an approximate ratio of cumulative duration of symptom activity to the duration of disease. That is, if a patient has been suffering from dermatitis for one year and the episodes of symptom activity added up to a total of approximately 90 days, the percent disease activity is recorded as 25%.

A validated DSQL* instrument was used to evaluate the life quality of the subjects who were enrolled in the study at baseline and at 6 and 12 months after enrollment. Data collected at baseline were summarized to build this profile for life quality. The DSQL instrument consisted of 52 items and included subscales for physical symptoms, activities of daily living, social functioning, vitality, mental health, work/school functioning, self-perception and a global assessment of intensity of impacts of dermatitis on each of the QOL domain. The scale items under each domain were rated on a 5-point scale (from 0 to 4) and the global items were evaluated on a

* Copies of the DSQL instrument may be obtained, under agreement, from R. Rajagopalan, Glaxo Dermatology, a division of Glaxo Wellcome Inc., 5 Moore Drive, Research Triangle Park, North Carolina, 27709.

10-point scale. Also assessed were general vitality and emotional well-being using component scales of the SF-36 (4), the popular quality-of-life scale developed by Medical Outcomes Trust to evaluate the quality of life of a general population with no specific disease connotation. Its subscales on vitality and emotional well-being are intended to assess the level of emotional well-being in general from all causes.

RESULTS

Practice Characteristics of the Investigators

The investigators in this study had differing experience with patch-testing. Of 10 investigators, 2 were members of the North American Contact Dermatitis Group, who provided tertiary dermatological care, and one of these patch-tested almost 100% of the subjects sent to him for treatment of suspected allergic contact dermatitis. Four of the investigators have had intense experience in patch-testing, and the other four have recently started patch-testing.

History, Demographics, and Disease Characteristics

A total of 10 investigator sites enrolled subjects ranging from 30–72 per site to a total of 569 subjects. The present report will be based on 566 patients only for whom the baseline data on patient characteristics and quality of life were completed. Seventy-one percent of the subjects were female, and 87.5% were Caucasian. The mean age of the subjects was 46.0 (S.E. = 0.7).

About 43% of the subjects had moderate disease, and the rest were classified severe (according to Table 2). The mean percent disease activity was 66.0 (S.E. = 1.3). Percent disease activity is shown in Table 3 distributed by number of visits within each group. For 216 subjects (38.2%), this was the first visit to a physician for the condition, and the others had visited as many as five physicians during the previous 6 months. The average number of visits was 2.4 (S.E. = 0.15) with a maximum of 32 for the current skin condition.

From these data it is apparent that there is little relationship between severity and number of previous visits to a dermatologist. For example, the proportion of subjects having no dermatologist visits in the previous 6 months ranged from approximately one half (51.6%) for those with mild disease activity (<25%) to one third (34.8%) with severe disease activity (≥75%). Similarly, between 8.7 and 21.7% of subjects had five or more visits.

The mean duration of disease for all the patients when they enrolled in the study was 45.1 months (S.E. = 3.5 months). The duration of disease was

Table 3 Distribution of Patients in the Study by Percent Disease Activity and Number of Dermatologist Visits in the Past 6 Months for the Current Disease Condition

Number of visits	Disease activity (%) <25		25–49		50–74		≥75%		Missing	
	Number	Percent	Number	Percent	Number	Percent	Number	Percent	Number	Percent
0	33	51.6	37	46.3	58	34.5	88	34.8		
1	10	15.6	17	21.2	33	19.6	45	17.8		
2	7	10.9	5	6.3	25	14.9	23	9.1		
3	2	3.1	6	7.5	17	10.1	21	8.3		
4	3	4.7	8	10.0	15	8.9	20	7.9	1	100.0
5+	8	12.5	7	8.7	20	11.9	55	21.7		
Invalid/Missing	1	1.6					1	0.4		
Total	64		80		168		253		1	

Table 4 History of Suspected Allergic Contact Dermatitis

Duration of disease	Number	Percent
<2 months	82	14.5
2 months to 1 year	229	40.5
Over 1 year	255	45.1

also classified as in Table 4. Nearly one half (45.1%) of the subjects had their disease for longer than one year.

Multiple preliminary diagnoses were recorded for the subjects at enrollment. Allergic contact dermatitis is not recorded as preliminary diagnosis because a dermatologist has to diagnose that based on the history, physical examination, and with/without a patch-test. Therefore all contact dermatitis is recorded as "contact dermatitis with unknown etiology." The description and the frequencies are recorded in Table 5. Acute/Chronic/Recurring dermatitis of unknown etiology were the predominant preliminary diagnoses (32–38%). However, chronic/recurring hand eczema stands out as the largest definite diagnosis, with 25% of the subjects. Most (344, or 60.8%)

Table 5 Classification of Preliminary Diagnoses

	Number	Percent
Preliminary diagnosis (description)		
Patchy eczema	26	4.6
Atopic dermatitis	35	6.2
Shoe or foot dermatitis	15	2.7
Acute dermatitis	218	38.5
Chronic dermatitis—unknown etiology	185	32.7
Recurring dermatitis—unknown etiology	217	38.3
Chronic/Recurring hand eczema	143	25.3
Chronic/Recurring stasis eczema	5	0.9
Chronic/Recurring pruritus	17	3.0
Preliminary diagnosis (multiplicity)		
1	344	60.8
2	155	27.4
3	45	8.0
4	14	2.5
5 or more	3	0.5

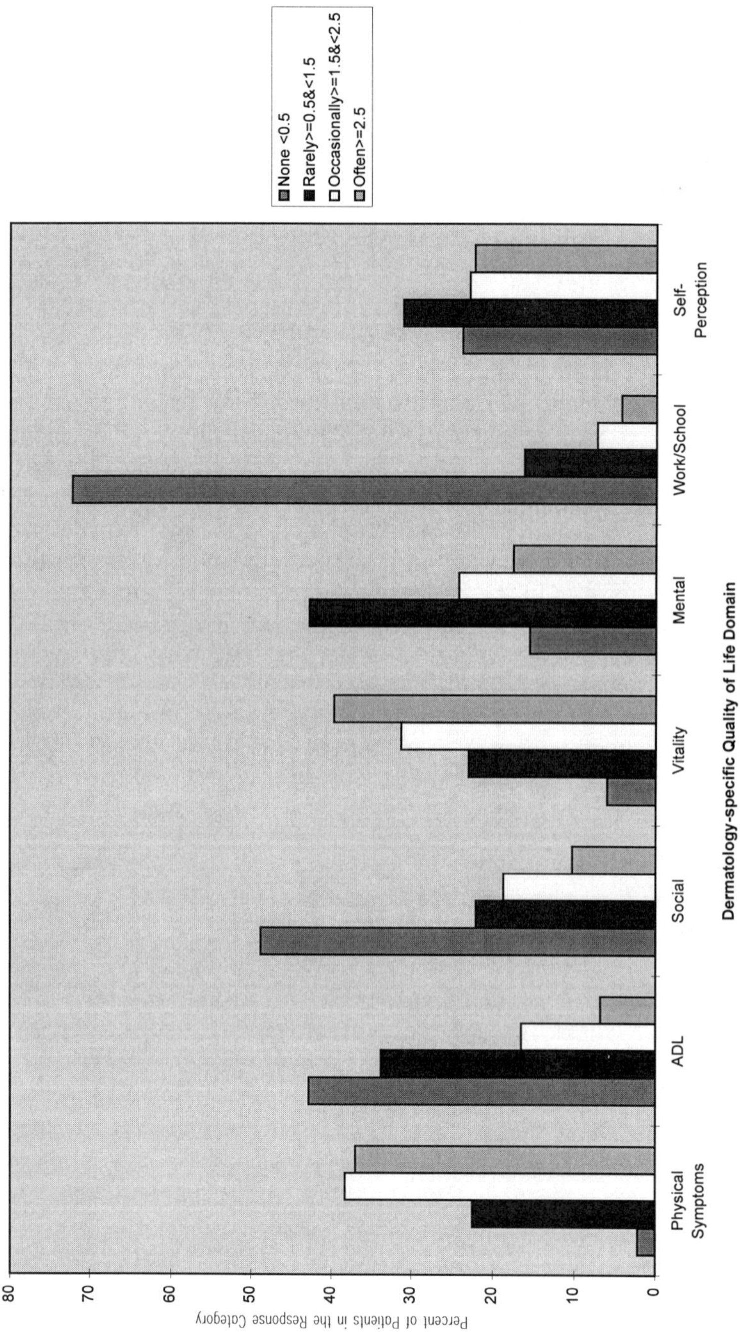

Figure 1 Percent distribution for mean DSQL subscale scores grouped by response categories. ADL = Activities of daily living.

had a single preliminary diagnosis, and about 40% of the subjects had multiple diagnoses documented to a maximum of 6 and a mean of 1.5 (S.E. = 0.03) at the time of enrollment in the study.

Quality of life

The areas of life quality showing the largest impacts in this population were physical symptoms, vitality (SF-36 scale), and self-perception. Lesser impacts were observed for activities of daily living, social functioning, and work/school activities. Figure 1 shows the percentages of subjects whose DSQL in each domain had been affected by their disease "not at all," "rarely," "occasionally," or "often/most of the time." Approximately 75.3% of subjects had a mean DSQL score that corresponded numerically as at least "occasionally" experiencing salient symptoms associated with ACD such as dryness, soreness, pain, itch, or burning. Approximately one quarter of subjects (24% and 23.3%) had reported at least occasional interference with social functioning and activities of daily living, respectively.

In addition to frequency of DSQL impacts in the areas of physical symptoms and negative self-perceptions, these impacts were also rated as most bothersome in intensity. Approximately 60% (322) of subjects experienced considerable distress due to contact dermatitis (scoring 7 or more on a 10-point scale) (Table 6). The self-perceived intensity of contact dermatitis was rated as very severe (scoring 7 or higher) in 317 (57.2%).

The responses to the global items on the degree of distress due to contact dermatitis and the perceived intensity of contact dermatitis were significantly correlated with the mean score of each domain (Figs. 2 and 3). The subjects who admitted to the highest degree of distress due to contact dermatitis and perceived their disease to be of the highest intensity also responded that their quality of life was affected the most on each domain. For example, in Fig. 2, DSQL mean subscale scores ranging from 0 ("no limitations from disease") to 4 ("constantly limited by disease") are plotted by self-rated symptom intensity grouping: mild, moderate, and severe. It is

Table 6 Mean (S.E.) Score for DSQL Global Items and Number and Percent of Subjects Demonstrating Severe Intensity of Disease

Global item	Mean (S.E.) score	No. (%) of subjects with severe intensity
Physical symptoms	6.8 (2.6)	322 (59.5)
Severity on baseline visit	6.0 (2.7)	247 (44.7)
Severity in previous month	6.8 (2.5)	317 (57.2)

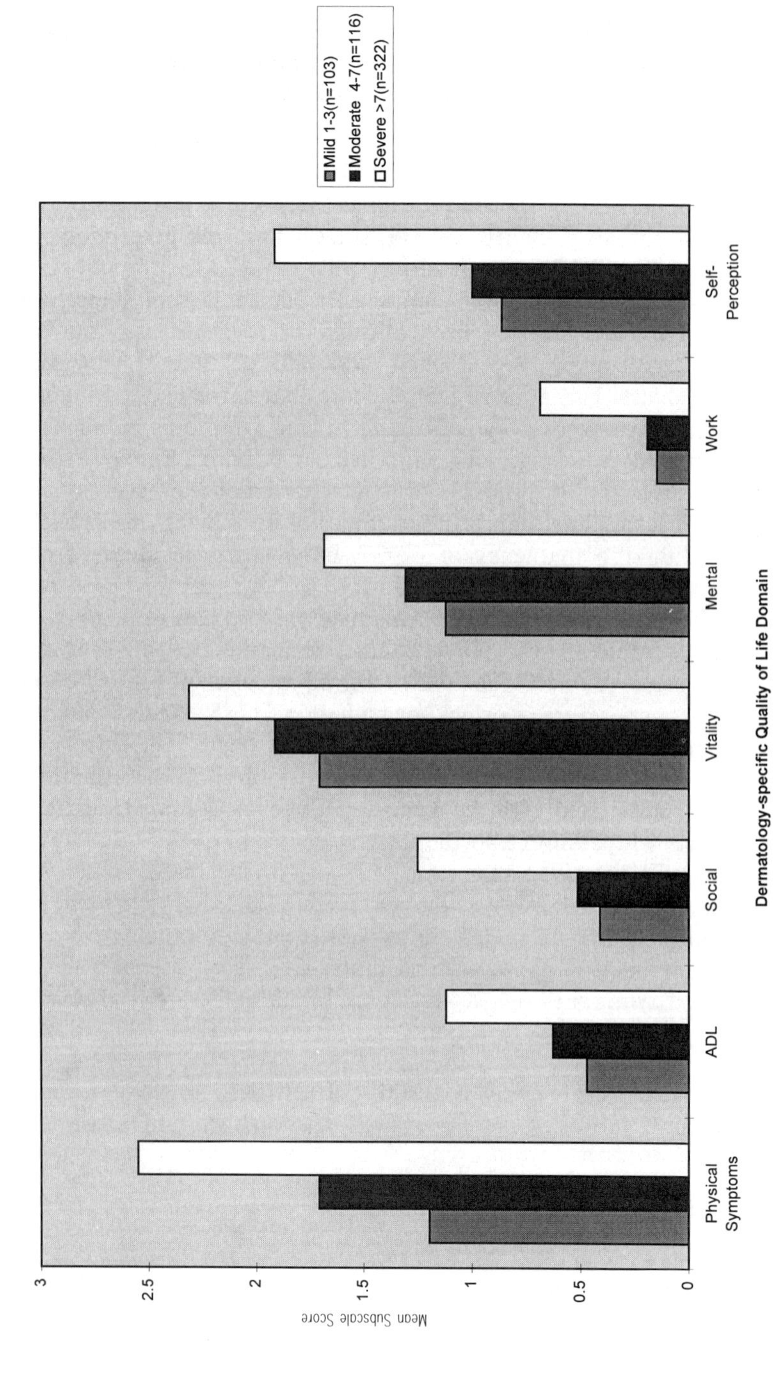

Figure 2 Mean DSQL subscale score by degree of distress due to contact dermatitis. ADL = Activities of daily living.

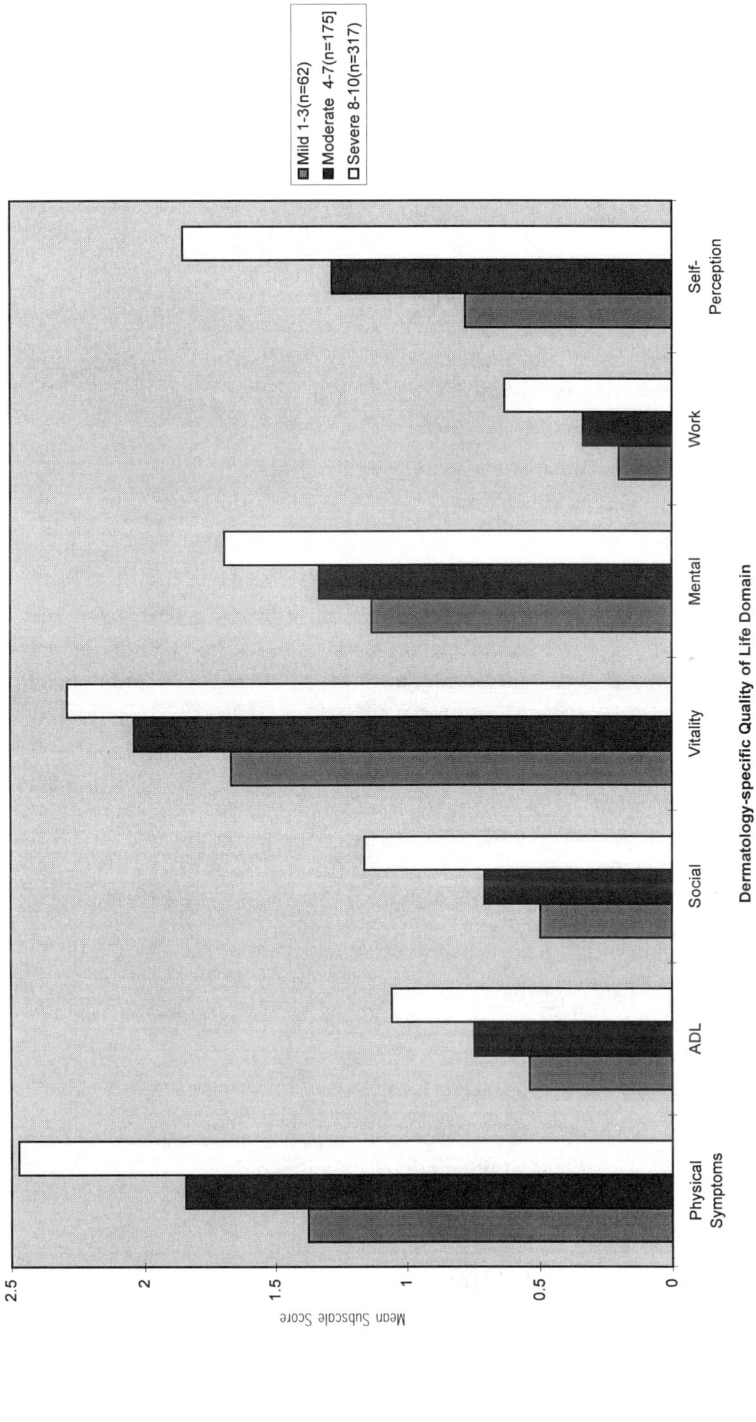

Figure 3 Mean DSQL subscale score by self-perceived degree of contact dermatitis intensity. ADL = Activities of daily living.

Table 7 Correlation* of DSQL Subscales with Selected Global Items

Subscales	Distress due to contact dermatitis	Disease intensity perceived by patient
Physical symptoms	0.6728	0.5413
ADL	0.3772	0.2848
Social functioning	0.4118	0.3322
Vitality	0.2484	0.2187
Mental	0.2656	0.2346
Work/School	0.3782	0.2851
Self-perception	0.4506	0.4319

* All correlation coefficients are statistically significant at $p < 0.05$.

evident that 103 (19%) subjects who had mild distress due to contact dermatitis had the lowest average score on each domain and the score gradually increased with moderate and severe distress. Similar trends were found for the perceived intensity of disease (Fig. 3). The distress due to contact dermatitis symptoms was highly correlated to the perceived intensity of the disease ($r = 0.5765$) and was statistically significant. The Pearson product-moment correlation coefficient with the domain mean scores ranged from 0.2484 to 0.6728 for distress due to the disease and from 0.2187 to 0.5413 for the perceived intensity of the disease (Table 7). The subscale scores for Mental Health and Vitality (SF-36) were less for the ACD cohort

Table 8 Comparison of SF-36 Subscale Scores Between U.S. General Population and a Cohort of Subjects with Suspected Allergic Contact Dermatitis

Subscales	General population mean (S.D.) score ($N = 2474$)	Contact dermatitis cohort mean (S.D.) score ($N = 547$)
Mental health	74.74 (18.05)	70.00 (20.6)
Vitality	60.86 (20.96)	57.68 (23.99)

than the U.S. general population, demonstrating a moderate effect of the disease on these factors (Table 8).

CONCLUSION

The profile of patients with allergic contact dermatitis has been mapped out in terms of their history and physical characteristics and their quality of life to apprise the PCPs of the nature of care these patients require and are looking for. They may very well appear to be healthy and independent in their daily activities and work environment. However, a sizable number of them are in great distress due to the physical symptoms, their vitality is impaired, and their self-perception diminished.

Considering that contact dermatitis may be effectively treated with appropriate screening, referral, and application of established pharmacological and nonpharmacological regimes (5), the often bothersome distress in identified areas affecting life quality is avoidable for many. Our results revealed that a substantial proportion of patients who sought care for contact dermatitis had their skin disease for more than one year. Thus, for many patients, the effects of contact dermatitis on quality of life may be considerable as well as longstanding. It is remarkable that many patients with moderate or severe contact dermatitis had no dermatologist visits in the previous 6 months. Given that quality of life impacts increase with contact dermatitis severity, an underutilization of dermatological care suggests that health care resources to manage contact dermatitis may be inefficiently accessed by primary care physicians. PCPs would be well advised to reach a prompt diagnosis or refer the patients to dermatologists who are proficient in the diagnostics for allergic contact dermatitis. As more and more health care is included under managed care, the patient profile will be a well-sought-out tool for developing guidelines for appropriate referrals.

REFERENCES

1. National Center for Health Statistics, Bethesda, MD. Advance Data, 1994.
2. Rietschel RL. Is patch-testing cost-effective? J Am Acad Dermatol 1989; 4(2):885–887.
3. Marks JG Jr, Belsito DV, DeLeo VA, et al. North American Contact Dermatitis Group standard tray patch results (1992 to 1994). Am J Contact Derm 1995; 6(3):160–165.
4. Ware, JE Jr. SF-36 Health Survey. Boston: The Health Institute, New England Medical Center, 1993.
5. Rietschel RL. Human and economic impact of allergic contact dermatitis and the role of patch-testing, J Am Acad Dermatol 1995; 21:812–815.

14

The Impact of Atopic Dermatitis on the Quality of Life of Children, Adolescents, and Adults

Patricia O'Hare and Daniel P. Krowchuk *Bowman Gray School of Medicine of Wake Forest University, Winston-Salem, North Carolina*

INTRODUCTION

Atopic dermatitis (AD) is a cutaneous inflammatory condition characterized by pruritus, typical morphology and distribution of lesions, a chronic or relapsing course, and a personal or family history of other atopic diseases (e.g., asthma or allergic rhinitis) (1). It is a common skin condition in children, with an estimated incidence of 3–5% in those 5 years of age or less (2). Recent studies suggest, however, that the frequency of AD is increasing. A study conducted in Denmark revealed an incidence to age 7 years of 3% for twins born between 1960 and 1964 compared with 12% for twins born between 1975 and 1979 (3,4). The etiology of AD is not known, although it is believed to be multifactorial with clinical expression dependent on both genetic and environmental factors (3,5).

AD is rarely present at birth and typically begins after 2 months of age (5). Rajka studied the onset of AD and noted manifestations within the first year in 57% of subjects and by 5 years of age in 87% of children (6). In adolescents and adults, therefore, AD generally represents an extension of disease that had its onset in infancy or childhood; after the age of 20 years, less than 2% of individuals experience initial signs or symptoms of AD (6). Although the outcome of AD is difficult to predict in a given individual, disease tends to resolve or improve with age. For example, of 955 children and teenagers (ages 0–14 years) with AD treated in the Department of Dermatology of the Karolinska Hospital in Stockholm, Sweden, 60% of those with moderate disease and 38% of those with severe disease were considered "healed" by adulthood (7). For those with AD as adults, 76% had experienced symptoms continuously since childhood, while in 24% the disease had been quiescent only to return later. AD was considered to have decreased in severity in 85–90% of those whose disease had not resolved (7). Similar, although somewhat less optimistic, prognostic information was provided by a longitudinal study of 801 patients with AD treated at the Turku University in Finland as adolescents (ages 12–16 years) and reevaluated at ages 22–41 years (8). Approximately 45% of patients with mild AD and 22% with severe AD were symptom-free as adults. A trend toward improvement of symptoms was exemplified by the observation that among those initially diagnosed as having severe AD, 85–90% had symptoms at follow-up but in only 12–15% was disease still considered severe (8).

The diagnosis of AD is made clinically based upon the appearance of typical symptoms and signs. A minimum set of diagnostic criteria for AD has been proposed and validated that includes a history of flexural involvement, history of dry skin, onset younger than 2 years of age, personal history of asthma, history of a pruritic eruption, and visible flexural dermatitis (9). Individuals with AD have chronically dry skin and experience pruritus that leads to scratching and resultant cutaneous damage. Acutely, the involved skin may appear erythematous with weeping and crusting, while in chronic states it may become thickened. In infants, the lesions of AD are generalized, but in children, adolescents, and adults a flexural distribution is typical.

Any chronic cutaneous condition that produces visible cutaneous lesions and intense pruritus would be anticipated to have an impact on the quality of life. This chapter reviews published studies that address quality-of-life issues in children, adolescents, and adults with AD. To identify publications in this area, a literature search using Medline was conducted for the years 1966 through 1996. Key words and phrases employed included atopic dermatitis, atopy, dermatitis, eczema, hobbies, occupation, quality of life, recreation, relationships, school, self-esteem, sexuality, and sleep. Empirical studies appearing in English-language journals were then reviewed. The impact of AD on quality of life will be discussed separately for children, adolescents, and adults. A final section of the chapter is devoted to a review of the effect of therapeutic measures on improving quality of life in patients with AD.

CHILDHOOD

AD in children may have significant effects on quality of life, interfering with sleep, school performance and activities, behavior, sports participation, vacations, and interactions with other children (10). Family relationships may be compromised, and sleep loss may extend to parents and siblings of the affected child (10). Despite the potential impact of AD on quality of life in children, only recently has this area received attention.

Effects on the Child

There have been relatively few attempts to address empirically the impact of AD on children. An important advance in this area has been the development of the Children's Dermatology Life Quality Index (CDLQI), a validated, 10-item questionnaire that provides a global assessment of quality of life (11). The maximum score on the CDLQI is 30, with higher scores reflecting greater perceived impact of the condition on one's life. In initial studies of the instrument, 233 children and teenagers 4–16 years of age with various inflammatory dermatoses and 102 controls completed the CDLQI with parental assistance. Children with skin disease had significantly higher mean scores than controls. Mean scores of children with AD (7.7), psoriasis (5.4), and acne (5.7) were all significantly greater than for those of subjects with moles and nevi (2.3). Among the 23% of subjects who had AD, mean CDLQI scores were exceeded only by those of patients with scabies (11).

Sleep Disturbance

Parents and health care providers are aware that the itching associated with AD may adversely affect sleep patterns in children. Inadequate sleep, in turn, may have an effect on a child's behavior and school performance. Three studies have examined specifically the impact of AD on sleep. Dahl et al. (12) studied 59 children ages 6–12 years with AD who were enrolled in an ongoing research program. Parents completed the Child Sleep Behavior Scale (CSBS), a 22-item standardized scale, and a specially designed 12-item questionnaire that addressed sleep-related habits associated with nighttime pruritus and scratching and daytime behavioral problems resulting from inadequate sleep. A control group was not employed; however, subjects' responses on the CSBS were compared with normative data. The authors found that children with AD had statistically significant differences from normative data in 9 of 22 CSBS items. Children with AD were more likely to have restless sleep, frequent waking during the night, sitting up in bed, difficulty falling asleep, fear of the dark, difficulty waking up in the morning, frequent waking to go to the bathroom, frequent complaints about difficulty falling asleep, and fewer hours of sleep. Disease activity demonstrated significant positive correlations with waking up during the night, difficulty falling asleep because of itching or scratching, observed scratching while sleeping, and waking up at night due to itching or scratching. An important finding was that sleep difficulties correlated with daytime symptoms. For example, difficulty falling asleep because of itching was negatively correlated with ease of morning waking and positively correlated with unspecified major discipline problems. Night awakening due to itching or scratching was positively correlated with difficulty staying awake in the afternoon and major discipline problems (12).

Reid and Lewis-Jones (13) employed structured interviews of parents of 39 children with AD to assess the relationship between AD flares and sleep disturbances in both the child and family members. Data were examined with respect to disease activity and were compared to existing epidemiological information on sleep difficulties in normal children. During AD flares, parents were significantly more likely to report that children experienced difficulty getting to sleep (76% vs. 26%), required a longer median time to settle (24.3 minutes vs. 9.4 minutes), and had night waking (84% vs. 41%). During times when AD was quiescent, however, the proportion of children with AD who experienced difficulty getting to sleep or night waking did not differ significantly from data for normal children (13).

The effect of nighttime pruritus and scratching on objective sleep parameters was studied in nine children with AD by Monti et al. (14). The children had an "unremitting history of nighttime pruritus" and discontinued systemic and topical medications 7 days prior to study. Investigations conducted in a sleep laboratory included polysomnography (consisting of electroencephalography, electrooculography, and bipolar electromyography) and electrode monitoring of muscle potentials from the forearms to detect scratching movements. Scratching episodes occurred during rapid eye movement (REM) and non-REM (NREM) sleep. The total time spent scratching ranged from 11.0 to 84.6 minutes with a mean of 30.3 ± 7.4 minutes. Compared with existing data for normal children, study subjects experienced markedly increased total wake time, wake time after sleep onset and numbers of nocturnal wakenings (14).

Although limited by the lack of a control group and, in some cases, the use of unvalidated instruments, these studies support the commonly held belief that children with AD often experience disrupted sleep, particularly when their disease is flaring. Inadequate sleep is associated with difficulty staying awake during the afternoon and with behavioral difficulties. Clearly, improving sleep should be a major focus of the management of children with AD. Further research is needed, however, to examine the relationship between sleep disturbances and behavior problems and to characterize the nature of these abnormalities. In addition, it will be important to determine whether sleep disturbances in children with AD have an impact on academic achievement or an interactional effect with other conditions that affect school performance, including attention deficit–hyperactivity disorder and specific learning disabilities.

Behavior, Activities, and Social Interaction

Three studies have examined the effect of AD on children's behavior, participation in sports, school, and interaction with peers. Long et al. (10) mailed a questionnaire to all members of the National Eczema Society, an AD support group located in the United Kingdom. A response rate of 29% was achieved that included data from 1972 adults and 1944 parents of affected children. The majority of children (87%) ranged in age from 1 to 16 years. Activities affected by AD were sleep (60%), sports (27%), vacations (25%), school (in those over 4 years of age) (27%), and playing and meeting other children (14%) (10). Whether these data can be generalized is not clear since subjects were members of a support group and it could be hypothesized, therefore, that the children had relatively severe disease or that their parents had greater concern about their children's disease. Lawson et al. used a structured questionnaire to study 34 families of 35 children with moderate to severe AD (15). Although the study was not controlled and details of the design were limited, unspecified behavioral problems were reported by parents of 54% of children (15).

In a comprehensive assessment of the psychosocial effects of AD, Daud et al. used semi-structured interviews to evaluate psychiatric adjustment and mother-child attachment in 30 children with AD between the ages of 18 and 48 months and 20 unaffected children matched for age, gender, socioeconomic status, and parental marital status (16). Subjects had involvement of at least 10% of skin surface area and required outpatient visits every 3 months. Children with AD had more behavioral problems than controls. Those with AD were significantly more likely than controls to exhibit excess dependency/clinginess (50% vs. 10%) and fearfulness (40% vs. 10%) and to be characterized as "difficult" by their mothers (20% vs. none of the controls). No differences between subjects and controls were found with respect to eating difficulties, difficulties with activities and concentration, tantrums, manageability, mood changes, or relationships with siblings or peers. In addition, scores on the Denver Developmental Screening Test were comparable for both groups of children (16).

Based on limited data, AD appears to have the potential to adversely affect several areas of a child's life, including sports participation, school, and social interaction with peers. In addition, there is evidence that AD may be associated with behavioral disturbances. Nevertheless, we lack an understanding of the nature, magnitude, and clinical relevance of these effects. Pending the outcome of additional controlled studies, clinicians should be aware of the potential impact of AD on children's lives and should review this area regularly with patients and parents. For children experiencing difficulties, referral for evaluation or therapy of behavioral difficulties may be offered.

Effects on the Family

There is little doubt that the effects of AD extend beyond the child. As Halbert (17) observes, parents often become frustrated by their child's discomfort caused by itching, the chronic course of the disease, the exacerbations that occur without apparent cause, the lack of sleep, the work of applying topical agents, and the cost of medications. Nevertheless, attempts to critically examine the effects of AD on families have been limited. In Lawson's study of the families of 34 children with moderate to severe AD cited above, 74% of parents reported problems with practical care issues, 71% experienced psychological pressures, 66% had a restriction of lifestyle, 29% had altered family relationships, 23% had restricted vacations, and 11% experienced financial pressures resulting from their child's AD (15). Unfortunately, a detailed description of these difficulties was not provided.

In the study of psychosocial effects of AD conducted by Daud et al. described previously, the impact of disease on parental stress and parenting was investigated (16). When compared with controls, mothers of children with AD were significantly more likely to report being highly stressed about their child (51% vs. 20%) and to have less support from their social life (65% vs. 35%). Global quality of parenting was assessed to be lower in mothers of children with AD, primarily in the area of discipline. For example, mothers of children with AD were more likely than controls to acquiesce to children's demands. Significantly more mothers in the AD group reported feeling distressed (related to feeding the child and the child's attention seeking behavior, 30% vs. 5%) and being tired and frustrated (40% vs. 10%). Importantly, however, there were no differences between groups with respect to the mothers' affective response to the child or empathy and acceptance of the child. Among mothers of children with AD, 66% reported that their child's disease had an influence on their marriage (negative in 43%, positive in 20%), 86% reported an effect on family life (negative in 83%), and 66% felt it had a substantial effect on their parenting of the child (16).

Thus, parents of children with moderate to severe AD commonly report adverse personal, familial, and economic effects stemming from the disease. Although further study of the significance of these consequences is needed, providers should be aware of the potential negative impact of AD on the family and should regularly address this issue during clinical visits.

Effects on Health Care Costs

The economic impact of AD is discussed in a separate chapter.

ADOLESCENCE

During adolescence, two important psychological processes are initiated that may influence the impact of cutaneous disease. The first is the emergence of self-awareness or egocentrism. Egocentrism causes adolescents to feel that the thoughts they generate about themselves are shared by others. As a result, teenagers are extremely self-conscious, believing that the impressions others develop about them are the product of close attention to physical appearance. The second process, characteristic of early and middle adolescence, is the strong need to be accepted by one's peer group. This acceptance requires conformity; social or physical differences are poorly tolerated. For these reasons, one would anticipate that cutaneous diseases, including AD, would have a negative impact on an adolescent's self-esteem and quality of life. Nevertheless, no studies of which we are aware have specifically addressed the impact of AD on teenagers. Those investigations that have included adolescents and adults did not stratify results by age and, therefore, will be discussed in the section addressing effects in adults.

In addition to the potential psychological consequences, AD might also be expected to have an influence on occupational selection or performance by older adolescents. Again, however, no studies have assessed these issues exclusively in teenagers, and those that have included adolescents and adults have not stratified results by age. Therefore, the effect of AD on occupation in adolescents will be reviewed in the section on adults.

ADULTHOOD

Although AD tends to improve with age, as noted previously, many adults continue to experience symptoms. The survey conducted by Long et al. of members of the National Eczema Society in the United Kingdom described previously illustrates the extent to which AD may affect quality of life in adults (10). Of those surveyed, 64% reported that social and leisure activities were affected, 54% reported that AD had an impact on their occupation, 14% believed that development of personal relationships had been impaired, and 19% felt that their sex lives were affected (10). Several investigators have attempted to further characterize these effects.

Psychological Impact

Shuster et al. studied the effect of skin disease on self-image in a group of patients with acne, eczema, and psoriasis (18). Details of the research design, including number of subjects and their ages, were not presented. Participants were asked to evaluate nine schematic faces for attributes of age, happiness, good looks, and likability. In addition, subjects were asked to select faces for a variety of attributes, including "like me," "what I'd like to be like," "like someone I like," "like someone I dislike," "likeable," and "like what other people think I'm like." For controls, there was good correlation between "like me" and desirable characteristics such as "likeable" and "good looking." In acne patients, as disease severity increased, there was a progressive and highly significant decrease in this correlation with a decline in self-image. At the same time, there was a significant correlation with attributes of "someone I dislike." In AD, the damage to self-image was reported to be "less severe" and, in the investigators' opinion, may have related to the different sites of involvement (18).

Jowett and Ryan (19) interviewed 100 patients 16–79 years of age who had AD, psoriasis, or acne for longer than 12 months. Interviews consisted of 52 questions addressing the history, extent, and severity of the condition, employment experiences, including any functional and interpersonal difficulties, family and social relationships, limitations on leisure activities, and participants' subjective responses to their disease. Of subjects enrolled in the study, 32 had AD (mean age 38 years). Forty percent of subjects with AD believed that their disease had negative effects on social relationships, 78% experienced shame or embarrassment as a result of AD, and 65% reported some impact on occupation (19).

A major advance in the study of the impact of skin disease on quality of life in adults was the development of the Dermatology Life Quality Index (DLQI) (20). The DLQI is a 10-item questionnaire that provides a global assessment of the effect of skin disease on a number of aspects of an individual's life. The index has a maximum score of 30; the higher the score, the greater the perceived effect of skin disease on quality of life. The DLQI has undergone initial validation studies including construct validity and test-retest reliability. In developing the DLQI, Finlay and Khan studied 200 consecutive patients aged 15–75 years with a variety of cutaneous diseases who were attending a dermatology outpatient clinic and 100 healthy controls (20). Thirteen subjects (ages 6–23 years) had AD, and their mean DLQI scores exceeded those of individuals with other dermatoses. Mean scores of patients with AD (12.5), generalized pruritus (10.5), psoriasis (8.9), viral warts (6.7), and acne (4.3) were significantly higher than for the control population (0.5). Those with AD, generalized pruritus, and psoriasis had

DLQI scores that were significantly higher than those reported by individuals with acne, basal cell carcinoma, and viral warts (20).

Finlay used the DLQI to specifically study the effect of severe AD on the quality of life of 92 adults (49 female, mean age 33.2 years) (21). The mean DLQI score for subjects was 18 (60% of the maximum possible score), exceeding values reported for other skin diseases. The highest subsection scores were obtained for questions that addressed symptoms and feelings about the disease and difficulties associated with treatment. Attesting to the impact of the disease, subjects reported that they would rather have diabetes or hypertension than AD. Eighty percent of patients reported that AD affected their family life, 57% believed that their sexual relationships were affected, and 52% reported that relationships with friends were impacted (21).

Not surprisingly then, adolescents and adults, like children, report that AD has negative effects on quality of life. Further study is indicated, however, to better understand the nature and magnitude of these effects and to determine the extent to which they impact daily activities.

Occupation

It is not surprising that AD may have significant effect on occupation. Although the disease tends to improve with age, approximately 25% of adults suffer recurrences that most often are localized to the hands (7). Furthermore, the hands are essential to the performance of many occupational activities and may be exposed to a variety of irritants in the work setting. Several studies document that atopy, in general, and AD, specifically, increase the risk of developing occupational skin disease. Shmunes and Keil (22) reviewed all closed cases of work-related skin disease processed by the South Carolina Industrial Commission between July 1, 1978, and June 30, 1979. Questionnaires were mailed to all identified patients, and 134 (13.9%) responded. Among this sample, 92% had an occupational contact dermatitis and 82% were atopic using a standard definition. The authors calculated that the relative odds of developing occupational skin disease are 13.5 times greater if one is atopic. In addition, if one has a work-related dermatosis and is also atopic, they concluded that 92.6% of the dermatoses could be attributed to being atopic. Direct costs of occupational skin disease totaled $142,925 for cases that were closed during fiscal year 1979. Compensation for lost time at work accounted for 36.1% of costs, physician fees for 29.8%, final settlements for 17.8%, and medications for 11.6% (22).

Lammintausta and Kalimo investigated the influence of occupation on 1008 individuals with atopic disease, 801 of whom had AD and 207 of whom had other atopic disorders (e.g., allergic rhinitis, allergic conjunctivitis, or asthma) (23). Subjects were stratified by severity of AD (e.g., severe, moderate, mild, none) and were compared with 626 age- and sex-matched controls with respect to the course and severity of dermatitis, occupation, and sick leave over a 6-year period. Hand dermatitis demonstrated an association with occupation. Among atopic patients exposed to "wet" work (e.g., nursing, food handlers, hair dressers, domestic workers, etc.) or mechanically skin-irritating factors for 2 or more hours daily, for example, 90% had hand dermatitis compared with 50% of those who had little or no such exposure. The frequency of sick leave was similar for subjects and controls, although absences due to dermatitis lasted longer than those resulting from other diseases. In this study, atopic patients were not more likely than controls to change occupation. Eighty-three percent of those with AD; 76% of those with asthma, allergic rhinitis, or allergic conjunctivitis; and 80% of controls reported occupation changes. The reason for job change was dermatitis in 8% of atopic patients and in 18% of controls who had a history of dermatitis. The authors concluded that the majority of individuals with AD had "learned to work and live with their skin symptoms" (23).

These findings are similar to those of Rystedt, who studied 1376 persons, of whom 955 had AD, 222 were atopic but did not have AD, and 199 were nonatopic controls (7). Hand eczema was 4–10 times more likely to occur in individuals who had AD during childhood than in those who did not and was more common in those occupationally exposed to chemicals, water, soil, or wear. The frequency of hand eczema, for example, was 81% for food handlers, 76% for ladies hair dressers, 75% for nurses' assistants, and 68% for domestic workers. Importantly, however, 25–40% of those in high-risk occupations had no disease. Also, among office workers with no exposure to water or chemicals, hand eczema occurred in 62% of those with a history of AD, 37% of those who were atopic but had no history of AD, and 17% of controls. Occupational changes attributed to hand eczema were reported by 10% of those with a history of AD, 8% of atopic subjects without AD, and none of the controls (7).

Although the results of these studies are generally encouraging, some patients with AD experience a significant negative impact of AD on occupation. Among the 92 patients with severe AD studied by Finlay and cited previously (21), 32% reported a loss of income and a median of 5 days of work lost due to their disease in the year preceding the study. Fifty-three percent of the subjects who were not working or retired attributed this status to AD (21). In the study of Jowett and Ryan (19) discussed previously, 94 patients with acne, psoriasis, or AD were surveyed regarding the impact of skin disease. Of the 31 subjects with AD, 65% reported and adverse effect of their disease on occupation (16% believed that their opportunities were limited, 42% experienced functional difficulties, and 19% had interpersonal difficulties) (19).

Meding and Swanbeck examined the consequences of various forms of hand eczema in 1238 individuals drawn from a random sample of residents of Gothenberg, Sweden (24). Of these, 169 had confirmed atopic hand eczema. A minimum of 7 days sick leave because of AD was reported by 17.7% of patients with a mean total time on leave of 11.8 weeks. A change in occupation due to skin disease was reported by 5.9% of those with atopic hand eczema. Among all subjects, occupational changes were most frequently observed in hairdressers, bakers, cleaners, kitchen maids, machine tool operators, and practical nurses. Occupational changes were less common among those employed in administration, education, and engineering (24).

In summary, AD may have a significant effect on occupation and it is the single most important risk factor for the development of work-related skin disease (25). The nature of one's occupation, however, influences this risk. For those with AD, vocations or professions that require frequent hand washing, immersion in water, or exposure to irritants or sensitizing agents increase the likelihood of hand eczema. The results of large studies suggest, however, that most individuals are able to accomplish their responsibilities without significant difficulty. Nevertheless, it seems prudent to counsel adolescents and young adults contemplating career choices about the potential exacerbations of AD possible in certain high-risk vocations.

THE INFLUENCE OF TREATMENT ON QUALITY OF LIFE

Only recently has the effect of therapy for AD on quality of life been critically examined. Salek and colleagues enrolled 33 adults with severe refractory AD in a randomized, double-blind, placebo-controlled crossover trial of cyclosporin (26). Outcome measures included the United Kingdom Sickness Impact Profile (UKSIP), the Eczema Disability Index (EDI), and a global clinical assessment that included measures of disease activity, extent, sleep, and itch and tolerability and efficacy of treatment (26). Subjects were evaluated at baseline, 8 weeks, and 16 weeks. Significant improvements in quality of life, as reflected by UKSIP and EDI scores, were observed in both treatment sequences, although the magnitude of the effect was greater in those who received placebo followed by cyclosporin. Interestingly, there was no or very poor correlation between the quality-of-life parameters and objective assessments of the severity and extent of disease. However, there was a close association between quality-of-life measures and visual analog scores for sleep and itch. Both loss of sleep and pruritus improved during cyclosporin therapy (26). Thus, improvement in quality of life may accompany control of symptoms of AD in the absence of apparent improvement in the appearance of the eruption.

To evaluate the effect of inpatient management on quality of life, Kurwa and Finlay surveyed all patients admitted to the dermatology service of the University Hospital of Wales over a 6-month period (27). Subjects completed the DLQI on admission and 4 weeks following discharge. There was no control group, and measures of disease extent and severity were not employed. Of the 230 patients eligible to participate, 181 (83.4%) completed both questionnaires and 67 of these had AD. Mean DLQI scores for patients with AD declined from 16.2 (S.D. 6.3) on admission to 9.6 (S.D. 7.6; $p < 0.001$) at follow-up, reflecting improved quality of life (27).

The results of these two studies indicate that therapy for AD may be associated with measurable changes in quality of life. This is an important area of ongoing investigation since quality of life will likely be employed, in conjunction with other variables, to assess the relative merit of various forms of treatment for AD and other cutaneous disorders.

CONCLUSIONS

Assessment of quality of life in patients with AD is a relatively new area of investigation, and only recently have validated instruments for measurement been developed. Nevertheless, available data suggest that AD may have profound consequences. In children, the adverse effects of AD on sleep have been documented, and there is preliminary evidence that disturbed sleep is associated with behavioral difficulties. Furthermore, the disease affects the entire family because of concern about the patient, lost sleep, disturbance of relationships, and financial difficulties. Adolescents and adults report changes in self-image and social relationships, financial concerns, and, in some cases, occupational difficulties. The studies reviewed in this chapter provide an initial understanding of the potential effects of AD on quality of life. However, additional investigation is needed to define the nature, magnitude, and significance of these effects. Furthermore, it remains to be determined whether global measures of quality of life such as the CDLQI and DLQI will provide comprehensive information about the physical, social, psychological, and general functioning of children, teenagers, and adults with AD.

REFERENCES

1. Hanifin JM, Rajka G. Diagnostic features of atopic dermatitis. Acta Dermatovener (Stockh) 1980; 92(suppl):44–47.
2. Rabinowitz LG, Esterly NB. Atopic dermatitis and ichthyosis vulgaris. Pediatr Rev 1994; 15:220–226.

3. Schultz Larsen F, Holm NV, Henningsen K. Atopic dermatitis. A genetic-epidemiologic study in a population-based twin sample. J Am Acad Dermatol 1986; 15:487–494.
4. Schultz Larsen F. Atopic dermatitis: a genetic-epidemiologic study in a population-based twin sample. J Am Acad Dermatol 1993; 28:719–723.
5. Hanifin JM. Epidemiology of atopic dermatitis. Monogr Allergy 1987; 21:116–131.
6. Rajka G. Atopic Dermatitis. London: W.B. Saunders, 1975.
7. Rystedt I. Hand eczema in patients with a history of atopic manifestations in childhood. Acta Derm Venereol (Stockh) 1985; 65:305–312.
8. Lammintausta K, Kalimo K, Raitala R, Forsten Y. Prognosis of atopic dermatitis. A prospective study in early adulthood. Int J Dermatol 1991; 30:563–568.
9. Williams HC, Burney PGJ, Hay RJ, et al. The U.K. Working Party's diagnostic criteria for atopic dermatitis. I. Derivation of a minimum set of discriminators for atopic dermatitis. Br J Dermatol 1994; 131:383–396.
10. Long CC, Funnell CM, Collard R, Finlay AY. What do members of the National Eczema Society really want? Clin Exper Dermatol 1993; 18:516–522.
11. Lewis-Jones MS, Finlay AY. The Children's Dermatology Life Quality Index (CDLQI): initial validation and practical use. Br J Dermatol 1995; 132:942–949.
12. Dahl RE, Bernhisel-Broadbent J, Scanlon-Holdford S, Sampson HA. Sleep disturbances in children with atopic dermatitis. Arch Pediatr Adolesc Med 1995; 149:856–860.
13. Reid P, Lewis-Jones MS. Sleep difficulties and their management in preschoolers with atopic eczema. Clin Exper Dermatol 1995; 20:38–41.
14. Monti J M, Vignale R, Monti D. Sleep and nighttime pruritus in children with atopic dermatitis. Sleep 1989; 12:309–314.
15. Lawson V, Lewis-Jones MS, Reid P, Owens RG, Finlay AY. Family impact of atopic eczema. Br J Dermatol 1995; 133(suppl 45): 19.
16. Daud LR, Garralda ME, David TJ. Psychological adjustment in preschool children with atopic eczema. Arch Dis Child 1993; 69:670–676.
17. Halbert AR. The practical management of atopic dermatitis in children. Pediatr Ann 1996; 25:72–78.
18. Shuster S, Fisher GH, Harris E, Binnell D. The effect of skin disease on self image. Br J Dermatol 1978; 99(suppl 16): 18–19.
19. Jowett S, Ryan T. Skin disease and handicap: An analysis of the impact of skin conditions. Soc Sci Med 1985; 20:425–429.
20. Finlay AY, Khan GK. Dermatology Life Quality Index (DLQI)-a simple practical measure for routine clinical use. Clin Exper Dermatol 1994; 19:210–216.
21. Finlay AY. Measures of the effect of severe atopic eczema on quality of life. J Eur Acad Dermatol 1996; 7:199–154.
22. Shmunes E, Keil JE. Occupational dermatoses in South Carolina: a descriptive analysis of cost variables. J Am Acad Dermatol 1983; 9:861–866.

23. Lammintausta K, Kalimo K. Does a patient's occupation influence the course of atopic dermatitis? Acta Derm Venereol (Stockh) 1993; 73:119–122.
24. Meding B, Swanbeck G. Consequences of having hand eczema. Contact Derm 1990; 23:6–14.
25. Mathias CGT. The cost of occupational skin disease. Arch Dermatol 1985; 121:332–334.
26. Salek MS, Finlay AY, Luscombe DK, et al. Cyclosporin greatly improves the quality of life of adults with severe atopic dermatitis. A randomized, double-blind, placebo-controlled trial. Br J Dermatol 1993; 129:422–430.
27. Kurwa HA, Finlay AY. Dermatology in-patient management greatly improves life quality. Br J Dermatol 1995; 133:575–578.

15

Impact of Skin Cancer on Quality of Life

Christine J. Hashem and Barry Leshin *Wake Forest University Medical Center, Winston-Salem, North Carolina*

INTRODUCTION

Skin cancer is the most common type of cancer, affecting one out of 10 individuals in the United States. Between 900,000 and 1.2 million new cases of nonmelanoma skin cancers (NMSC), i.e., basal cell carcinomas (BCC) and squamous cell carcinomas (SCC), are diagnosed in the United States each year (1). The aging of America's baby boomer population combined with the fact that the incidence of BCCs and SCCs rises with each decade of life (2) will likely cause the prevalance of NMSC to continue to soar.

Despite this high prevalence of disease, very little information has been documented on the effect of NMSC on quality-of-life issues. The impact of NMSC on quality of life is both immediate and long term. Immediate quality-of-life issues include a patient's initial psychological adjustment in dealing with the diagnosis of having cancer and the preconceived implications that may go along with this word. In addition, selecting an appropriate treatment plan for NMSC in any given patient requires attention to the patient's own quality-of-life priorities. The effect of treatment on work and/or social activities as well as the expense of the treatment need to be considered as well. Long-term quality-of-life issues encompass not only the above-noted short-term concerns, but also potential cosmetic/functional impairments due to treatment, concern regarding additional NMSC formation, and the need to institute lifestyle changes to minimize further sun damage. Based upon our own observations culled from the management of thousands of patients with NMSC, this chapter will focus on the psychosocial effects of these usually nonlethal tumors.

IMMEDIATE EFFECTS

Diagnosis

Cancer diagnosis carries with it great significance. We hear in patients' voices their concerns about the dreaded "c word." *Cancerphobia* has worked its way into the medical lexicon. Even though NMSC is only very rarely life threatening, becoming a cancer patient can be a life-changing event. A study of the psychosocial management of patients with skin cancers revealed that patients connect the word "cancer" with feelings of shame, guilt, contagion, and loss of control (3). The spectrum of patient responses to the diagnosis of skin cancer is vast. Some immediately trivialize the event and attribute minimal significance to it because of slow growth and lack of associated pain. On the other hand, some patients are overwhelmed by the prospects of suffering and even death. It is essential in discussing a diagnosis of NMSC to anticipate such a variation in response and to be attentive to the potential for immediate and long-term impacts on patients' quality of life.

Several critical elements can mollify patient apprehension and should be a part of the patient-physician interaction. The physician should:

- Emphasize that these tumors are rarely life-threatening or health-threatening
- Emphasize that the cancer is typically slow-growing
- Discuss the reasons that treatment is recommended—the cancers destroy/replace normal tissue and thereby may encroach upon critical anatomical structures if left untreated; moreover, continued growth increases the risk for significant cosmetic or functional impairment
- Emphasize that there are a number of different effective treatment modalities

Treatment

Certainly treatment options must be thoroughly discussed with patients as a matter of course when obtaining informed consent. But as one considers making a treatment recommendation, it is important to outline recommendations for treatment based not only on important tumor parameters, but also on quality-of-life issues such as patients' concerns, expectations, health, and occupation. Whereas issues such as tumor location, size, histological characteristics, etc., are vital elements of the medical decision-making process, human issues should not go unheeded.

A couple of examples might be illuminating:

> F.G. is an 88-year-old woman with a heme-crusted lesion on the nasal tip. She lives in a nursing home and suffers with dementia. She occasionally picks at the lesion and causes some bleeding. This frightens the nursing staff and her family, who request consultation from a physician. The physician biopsies the site and confirms his clinical diagnosis of basal cell carcinoma. Because of the ill-defined clinical margins of the lesion and its location at a high-risk (for recurrence) site, he refers her for Mohs micrographic surgery.

The treatment recommended for F.G.'s skin cancer is considered to be the gold standard of NMSC treatment. Mohs surgery has the clear advantages of an extremely high cure rate with maximal conservation of normal tissue. But is it the most appropriate treatment option? It is important to consider quality-of-life issues in choosing a treatment specifically tailored toward an individual's life situation. In the above example, consider that the recommended technique is time-consuming and tedious, often requiring several hours or more; the surgery will result in a wound of significant breadth and depth; wound healing by second intention would likely be impeded by F.G.'s picking at the site (a graft or other reconstructive techniques would also be undone by the patient's manipulation); the technique is a highly specialized one, and arrangements for travel to the nearest surgeon will be impossible for her elderly children, and expensive if by ambulance. And who will manage the patient postoperatively, particularly if complications arise? All of these factors would on balance favor a lesser treatment such as electrosurgical or cryosurgical ablation, or even no treatment at all.

> R.T. is a 33-year-old woman who presents to her primary care physician for evaluation of a pimplelike lesion on the nose. The lesion has steadily grown over the past 3 weeks and is tender when touched. An inflammatory etiology is suspected, but incision and drainage yielded no pus. A biopsy was performed and a diagnosis of well-differentiated SCC was made. Ms. T is a flight attendant and is anxious about the impact of treatment on her appearance. The physician recommends a course of radiation therapy.

Radiation therapy is an effective treatment modality for this type of tumor, carrying with it a cure rate of 90%. But is it the most appropriate for this patient? R.T. has a hectic travel schedule and is typically away from home 4 days of the week. Although she has accrued 6 weeks of sick leave, she is not anxious to use this due to her plans for starting a family in the near future. Consider that a course of radiation therapy will require 3–4 weeks of daily therapy, and that unsuccessful treatment may result in an extremely difficult-to-treat recurrent tumor (4). These factors would favor referral for Mohs micrographic surgery with immediate postoperative wound repair.

Socioeconomic Impact

In this era of emphasis on cost containment, we cannot neglect the impact of cost associated with treatment. Should we choose therapy with consideration given to the economic impact on the patient, as in the case described above? A patient in a capitated managed care system would be costly to refer for Mohs surgery or even radiation therapy. Is he or she capable of paying for such services out of pocket?

Consider also that the patient's recovery period following treatment is often centered around pain control, minimizing stresses that might provoke postoperative bleeding and swelling, cleaning and care of the surgical site, and adjustment to the immediate cosmetic outcome. In one survey, 11.5% of patients surveyed after Mohs micrographic surgery reported "significant pain" in the first few days after surgery (5). This level of discomfort requires the patient to make adjustments to his or her daily routine, often necessitating help from family members or friends to perform daily living functions.

Quality of life is also affected by time lost from work, which is often costly for a patient or for the patient's employer. The interface of these economic issues with medical decision making may be difficult to reconcile. It is imperative to assess a patient's lifestyle and individual circumstances when deciding on a treatment plan that often includes postoperative adjustments in one's daily routine. For instance, an individual who is self-employed and involved in work requiring physical exertion may be economically compromised by limitations on activity. Heavy lifting may actually put direct undue tension on a sutured wound and be counterproductive to wound healing. Such lifting may increase central venous pressure and cause postoperative bleeding, which can also have a deleterious impact on wound healing. How much weight is too much, and for how long should there be restriction on activity? If it is valuable to defer elective surgery until after a busy season, this would be an appropriate consideration. Similarly, consideration should be given to a patient's ability to adjust his or her usual work routine. Can the patient's employer find a less physically taxing job? Aside from exertion, it is prudent to inquire as to whether the patient works in a dirty or dusty environment, which may increase the risk of wound infection. Additionally, if the person interfaces with the public, the presence of a wound dressing, sutures, bruising, or edema on the face may be disconcerting for both the patient and others.

LONG-TERM EFFECTS

A skin cancer may have lifelong implications for affected individuals. Because NMSC's arise most frequently on sun-exposed skin, cosmetic and functional implications are paramount. In a study that assessed the psychosocial impact of having a BCC, cosmetic concerns were the most common cancer-related concerns reported (6) and are important irrespective of occupation or social class. A prominent scar or facial asymmetry might jeopardize the career of a flight attendant whose image is critical. A trial attorney may fear that an obvious scar will be a distraction to a jury or judge, and thereby compromise his or her clients' cases. Distortion of facial anatomy following cancer treatment may cause some functional abnormalities and be quite disconcerting. Malposition of the lower eyelid, for instance, may result in epiphora, or keratitis. Scarring on the lower nose may affect function of the nasal valve; an inability to flare the nostril with inspiration may result in a sensation of shortness of breath. These long-term effects of treatment may have a significant negative impact on quality of life.

Lifelong concerns regarding the potential of recurrent, additional, or metastatic cancer are not unusual. In fact, the risk of metastases from NMSC is sufficiently small that reassurance about this rarity can allay fears. The initial patient education at the time of skin cancer diagnosis should continue through the follow-up period. Discussion of sun protection, reassurance about lack of evidence of tumor recurrence, and education about warning signs of new or recurrent tumors should be integrated into each follow-up visit. Patients should be advised that although there is a 33–45% chance for developing an additional BCC within 5 years (7,8), should that happen, regular surveillance should ensure that such cancers will be diagnosed and treated at an early stage.

Up to three quarters of our lifetime ultraviolet light exposure occurs before the age of 18. However, use of a broad-spectrum SPF 15 sunscreen has been reported to reduce the development of solar keratoses, a known risk factor for BCCs and a precursor of SCCs (9). Patients should be advised that although diligent sunscreen use and prudent sun-exposure habits will not eliminate the risk of future skin cancers, such preventive behaviors may decrease this risk. The use of daily sunscreens appears to be a relatively easy lifestyle adjustment for skin cancer patients, with nearly three fourths of patients surveyed after Mohs micrographic surgery reporting frequent sunscreen use (5). Emphasis should be placed on sun-smart behavior, such as:

Avoidance of direct sun exposure between 10 a.m. and 3 p.m., even on cloudy days
Use of sun-protective apparel
Caution about reflectance of ultraviolet light from snow or sand.

Many skin cancer patients work outdoors. Financial constraints may weigh heavily against avoiding sun exposure in the work arena, and it is not feasible for many patients to change careers. But counseling the farmer to shade the tractor seat with an umbrella or cab, recommending to the mail carrier to change from foot to truck delivery, or encouraging the construction worker to keep his shirt on during the day are worthwhile endeavors. Avid recreational outdoorsmen should be similarly educated. Quality of life after skin cancer diagnosis may therefore be affected by changes in work and/or recreation habits.

SUMMARY

Despite being the most common type of cancer in the United States today, there is little information regarding skin cancer's impact on quality of life. Short- and long-term effects of skin cancer on quality of life encompass issues such as anxiety, possible functional impairments, cosmesis, cost, and necessary lifestyle adjustments. The effect of skin cancer and skin cancer treatment on patients' quality of life should not be ignored. A compassionate and informative doctor-patient relationship is critical to maximizing patients' quality of life. Further studies specifically focusing on the quality-of-life issues associated with NMSC are needed. The extent to which treatment for NMSC affects patients' lives as well as the societal costs incurred, either directly or through loss of productivity, deserves more thorough exploration. The management of skin cancer may also be improved by analyzing quality-of-life assessments in relation to patient outcomes, keeping in mind that all treatment decisions need to be individualized. Fortunately, the development of more reliable clinically useful indices for measuring the effect of skin disease in general, and skin cancer specifically, on a patient's quality of life is currently underway (10,11).

REFERENCES

1. Miller DL, Weinstock MA. Nonmelanoma skin cancer in the United States: incidence. J Am Acad Dermatol 1994; 30:774–778.

2. U.S. Public Health Service. Incidence of Nonmelanoma Skin Cancer in the United States. Washington, DC: National Institutes of Health, U.S. Department of Health and Human Services, 1983.
3. Friedenbergs I. Psychosocial management of patients with cutaneous cancers: a preliminary report. J Dermatol Surg Oncol 1981; 7:828–830.
4. Smith SP, Grande DJ. Basal cell carcinoma recurring after radiotherapy: a unique, difficult treatment subclass of recurrent basal cell carcinoma. J Dermatol Surg Oncol 1991; 17:26–30.
5. Sherertz EF, Pollack SV. Response of 156 patients to the chemosurgery "experience" (letter). J Dermatol Surg Oncol 1982; 8:4.
6. Holfeld KI, et al. A psychosocial assessment of patients with basal cell carcinoma. J Dermatol Surg Oncol 1990; 16:750–753.
7. Robinson JK. Risk of developing another basal cell carcinoma: a 5-year prospective study. Cancer 1987; 60:118–120.
8. Marghoob A, et al. Risk of another basal cell carcinoma developing after treatment of a basal cell carcinoma. J Am Acad Dermatol 1993; 28:22–28.
9. Thompson SC, et al. Reduction of solar keratoses by regular sunscreen use. N Engl J Med 1992; 329:1147–1151.
10. Chren M-M, et al. Skindex, a quality of life measure for patients with skin disease: reliability, validity and responsiveness. J Invest Dermatol 1996; 107:707–713.
11. Finlay AY, et al. Dermatology Life Quality Index (DLQI)—a simple practical measure for routine clinical use. Clin Exp Dermatol 1994; 19:210.

16

Impact of Hair Disorders and Pigment Disorders on Quality of Life

Amy J. McMichael Bowman Gray School of Medicine of Wake Forest University, Winston-Salem, North Carolina

INTRODUCTION

Morbidity from disorders such as cutaneous pigmentation abnormalities or hair loss usually cannot be measured in traditional ways, but they can cause significant psychosocial problems for those who suffer with them. There may be little physical pain or discomfort from these disorders, but the psychological pain can be devastating. In a society that puts great importance on beauty and youth, hair loss and pigmentary alterations are visible disorders that may signal loss of self or power in society. There is a body of literature examining the psychological ramifications of disease affecting body image (1), but very little has been published on the quality-of-life impact of either hair or pigmentation disorders. One factor contributing to this lack of information is the difficulty in assessing quality of life when so many different diseases can have the end outcome of either pigmentation or hair alteration. Another problem that exists is determining what instrument is best suited for testing populations with skin disease. Finally, there has previously been an emphasis on diseases causing significant morbidity and mortality. Since neither hair loss nor pigmentation alteration frequently cause these outcomes, they have been relatively ignored as research subjects. To help understand what has been studied in the field of quality of life for these disorders, hair and pigmentation disorders are best classified by the health states leading to disease outcome, treatment success, and then success of designing valid quality-of-life testing instruments. Only analysis of these results can improve treatment planning and identify resources needed for treatment and patient support, which in turn will help determine necessary resource costs.

Newton describes generic and specific quality-of-life measurement instruments used in dermatology (2). The generic instrument usually tests quality of life for all underlying diseases in a given population but may be difficult to analyze for a specific conditions. A second approach has been to use an already validated dermatology-specific instrument, but generalization of results may not possible. An alternative would be to design a new disease-specific instrument, validate it, and then apply it in the population of interest. Most of the literature examining quality of life in hair and pigment disorders use a combination of instruments to improve capture of psychosocial problems because of the lack of all-inclusive hair loss or dyspigmentation instruments. In this chapter, disease processes leading to hair and pigment disorders will be discussed. Treatments for these disorders will be discussed briefly as well as measured impairments in quality of life.

HAIR DISORDERS

Classification

Classification of hair disorders, or more specifically hair loss (alopecia), is a feat in itself, for there are at least 30 diseases that can cause permanent or long-term hair loss. Thus, most of the existing data on quality of life examines hair loss by cause. This approach has been helpful, but not comprehensive, since many factors that impact quality of life—severity, underlying disease process, duration, and availability of treatment—can vary for patients with the same diagnosis. The most common forms of alopecia studied for impact of quality of life include androgenetic alopecia, alopecia areata, trichotillomania, and chemotherapy-induced alopecia. In challenging cases, different forms of alopecia can occur together in the same patient, which underscores the importance of a quality-of-life evaluation for alopecia in general. Many forms of hair loss have not yet been examined for their psychosocial impact, perhaps due to low prevalence or incomplete disease pathogenesis.

Hair plays a major role in defining individuality and appearance. As a result, alopecia can negatively influence self-esteem and cause tremendous psychological upheaval. In the American society, hair embodies the concept of a complete, attractive person, often symbolizing youth and femininity for women and virility for men (3). While no general studies of quality of life for all-cause alopecia exist, many studies reiterate the impact of hair loss on approach to life (4,5). Qualitative studies of hair loss have shown that hair loss can represent a loss of self and illuminate societal failure (3). The trauma related to hair loss can be the most devastating side effect of cancer treatment for some patients (6).

Androgenetic Alopecia

The most common form of alopecia is androgenetic alopecia (AGA), also termed male- or female-patterned hair loss. It is an androgen-dependent disorder that affects at least 50% of adult men and perhaps as many women (7). This form of alopecia is thought to be clinically distinct from the progressive thinning of scalp hair that occurs in all adults by the seventh or eighth decade (8). Clinically, patients present with diffuse nonscarring hair loss on the scalp, with minor differences between men and women. Men have vertex thinning and recession of the hairline, while women tend to have frontal and vertex thinning with minimal recession of the hairline (9). Severity of disease has also be classified by several authors to help establish potential treatment plans and follow progression of disease (7,9,10). Histopathologically, biopsy reveals terminal follicles becoming progressively miniaturized due to a shortening of anagen phase.

Treatments for this form of progressive alopecia include topical, oral, surgical, and cosmetic interventions. The least invasive treatment is topical minoxidil, which has some efficacy in both women and men (11,12). Oral therapies include hormonal manipulation with various single agents and combinations of agents, including spironolactone, flutamide, cyproterone acetate (8,13,14) and finasteride (8), although many of these drugs must be monitored closely for side effects. Surgical treatments for AGA include transplant grafting of hair and flap rotation grafts, which have been successful in many patients when costs of treatment, patient expectation, and surgical proficiency are considered prior to treatment (15). While many of these drugs and procedures can cause objective and subjective improvement in balding, there is no therapy that can completely abrogate the effects of time and heredity. For this reason, quality of life during treatment for AGA is as important as the study of baseline disease states.

Much of the groundwork for quality-of-life literature on AGA has been based on psychiatric and psychologic data. In a study examining the relationship between AGA and personality disorders, Maffei et al. revealed an increased prevalence of personality disorders in subjects with AGA compared to that observed in the general population (16). The study enrolled consecutively admitted patients to a psychology and psychiatric treatment facility who received a diagnosis of AGA. None of the subjects had a history of psychopathological symptoms previous to the development of AGA. The results were compared to the rates of personality disorders in the general population found by the authors in a previous study (17). There was also an observable increase in prevalence of personality disorders in women as compared to men, but this difference was not found to be significant. Van der Donk and colleagues examined 168 men participating in a minoxidil trial for improvement in social and psychological well-being after treatment (18). Using a combination of instruments, these researchers found no evidence of psychological malfunctioning at baseline with no change in psychosocial well-being with perceived hair regrowth (18).

Both studies were conducted with small sample sizes which could contribute to bias in already complex results; for example, sample size problems may have distorted differences between men and women in the Maffei study. Generalizabilty also becomes a problem in both studies since van der Donk et al. examined a self-selected population of AGA patients who may be different from all patients with AGA. Similarly, the study of patients by Maffei and colleagues includes only patients seeking help for psychologic disorders which may be associated with increased distortion in body-image as compared to the general population. At the least, the contradictory results of these two studies suggests the need to find the true effect of alopecia on quality of life.

Quality of life for patients with AGA has been studied for men and women separately and in combination. Again, a mixture of testing instruments has been utilized, often in a patchwork manner, splicing together modified parts of different questionnaires. Well et al. studied 182 men of varying ages and severity of hair loss with a modified combination instrument and demonstrated that there was a significant loss of self-esteem with increasing hair loss independent of age (19). Introversion was also associated with increasing severity of AGA, while hair loss and young age together showed significant association with increased introversion. Feelings of unattractiveness were significantly associated with increasing baldness with particularly adverse affects in younger men (19). A study examining 145 men referred from barber shops found preoccupation, moderate stress, or distress from AGA, with balding men showing less body-image satisfaction relative to controls (20), but there appeared to be no overall alteration of personality function for the majority of men (20). In contrast, a study of 58 women with mild to moderate AGA questioned during a minoxidil clinical trial reported that daily behavior was affected in 88% of the women, with 72% reporting loss of self-esteem (21). Several patients reported tense feelings in public places with complaints of neck cramps from holding their head to prevent others from discovering the hair loss. Most women stayed at home when it was raining or very windy. Over half (57%) of the women felt less attractive as a result of their hair loss. In a study comparing men and women with AGA and women without AGA, Cash and colleagues found that AGA was significantly more distressing for women than for men (22). There was a pattern of less adaptive functioning among women with women with AGA reporting higher social anxiety, poorer self-esteem and well-being, and less life satisfaction than men with AGA and female controls (22).

Overall, most studies support the finding of loss of self-esteem in patients with AGA, which ultimately affects their quality of life (23). There is still a need for studies that examine how these effects manifest concretely, such as divorce rate, loss of job, or lost of workdays related to this form of hair loss. Presumably the self-esteem variables have wide-reaching effects on productivity and relationships, but more information is needed before recommendations can be made as to how to improve quality of life. While perceived improvement in hair loss may be part of the puzzle for patients with AGA, these clinical trial studies show that treatment alone does not address all quality-of-life and psychosocial issues for these patients.

Alopecia Areata

Alopecia areata is a nonscarring, recurrent, sometimes treatment-refractory disease causing hair loss in any hair-bearing area of the body. The etiology of the disease is unknown, but an autoimmune pathogenesis with a genetic component has long been suspected. Overall prevalence of the disease has been estimated at approximately 0.1–0.2% of the population, with a prevalence rate of 122 per 100,000 as determined by the first National Health and Nutrition Examination Survey (24). Cumulative lifetime incidence has been estimated at 1.7% (25). Scalp involvement has been estimated to occur in 95% of cases (26). Frequently, patients may have involvement of other body sites but notice only the affected areas of the scalp. Typically, there are no symptoms that occur along with the shedding of hair, but some patients do experience paresthesias or pruritus just before or concurrent with hair loss (27). Though some patients have complete or partial spontaneous hair growth weeks, months, or years after loss, it is not predictable in whom this will occur. Muller et al. found that in a group of 736 patients with alopecia areata, 44% of children and 34% of adults who developed total loss of scalp hair had subsequent significant periods of normal or near-normal hair growth (26). Pathogenesis is still not well understood for the disease, but there is evidence to support an autoimmune cause (28).

Treatments for alopecia areata have been disappointing. Treatments include oral and intralesional steroids (29), topical sensitizing agents (30,31), ultraviolet light therapy (32), systemic immunotherapy (33), and dapsone (30). There are varying reports of efficacy for each of these treatments, but none of the treatments are thought to cure the disease. Recently there has been interest in topical sensitizing agents because of their low side effect profile and ease of application. Efficacy of topical sensitizers is thought to be the highest of all treatments modalities for chronic severe alopecia areata (33), though most of this data has come from small studies in separate institutions (34,35).

With extensive alopecia areata can come a significant loss of identity, especially if the disease affects eyebrows and lashes, which help to define appearance and individuality. Not only has the stress of having the disease been examined, the role stress plays in triggering the disease has also been studied. An uncontrolled evaluation of 178 patients with extensive hair loss revealed no evidence of a role of emotional stress in the causation of disease (36), although there is a published case of a 16-year-old whose alopecia areata was treated with massage, relaxation, and reward with measured improvement (37). Since alopecia areata can spontaneously remit and recall bias can increase the likelihood of an association between stress and alopecia areata, results of studies regarding stress and causation must interpreted with caution.

More important is the quality of life associated with the disease process once the disease is visible. Much less research has been done on quality of life in alopecia areata patients than in AGA patients. While there are few studies examining quality of life, the need for patient support was recognized and acted upon with the organization of the National Alopecia Areata Foundation in 1981. This group raises funds for research, provides education about the disease, and creates local support groups for patients, Despite the good works of the foundation, many patients have described feelings of lowered self-esteem and difficulty coping with the public and family members because of the disease (38). In response to a survey, 294 patients with alopecia areata self-reported presence or absence of psychiatric disease in their past or present medical history (39). Results of this survey revealed that major depression, generalized anxiety disorder, social phobia, and paranoid disorder were present at significantly higher rates than reported for the general population (39). Recall bias could have increased reported psychiatric disease in patients with alopecia areata, and no conclusions can be drawn about causation, but the reported differential in rates of psychiatric disease is a startling finding that should be examined further. It also echoes findings of a much earlier study in which alopecia areata patients seeking treatment were found to have increased mental and emotional disturbances (40). Initial work using quality-of-life instruments in alopecia areata patients has shown that there is an effect on daily activities as measured by a adjustment-to-illness scale (41). There is a need for further evaluation of quality of life with this relatively common disease using controlled studies to eradicate self-selection bias and to understand the relationship between quality of life and causation of disease and treatment effect.

Chemotherapy-Induced Alopecia

Chemotherapy-induced alopecia is a special case of alopecia that is predictable and temporary, but still devastating to self-esteem. It is a striking reminder of the cancer diagnosis to patients and all people with whom they have contact. Pathophysiologically, many but not all chemotherapeutic agents affect the anagen phase of the hair growth cycle, causing near or total alopecia. Various therapies have been used to prevent this disorder, including scalp tourniquets, scalp hypothermia (42), and topical minoxidil. Much of the practice of tourniquet and hypothermia use has ceased because of the theoretical risk of scalp metastases (6). Minoxidil has not shown effectiveness in the prevention of alopecia after chemotherapy, but does show a significant increase in regrowth compared to controls if the medication is continued up to 4 months after treatment (43). While this is boon to those who can afford and feel well enough to use minoxidil soon after treatment, it does not prevent alopecia or the psychosocial impact that can ensue. Freedman's qualitative examination of a group of 10 women who had undergone chemotherapy for breast cancer revealed impact in three main areas: the loss of privacy because of visible hair loss, the loss of self because the patient has no control over her appearance, and reminder of the societal failure of becoming ill (3).

Suggested interventions have included allowing patients to discuss their concerns openly with health care providers and the development of scalp prosthesis resources and self-care regimens to restore appearance and self-image (6). While extensive quality-of-life evaluations in this population for hair loss may not be a helpful use of resources due to the short-lived nature of the alopecia, these patients can certainly benefit from what has been learned about the quality of life of patients with other forms of alopecia. Also, this may be a population in whom interventions can be tested because of the large number of patients undergoing cancer chemotherapy treatment.

Trichotillomania

Trichotillomania is a primary psychiatric disorder that deserves mention in the discussion of quality of life and alopecia. The disorder is a form of repetitive hair pulling that is poorly understood, and many patients with this illness are unaware of their own part in the disease (44). There are severity and impairment scales specific to the disease, and these have been used in clinical trials for the disease (44). Trichotillomania is another disorder where there may be an interaction between preexisting psychological issues and those that result from the disease. In a survey of 62 women who had trichotillomania, self-esteem did not appear to be associated directly with age at onset of hair pulling or severity of disease. Disease was related to level of depression, frequency of hair pulling, level of anxiety, and body dissatisfaction (unrelated to hair pulling) (45). There was no control group in this study and possible confounders were not addressed in the results, such as those that might cause depression in young women unrelated to hair pulling. Despite the lack of controlled studies, there is a quality-of-life impact on these patients that may be lessened with more knowledge of quality of life for alopecia in general.

PIGMENTATION DISORDERS

Definition and Classification

The diversity of skin color among humans is the result for the most part of melanin pigment distribution in the skin. Melanin is contained in membrane-limited organelles called melanocytes. In lighter-skinned individuals, melanosomes are small, spherical, and aggregated in groups of two or three, whereas those in darkly pigmented individuals are larger, oval, and individually dispersed (46). There can be normal changes in pigmentation in response to ultraviolet light, which is thought to be a protective mechanism of the skin (47). Also, many individuals have a normal pigmentary variation in the skin depending on site of the body. Most other changes in pigmentation, even if not bothersome to the individual, are classified as pathological states or diseases (47). Common disorders of the pigmentary system causing significant variation from normal include vitiligo, albinism, chemical leukoderma, postinflammatory hyper- and hypopigmentation, and melasma. Of these disorders, vitiligo is the most well studied in terms of quality of life, but the issues that patients with vitiligo face are often the same as those faced by patients with other causes of significant visible pigmentary alteration.

Similar to alopecia, skin lesions of pigmentary disorders often occur in places noticeable by casual observers, affecting self-esteem because skin lesions often imply imperfection, both to the patient and to others (48). In our society where perfection is the ideal, pigmentation abnormalities can affect interpersonal relationships as well. Often the "affected person symbolizes our own vulnerability and imperfection, our defectiveness and our lack of autonomy" (48). Unlike alopecia, pigment disorders often result from other skin disorders that cause significant discomfort, pruritus, or pain, for example, severe atopic dermatitis, infection, or cystic acne. This is one reason why quality-of-life determination is so difficult to test in patients who have a postinflammatory pigmentation alteration—it is difficult to separate the impact of the underlying skin disorder from the pigmentary process. Also, there are so many things that can ultimately lead to pigmentary alteration, there is undoubtedly no complete list in existence. For the scope of this review, impact on quality of life for patients with vitiligo will be discussed as the prototypical disease process, but special mention of melasma and postinflammatory disease will be made. Also, the particular quality-of-life issues in deeply pigmented patients will be given special attention for all disorders.

Vitiligo

Vitiligo is an acquired, sometimes familial, depigmenting disorder of the skin that affects 1% of the general population (49). An autoimmune etiology is favored in this disease (47). It can effect children and adults and usually has a unpredictable course. Although not thought to be more common in deeply pigmented patients, it is more noticeable in this group (50). Treatments for the disease include topical, intralesional, and oral steroids, ultraviolet light with or with topical or oral psoralen (PUVA) (51), modified skin grafting (52,53), complete depigmentation with bleaching agents, or cosmetics. There is no cure among these many treatments, but topical steroids and PUVA have been the most successful in reports of treatment response (54). Unlike many disorders in which crude, mechanical or costly prostheses must be used, reasonably priced cosmetic coverage with make-up is quite advanced and acceptable for patients of almost every skin tone (55).

The psychosocial effects of vitiligo have been examined in African Americans, Caucasians, and in a controlled manner with comparison groups of patients with psoriasis and those with other pigmentary disorders. In one of the largest reports of social and psychological effects of the disease, 614 patients with vitiligo were surveyed (56). Results showed that the majority of respondents (59%) felt their vitiligo had affected their lives during the previous 3 weeks. Qualitative data results showed that there was significant distress related to specific types of social encounters. In this self-selected population, one must question if these data reflect the concerns of those who are so bothered by their disease that they are interested in completing the study, but the large sample size would argue against this bias. In a controlled study, vitiligo patients scored lower on a self-esteem scale as compared to controls without skin disease, but scored better on adjustment than patients with psoriasis (57). There was significantly more use of make-up to conceal disease in patients with vitiligo vs. psoriasis, which may be due to the flat nature of skin lesions in vitiligo vs. thick, scaly lesions in psoriasis. This ability to cover lesions effectively may also reflect the observed better adjustment in vitiligo patients. There were no significant differences between the patients with vitiligo and those with other pigmentary skin disorders (57). These studies show that intervention and adjustment are closely linked to quality of life, which lends further credence to testing quality-of-life issues. Still, there is a need to unravel which interventions may work for which skin diseases. Questions remaining include:

How does one best measure the impact of family support in vitiligo?
Does family support affect adjustment?
Is a flat, but very apparent skin disorder like vitiligo more acceptable to patient or others or both?
Which adjustments to vitiligo are most likely to be reproducible in other skin diseases?

A better understanding of feelings of disfigurement and coping mechanisms in vitiligo is needed to help patients better cope with their disease and maintain social interaction.

When racial variation among patients with vitiligo was studied for reaction to physical stigma, findings revealed that African Americans perceived significantly more stigmatization from others than did Caucasians, but there was no racial difference in degree of disturbance (58). Psychological resources, such as family, friends, and caregiver interaction, may have mitigated the effects of the perceived stigma (58). This suggests an important role for improving psychological support to patients with visible skin disease in the hope of improving coping mechanisms for the long term.

Postinflammatory Pigmentation Disorders and Melasma

Pigment lability has been described as the problem of dyschromia in patients after inflammatory skin diseases, especially in deeply pigmented patients. Postinflammatory disorders differ from vitiligo in that patients may have partial loss of pigment in affected areas or slight to severe darkening in affected areas. While there is no clear understanding of why this dyschromia occurs, it has been a distressing problem to all practising dermatologists (59). There can be persistent hyperpigmentation as well as persistent hypopigmentation as a result of the inflammatory process. Treatment of patients for hyperpigmentation has been more satisfying than for hypopigmentation and can consist of azelaic acid, hydroquinone (60), topical tretinoin, laser (61), topical steroids, and mixtures of the above therapies. The study of mechanisms of pigmentation has become a science of its own, but this devastating problem has largely been ignored in the quality-of-life literature.

Melasma is a common, acquired condition consisting of symmetrical, hyperpigmented patches over the face with a predilection for the sun-exposed areas of the face, usually in women (62). It can be a very disfiguring disorder, especially when from a distance there is simulation of facial hair in the darkened areas of skin. The therapies listed above for the treatment of hyperpigmentation are standard treatments of melasma, but there has been particular interest in tretinoin cream, with two clinical trials showing efficacy in melasma patients (63,64). Still, therapies are only partially efficacious, and there remains a need for support systems for patients who will have long-term disfigurement from dyschromia. Only careful, controlled trials of quality-of-life studies can provide these necessary data.

SUMMARY

Quality-of-life studies are truly in their infancy in alopecia and pigmentary disorders. There has been some overlap with psychological interest in daily life activities, self-esteem, adaptation to disease, and success of interventions other than therapy for the disease itself. The instruments used run the gamut of multiple specific questionnaires to very general personality analyses, making the comparison of studies difficult. Finally, each disorder has its own intervention culture, which is determined mostly by the health-care provider team instead of patients, family, and support organizations. Most of the work done on quality of life in these two areas of dermatology leaves significant unanswered questions about quality-of-life issues, perhaps because quality of life may mean something different for each patient, for each disorder, and for each health care provider. There is a need for well-validated instruments to assess quality-of-life impact from alopecia and pigmentation disorders. Our goals, then, must include continued classification of disease with clear treatment goals. Then controlled trials of quality of life in patients with these diseases must be planned with longitudinal follow-up before, during, and after treatment, with emphasis on measurement of efficacy of these treatments. This will be the only way to allow patients, other health care providers, insurers, and granting agencies to see the deleterious effects on psychosocial life that a painless but extremely visible disease can have.

REFERENCES

1. Kalick SM. Psychological characteristics of alopecia patients. Arch Dermatol 1994; 130:907–908.
2. Newton JN. Evaluating services. In: Williams HC, Strachan DP, eds. The Challenge of Dermatoepidemiology. Boca Raton, FL: CRC Press, 1997:116–117.

3. Freedman TG. Social and cultural dimensions of hair loss in women treated for breast cancer. Cancer Nursing 1994; 17:334–341.
4. Parkinson RW. Hair loss in women: what to say and do to ease these patients' distress. Post Grad Med 1992; 91:417–431.
5. Davidhizar R, Bartlett D. When your patients lose their hair. Today's OR Nurse 1993; 15:39–42.
6. Pickard-Holly S. The symptom experience of alopecia. Sem Oncol Nurs 1995; 11:235–238.
7. Hamilton JB. Patterned Loss of hair in man: types and incidence. Ann NY Acad Sci 1951; 53:708–728.
8. Kaufman KD. Androgen metabolism as it affects hair growth in androgenetic alopecia. Dermatol Clin 1996; 14:697–711.
9. Ludwig E. Classification of the types of androgenetic alopecia occurring in the female sex. Br J Dermatol 1977; 97(3):247–254.
10. Norwood OT. Male pattern baldness: classification and incidence. South Med J 1975; 68:1359–1365.
11. Devillez RL. Topical minoxidil therapy in hereditary androgenetic alopecia. Arch Dermatol 1985; 121:197–202.
12. Olsen EA. Topical minoxidil in the treatment of androgenetic alopecia in women. Cutis 1991; 48:243–248.
13. Olsen EA. Androgenetic alopecia. In: Olsen EA, ed. Disorders of Hair Growth: Diagnosis and Treatment. New York: McGraw-Hill, 1994:195–197.
14. Callan AW, Montalto J. Female androgenetic alopecia: an update. Australas J Dermatol 1995; 36:51–57.
15. Griffin EI. Hair transplantation. Dermatol Clin 1995; 13:363–386.
16. Maffei C, Fossati A, Rinaldi F, Riva E. Personality disorders and psychopathologic symptoms in patients with androgenetic alopecia. Arch Dermatol 1994; 130:868–872.
17. Fossati A, Rinaldi F, Maestroni L, Cappio F, Maffei C. Trichologic consultation and personality disorders. G Ital Dermatol Venereol 1993; 128:101–108.
18. van der Donk J, Passchier J, Dutree-Meulenberg ROGM, Stolz E, Verhage F. Psychologic characteristics of men with alopecia androgenetica and their modification. Int J Dermatol 1991; 30:22–28.
19. Wells PA, Willmoth T, Russell RJ. Does fortune favour the bald? Psychological correlates of hair loss in males. Br J Psychol 1995; 86:337–344.
20. Cash TF. The psychological effects of androgenetic alopecia in men. J Am Acad Dermatol 1992; 26:926–931.
21. van der Donk J, Hunfield JAM, Passhier J, Knegt-Junk KJ, Nieboer C. Quality of life and maladjustment associated with hair loss in women with alopecia androgenetica. Soc Sci Med 1994; 38:159–163.
22. Cash TF, Price VH, Savin RC. Psychological effects of androgenetic alopecia on women: comparisons with balding men and with female control subjects. J Am Acad Dermatol 1993; 29:568–575.
23. van der Donk J, Passchier J, Knegt-JUnk C, can der Wegen-Keijser MH, Niebor C, Stolz E, Verhage F. Psychological characteristics of women with androgenetic alopecia: a controlled trial. Br J Dermatol 1991; 125:248–252.

24. Safavi K. Prevalence of alopecia areata in the First National Health and Nutrition Survey. Arch Dermatol 1992; 128:702.
25. Safavi KH, Muller SA, Suman VJ, Moshell AN, Melton LJ. Incidence of alopecia areata in Olmstead County, Minnesota, 1975 through 1989. Mayo Clin Proc 1995; 70:628–633.
26. Muller SA, Winkleman RK. Alopecia areata: an evaluation of 736 patients. Arch Dermatol 1963; 88:290–297.
27. Hordinsky MK. Hair. In: Sams WM, Lynch PJ, eds. Principles and Practice of Dermatology. New York: Churchill-Livingstone, 1990:761–762.
28. McMichael AJ. The genetic epidemiology of alopecia areata. J Eur Acad Dermatol Venereol. In press.
29. Ro BI. Alopecia areata in Korea (1982–1994). J Dermatol 1995; 22:858–864.
30. Van Barr HMJ, van der Vleuten CJM, van der Dekerkhof. Dapsone versus topical immunotherapy in alopecia areata. Br J Dermatol 1995; 133:270–274.
31. Schuttelaar M-LA, Hamstra JJ, Plinck EPB, Peereboom-Wynia JDR, Vuzevski VD, Mulder PGH, Oranje AP. Alopecia areata in children: treatment with diphencyprone. Br J Dermatol 1996; 135:581–585.
32. Taylor CR, Hawk JLM. PUVA treatment of alopecia areata partialis, totalis, and universalis: audit of 10 years' experience at St. John's Institute of Dermatology. Br J Dermatol 1995; 133:914–918.
33. Shapiro J. Alopecia areata: update on therapy. Dermatol Clin 1993; 11:35–46.
34. van der Steen PHM, Boezeman JBM, Happle R. Topical immunotherapy for alopecia areata: re-evaluation of 139 cases after an additional follow-up period of 19 additional months. Dermatology 1992; 184:198–201.
35. Orecchia G, Malagoli P, Santagostino L. Treatment of severe alopecia areata with squaric acid dibutylester in pediatric patients. Pediatr Dermatol 1994; 11:65–68.
36. van der Steen P, Boezeman J, Duller P, Happle R. Can alopecia areata be triggered by emotional stress? Acta Derm Venereol (Stockh) 1992; 72:279–280.
37. Putt SC, Weinstein L, Dzindolet MT. A case study: massage, relaxation, and reward for treatment of alopecia areata. Psychol Rep 1994; 74:1315–1318.
38. Beard HO. Social and psychological implications of alopecia areata. J Am Acad Dermatol 1986; 14:697–700.
39. Koo JYM, Shellow WVR, Hallman CP, Edwards JE. Alopecia areata and increased prevalence of psychiatric disorders. Int J Dermatol 1994; 33:849–850.
40. Greenburg SI. Alopecia areata: a psychiatric survey. AMA Arch Dermatol 1955; 72:454–457.
41. Berfeld WF, Remzi BK. A quality of life investigation in patients with alopecia areata. Poster presentation, 55th Annual Meeting of the Academy of Dermatology, San Francisco, 1997.
42. Smith FP, McCabe MS. Preventing chemotherapy-induced alopecia. Arch Fam Pract 1983; 28:182–184.
43. Duvic M, Lemak NA, Valero V, Hymes SR, Farmer KL, Hortobagyi GN, Trancik RJ, Bandstra BA, Compton. A randomized trial of minoxidil in chemotherapy-induced alopecia. J Am Acad Dermatol 1996; 35:74–78.

44. Rothbaum BO, Ninan PT. The assessment of trichotillomania. Behav Res Ther 1994; 32:651–662.
45. Soriano JL, O'Sullivan RL, Baer L, Phillips KA, McNally RJ, Jenike MA. Trichtillomania and self-esteem: a survey of 62 female hair pullers. J Clin Psychiatry 1996; 57:77–82.
46. Szabo G, Gerald AB, Pathnak MA, Fitzpatrick TB. Racial differences in the fate of melanosomes in human epidermis. Nature 1969; 222:1081–1082.
47. Bolognia Jl, Pawelek JM. Biology of hypopigmentation. J Am Acad Dermatol 1988; 19:217–255.
48. Ginsburg IH. The psychosocial impact of skin disease. Dermatol Clin 1996; 14:437–484.
49. Lerner AB. Vitiligo. J Invest Dermatol 1959; 32:285–310.
50. Barsky s, Knapp DP, Levine M, Schuller-Goldman S. Vitiligo in a black population. Arch Dermatol 1979; 115:225.
51. Kenney JA. Vitiligo treated by psoralens. Arch Dermatol 1971; 103:475–480.
52. Falabella R. Arrunategui A, Barona MI, Alzate A. The minigrafting test for vitiligo: detection of stable lesions for melanocyte transplantation. J Am Acad Dermatol 1995; 32:228–232.
53. Bose SK. Modified thiersch grafting in stable vitiligo. J Dermatol 1996; 23:363–364.
54. Kenney JA, Grimes PE. How we treat vitiligo. Cutis 1983; 43:347–348.
55. Westmore MG. Make-up as an adjunct and aid to the practice of dermatology. Dermatol Clin 1991; 9:81–88.
56. Kent G, Al'Abadie M. Psychologic effects of vitiligo: a critical incident analysis. J Am Acad Dermatol 1996; 35:895–898.
57. Porter JR, Beuf AH, Lerner A, Nordlund J. Psychosocial effect of vitiligo: a comparison of vitiligo patients with "normal" control subjects, with psoriasis patients, and with patients with other pigmentary disorders. J Am Acad Dermatol 1986; 15:220–224.
58. Porter JR, Beuf AH. Racial variation in reaction to physical stigma: a study of degree of disturbance by vitiligo among black and white patients. J Health Soc Behav 1991; 32:192–204.
59. Laude TA. Approach to dermatologic disorders in black children. Sem Dermatol 1995; 14:15–19.
60. Bolognia JL, Sodi SA, Osber MP, Pawelek JM. Enhancement of the depigmenting effect of hydroquinone by cystamine and buthionine sulfoximine. Br J Dermatol 1995; 133:349–357.
61. Taylor CR, Anderson RR. Ineffective treatment of refractory melasma and postinflammatory hyperpigmentation by Q-switched ruby laser. J Dermatol Surg Oncol 1994; 20:592–597.
62. Newcomer VD, Lindberg MC, Sternberg TH. A melanosis of the face ("chloasma"). Arch Dermatol 1961; 83:284–299.
63. Kimbrough-Green CK, Griffiths CEM, Finkel LJ, Hamilton TA, Bulengo-Ransby SM, Ellis CN, Voorhees JJ. Topical retinoic acid (tretinoin) for melasma in black patients. Arch Dermatol 1994; 130:727–733.

64. Griffiths CEM, Finkel LJ, Ditre SM, Hamilton TA, Ellis CN, Voorhees JJ. Topical tretinoin (retinoic acid) improves melasma. a vehicle controlled, clinical trial. Br J Dermatol 1993; 129:415–421.

17

Pruritus and Health-Related Quality of Life

Alan B. Fleischer, Jr. *Bowman Gray School of Medicine of Wake Forest University, Winston-Salem, North Carolina*

INTRODUCTION

Since pruritus is the primary symptom of inflammatory skin disease, this symptom deserves special attention in any work on health-related quality of life (HRQOL) in dermatology. Pruritus, like pain, is a subjective symptom. Accordingly, the attributes of pruritus such as intensity, quality, and duration cannot be verified by physical or biophysical examination.

In order to address the issue of pruritus, we must first agree upon a definition. Malcolm Greaves stated that pruritus "can be defined subjectively as a poorly localized, non-adapting, usually unpleasant sensation which elicits a desire to scratch" (1). In affected individuals, pruritus may be minor or extremely severe; people affected can ignore pruritus, or it may occupy all of their thoughts and actions.

Little attention in dermatological research has been devoted to the issue of pruritus and HRQOL. Indirect reference has been made to the relationship between pruritus and HRQOL (2–6), but these reports fail to substantiate this association.

MEASUREMENT OF PRURITUS

One of the obstacles in addressing this issue remains the difficulty in objectively assessing pruritus severity. A great deal of scholarly activity has focused on the related symptom, pain (7), but less is available to review for pruritus (8–11). Nevertheless, due to the dedicated work of a number of investigators, our understanding of pruritus measurement has progressed significantly in the past decade. Note that pruritus is not a unidimensional sensation. Accordingly, measurement of pruritus must take into account qualities of severity and duration and subjective differences in the determination of pruritus threshold. Although not well studied, pruritus may have other qualities such as burning or stinging, which may add to the unpleasantness of the sensation (10).

Categorical Scales

Categorical scales are the most commonly employed research scales and consist of discrete divisions of the frequency of the measured dimension. This type of scale is intuitively easy for literate adults to use. For example, in assessing pruritus frequency, the following question may be used: "Over the past week, I itched: never, rarely, occasionally, frequently, or always." Pruritus severity may also be assessed in analogous fashion.

Categorical scales can also be employed to assess the impact of pruritus upon the life of the affected patient. Consider the behavioral rating scale developed by this author to assess the life-impact of pruritus and intended to transcend unidimensional intensity or frequency measures (12). As originated, this question reads: "Over the past week, how would you describe the effect your itching has had on you? no itching; itching present, but easily ignored; itching present, cannot be ignored, but does not interfere with everyday activities; itching present, cannot be ignored, interferes with all tasks except taking care of basic needs such as toileting and eating; itching present, cannot be ignored, it interferes with all daily activities." We assessed the intercorrelation between the behavioral rating scale with frequency and intensity categorical and visual analog scales (VAS). We found modest ($r = 0.5–0.78$) but statistically highly significant correlations. This finding suggests that pruritus intensity and frequency are overlapping but separate constructs.

A similar behavioral scale was developed by Pederson and colleagues to assess therapeutic response. This scale consists of the following points: "I itch never; I itch rarely but never complain; I itch occasionally with mild annoyance; I itch often, it may be severe, but I can be active or rest easily; I itch often; it may be severe, and it interferes with rest but not activity; I itch always, it is severe and it interferes with both rest and activity." Similar to the question developed by the author, this instrument attempts to assess life-impact.

A disadvantage of all types of categorical scales is that differences between response categories may be unequal (10). For instance, the difference in a pruritus frequency response question between "I itched never" and "I itched rarely" may differ from the responses "I itched frequently" and "I itched always." Accordingly, when evaluating the responses, great caution must be exercised in interpretation.

Interval Scales

Pruritus can also be described by choosing a number on a fixed or limited scale, such as 0 to 10. Unlike the categorical scales, numerical scales have the advantage of equidistant points between response categories.

This process can also be automated for providing more information about the time-course for pruritus. Ståhle-Bäckdahl et al. evaluated the Pain-Track, a computerized system with a 7-step-graded, fixed-point, nonverbal scale in experimental pruritus compared with the VAS (14). This method allows frequent sampling and surveillance of compliance and generates a large amount of data. The Pain-Track response was found to be related to pruritus duration and "total itch index" but not to other measured subjective variables. Additionally, this 7-point scale appeared to be useful in measuring clinical pruritus, supporting the validity of this approach (15). A benefit of continuous recording is that recall bias is likely to play only a small role when using the Pain-Track, while retrospective questions are likely to be subject to bias.

Ståhle-Bäckdahl et al. found that in patients undergoing maintenance dialysis, Pain-Track recordings showed that pruritus intensity was greater during dialysis days than on days following dialysis and that pruritus was worse at night (14). Fluctuations in pruritus were detected by the Pain-Track and VAS data. The Pain-Track has been successfully used in clinical studies to assess the comparative value of different antipruritic agents (11). These studies support the construct validity of the Pain-Track as a clinical measure.

Continuous Scales

The aforementioned VAS is the most common example in pruritus research (8). A VAS is a line of defined length (in most studies 100 mm) with descriptive anchors at the extremes, e.g., "no itching" and "itching as bad as it could be." This tool allows subjects to precisely describe the pruritus sensation without limitation to a few discrete categories. VAS measures enable investigators to produce continuous data for analysis, which can be analyzed using tests appropriate for these data, such as *t*-tests. Additionally it may represent the most sensitive approach to measuring pruritus intensity (14).

Subjects unfamiliar with the VAS may be confused by this unusual instrument and may require an example and/or detailed instructions. We have found that some patients mark above or below the VAS rather than intersecting the line, and others need careful personal instructions.

The Pain-Track instrument discussed above has also been modified to record VAS measurements over time, thus maximizing sensitivity and minimizing recall bias. It has yet to find widespread use in clinical trials, but this tool is relatively new.

Scratch-Behaviour Measurement

Scratch behaviour reflects, in some fashion, pruritus sensation, Clinicians may be able to subjectively rate the number of excoriations or lichenification (16). This rating is widely used clinically, but has not been validated and is not likely to be reproducible. Consider the fact that some intensely pruritic conditions such as urticaria rarely show lichenification or excoriation. Thus, the measurement of scratching behavior is problematic and has been addressed in a variety of ways.

Self-Report of Scratching Behavior

Patients can be provided with hand-activated counters to record their scratching (17). Although obsessive-compulsive patients may be able to easily record their scratches (18), the act of recording the behavior may influence the behavior itself. Moreover, nocturnal scratching behavior cannot be recorded in this fashion. Accordingly, other techniques have been developed.

Nocturnal Bed Movement

Felix and Shuster measured whole body movement at night by a vibration transducer on a bed leg as well as to measuring limb movement with movement-sensitive meters (19). They found that the subjective sensation of pruritus correlated with nocturnal scratching behavior. Moreover, increased pruritus severity is associated with an increase in the number of scratching episodes but not scratching duration. Most importantly, these motion-detection techniques demonstrate response to disease-specific therapy (20).

Limb Activity Meters

Itchy patients tend to move their arms more than their legs, and careful analysis of both arm and leg movements can allow discrimination. A number of approaches have been used, each with relative merits (21–24). For instance, Osifo monitored scratching behavior with limb activity meters that were modified self-winding watches (24). These watches are not likely to be equally sensitive to all scratching movements, and temporal sequence recording is not possible. Although these methods are not subjective, may be reproducible, and may demonstrate response to therapy, wiring and recording nightly using biophysical devices will always be intrusive and costly. One negative study used this technique to dissociate the etiology of pruritus in cholestatic liver disease from bile acid levels, a previously popular hypothesis (23).

Forearm Activity Meters

Rhythmic muscle potentials can be recorded at the same time that an electroencephalogram records sleep activity (25–27). This type of approach may be ideally suited to intensively studying a limited number of patients with night pruritus. Like limb-activity meters, wiring and nightly recording from biophysical devices will always be intrusive and costly.

Direct Observation

Cornbleet reported the results of his investigations in 1953 in which he directly observed patients and their scratching behavior (28). He found that scratching occurred in bouts of multiple rhythmic strokes. Given the intrusive nature and time requirements of this approach, this technique is unlikely to ever be repeated. Moreover, the act of observation may influence behavior and alter the expression.

Using different methods, Ebata and colleagues recorded the total scratch time of nocturnal pruritus using photographic monitoring sensitive down to zero ambient light levels (29). In atopic dermatitis, nightly scratching time was found to vary between 7 minutes to nearly 5 hours. Other studies on nighttime scratching have uncovered tremendous morbidity (30–32). Limitations of nighttime monitoring include the fact that observation may miss scratching behavior underneath covers and that these techniques are extraordinarily expensive.

PRURITUS AS PART OF HRQOL INDICES

Within medical research, conventional quality-of-life instruments such as the Brief Symptom Inventory (33) and SF-36 (34) fail to mention pruritus. Thus, despite their broad use within disease and normative populations, these instruments rarely meet the needs of dermatological investigators. More specific dermatological instruments have been developed that utilize pruritus as part of their construct.

Dermatology Life Quality Index (DLQI)

Finlay and Khan incorporated pruritus into this dermatology-specific instrument (35). In order to decrease the number of questions, this index includes the question: "Over the last week, how itchy, 'scratchy,' sore or painful has your skin been?" The categorical responses include "very much," "a lot," "a little," and "not at all." Obviously, this question measures global skin symptoms including pruritus, but it also includes skin soreness and painfulness. Nevertheless, the DLQI as a whole suggests that patients with pruritic dermatoses (atopic dermatitis, psoriasis, and generalized pruritus) have lower HRQOL than those with nonpruritic dermatoses (acne, basal cell carcinoma, and viral warts).

Children's DLQI (CDLQI)

This analogous instrument was subsequently developed by Lewis-Jones and Finlay and contains the same global symptom question as noted above (36).

Psoriasis-Related Stressor Scale

Based on focus group sessions with patients and physicians, our group developed a 20-item Psoriasis-Related Stressor Scale (PRSS), a measure of the stressful aspects of psoriasis (S. R. Rapp et al., unpublished). Unlike the DLQI, this psoriasis-specific instrument inquires about pruritus itself without mention of scratching, soreness, or pain. Accordingly, it may be more useful for psoriasis, which has pruritus as a major component. Unfortunately, because of its focus, the PRSS is likely less useful for nonpsoriatic skin disease. The PRSS has undergone validation studies on a large group of psoriasis patients and has been used to demonstrate HRQOL improvement in a clinical trial (A. B. Fleischer Jr. et al., unpublished).

SCORAD

The European Task Force on Atopic Dermatitis developed a scoring index (SCORAD) for their target disease combining extent, severity, and subjective symptoms (37). Unlike the Psoriasis Area Severity Index (PASI) (38), which describes cutaneous disease severity, this global score incorporates both skin symptoms and disease severity into one index. The pruritus question in this index is a VAS with anchors of 0 and 10. The VAS text asks the subject to describe the average pruritus severity for "the last 3 days or nights." Supporting the construct validity of the instrument, SCORAD has been subsequently used to show HRQOL improvement in a clinical trial (39).

Skindex

The Skindex is a 62-item self-administered study instrument designed to assess skin disease HRQOL that has had reliability and responsiveness validation (40). Pruritus is assessed as part of the physical discomfort component of the entire conceptual framework. The question about pruritus is similar to the 5-point Frequency Rating Scale described above. In one study, pruritus and other components including skin hurting only explained 5% of the variance in the response to this instrument, whereas embarrassment and being ashamed explained 46% of the variance. This study did not assess typical itchy conditions exclusively, so the contribution of pruritus in these conditions is likely to be greater than that observed.

SUMMARY

As Professor Malcolm Greaves has stated, research into pruritus "has barely scratched the surface" (41). Investigators interested in measuring clinical response to dermatological therapeutics and understanding the impact of skin diseases on HRQOL are especially interested in pruritus measurement. No single instrument has been demonstrated to capture all aspects of pruritus. Intensity and frequency scales are frequently used, and the VAS is likely to be the most sensitive technique. Intensity measures may be more reliable as they do not depend upon recall bias, but address pruritus only at the moment the patient completes the instrument. Behavioral rating scales can transcend symptom intensity and frequency and may thus be preferable as adjunct instruments. The author hypothesizes that a mixed approach; assessing intensity, frequency, and life-impact, is likely to be the most useful clinical HRQOL measurement approach. Scratching activity has been reported as a proxy for pruritus, but remains cumbersome and costly to measure. Nevertheless, we have learned a great deal about the amount of time spent scratching, a behavioral phenomenon associated with poor quality of life. Dermatology-specific HRQOL instruments for inflammatory dermatological seases should include questions about pruritus, and many recent instruments have recognized this need. SCORAD, PRSS, and Skindex specifically include this symptom in their constructs. Pruritus has been included as a symptom in dermatology-specific HRQOL instruments, but not in general HRQOL instruments. Some of the newer dermatology-specific instruments may offer insight into the relative contribution to morbidity from pruritus.

REFERENCES

1. Greaves MW. Pruritus. In: Champion RH, Burton JL, Ebling FJG. Textbook of Dermatology. 5th ed. Blackwell Scientific Publications, 1992: 527–536.
2. Turner IB, Rawlins MD, Wood P, James OF. Flumecinol for the treatment of pruritus associated with primary biliary cirrhosis. Aliment Pharmacol Ther 1994; 8: 337–342.
3. Ballinger AB, McHugh M, Catnach SM, Alstead EM, Clark ML. Symptom relief and quality of life after stenting for malignant bile duct obstruction. Gut 1994; 35: 467–470.
4. Finelli C, Gugliotta L, Gamberi B, Vianelli N, Visani G, Tura S. Relief of intractable pruritus in polycythemia vera with recombinant interferon alfa. Am J Hematol 1993; 43: 316–318.
5. Alarabi AA, Wikstrom B, Loof L, Danielson BG. Treatment of pruritus in cholestatic jaundice by bilirubin-and bile acid-adsorbing resin column plasma perfusion. Scand J Gastroenterol 1992; 27: 223–226.
6. Lauterburg BH, Taswell HF, Pineda AA, Dickson ER, Burgstaler EA, Carlson GL. Treatment of pruritus of cholestasis by plasma perfusion through USP-charcoal-coated glass beads. Lancet 1980; ii: 53–55.
7. Jensen MP, Karoly P, Braver S. The measurement of clinical pain intensity; a comparison of six methods. Pain 1986; 27: 117–126.
8. Wahlgren CF, Ekblom A, Hägermark O. Some aspects of the experimental induction and measurement of itch. Acta Dermato-Venereol 1989; 69: 185–189.
9. Wahlgren CF. Itch and atopic dermatitis: clinical and experimental studies. Acta Dermato-Venereol 1991; 165(suppl): 1–53.
10. Wahlgren CF. Measurement of itch. Sem Dermatol 1995; 14: 277–284.
11. Hägermark O, Wahlgren CF. Some methods for evaluating clinical itch and their application for studying pathogenic mechanisms. J Dermatol Sci 1992; 4: 55–62.
12. Fleischer AB Jr, McFarlane M, Hinds MA, Mittelmark MB. Skin conditions and symptoms are common in the elderly: the prevalence of skin symptoms and conditions in an elderly population. J Geriatr Dermatol 1996; 4: 78–89.
13. Pederson JA, Matter BJ, Czerwinski AW, et al. Relief of idiopathic generalized pruritus in dialysis patients treated with activated charcoal. Ann Intern Med 1980; 93: 446–448.
14. Ståhle-Bäckdahl M, Wahlgren CF, Hägermark O. Computerized recording of itch in patients on maintenance hemodialysis. Acta Dermato-Venereol 1989; 69: 410–414.
15. Wahlgren CF, Hägermark O, Bergström R, et al. Evaluation of a new method of assessing pruritus and antipruritic drugs. Skin Pharmacol 1988; 1: 3–13.
16. Savin J. The measurement of scratching. Sem Dermatol 1995; 14: 285–289.
17. Melin L, Frederikson T, Noren P, Swebilius BG. Behavioral treatment of scratching in patients with atopic dermatitis. Br J Dermatol 1986; 115: 467–474.
18. Savin J. Neurotic excoriations—a quantitative approach to the effect of treatment. Br J Clin Pract 1970; 24: 451–453.

19. Felix R, Shuster S. A new method for the measurement of itch and the response to treatment. Br J Dermatol 1975; 93:303–312.
20. Shuster S. Pruritus and its assessment as itch and scratch. Acta Dermato-Venereol 1991; 156(suppl):45.
21. Summerfield JA, Welch ME. The measurement of itch with sensitive limb movement meters. Br J Dermatol 1980; 103:275–281.
22. Mustakallio KK. Scratch radar for the measurement of pruritus. Acta Dermato-Venereol 1991; 156(suppl):44.
23. Bartholomew TC, Summerfield JA, Billing BH, Lawson AM, Setchell KD. Bile acid profiles of human serum and skin interstitial fluid and their relationship to pruritus studied by gas chromatography-mass spectrometry. Clin Sci 1982; 63:65–73.
24. Osifo NG. The antipruritic effects of chlorphenirimine, cyproheptadine and sulphapyridine monitored with limb activity meters on chloroquine induced pruritus among patients with malaria. Afr J Med Sci 1995; 24:67–73.
25. Savin JA, Paterson WD, Oswald I. Scratching during sleep. Lancet 1973; ii:296–297.
26. Monti JM, Vignale R, Monti D. Sleep and nighttime pruritus in children with atopic dermatitis. Sleep 1989; 12:309–314.
27. Brown DG, Kalucy RS. Correlation of the neurophysiological and personality data in sleep scratching. Proc Roy Soc Med 1975; 68:530–532.
28. Cornbleet T. Scratching pattern. 1. Influence of site. J Invest Dermatol 1953; 20:105–110.
29. Ebata T, Aizawa H, Kamide R. An infrared video camera system to observe nocturnal scratching in atopic dermatitis patients. J Dermatol 1996; 23:153–155.
30. Aoki T, Kushimoto HK, Hishikawa Y, et al. Nocturnal scratching and its relationship to the disturbed sleep of itchy subjects. Clin Exp Dermatol 1991; 16:268–272.
31. Aoki T, Kushimoto HK, Kobayashi E, et al. Computer analysis of nocturnal scratch in atopic dermatitis. Acta Derm Venereol Suppl 1980; 92:33–37.
32. Savin JA, Paterson WD, Oswald I, et al. Further studies of scratching during sleep. Br J Dermatol 1975; 115:297–302.
33. Derogatis LR, Spencer PM. The Brief Symptom Inventory (BSI): Administration, Scoring and Procedures Manual. Baltimore: Johns Hopkins University Press, 1982.
34. Julious SA, George S, Campbell MJ. Sample sizes for studies using the short form 36 (SF-36). J Epidemiol Comm Health 1995; 49:642–644.
35. Finlay AY, Khan GK. Dermatology Life Quality Index (DLQI)—a simple practical measure for routine clinical use. Clin Exp Dermatol 1994; 19:210–216.
36. Lewis-Jones, Finlay AY. The children's life quality index (CDLQI): initial validation and subsequent use. Br J Dermatol 1995; 132:942–949.
37. Severity scoring of atopic dermatitis: the SCORAD index. Consensus Report of the European Task Force on Atopic Dermatitis. Dermatology 1993; 186:23–31.

38. Fredriksson T, Pettersson U. Severe psoriasis—oral therapy with a new retinoid. Dermatologica 1978; 157:238–244.
39. Kowalzick L, Kleinheinz A, Weichenthal M, et al. Low dose vs. medium dose UV-A1 treatment in severe atopic eczema. Acta Dermato-Venereol 1995; 75:43–45.
40. Chren MM, Lasek RJ, Quinn LM, Mostow EN, Zyzanski SK. Skindex, a quality-of-life measure for patients with skin disease: reliability, validity and responsiveness. J Invest Dermatol 1996; 107:707–713.
41. Greaves MW. Itching—research has barely scratched the surface. N Engl J Med 1992; 326:1016–1017.

18

Quality-of-Life Study in Patients with Chronic Vulvar Dermatoses

Betty Bellman *University of Miami School of Medicine, Miami, Florida*

INTRODUCTION

Quality of life is a highly subjective, abstract concept encompassing an individual's perception of psychological, physical, and social well-being (1). The term is further influenced by a multitude of human experiences, emotions, pain tolerance, and interpersonal social interactions. Chronic vulvar dermatoses can be very distressing and disabling, often causing significant morbidity. This type of skin disease can affect the psychological, occupational, domestic, physical, and sexual lives of women of all ages. Patients often give up various activities in their usual lifestyle with significant detriment to their relationships, social interactions, and emotional well-being. Frequently, patients who suffer from vulvar symptoms visit countless physicians and gynecologists in search of a diagnosis and "cure." Many of these women are unable to discuss their private problem with their family or friends.

This chapter will attempt to first briefly define some of these vulvar dermatoses and discuss the chronic distressing symptoms of 43 women seen in a private dermatology office. This chapter will also evaluate the way their disease has affected the quality of their lives, their activities of daily living, their emotional well-being, and their sexual and interpersonal relationships.

CHRONIC VULVAR DERMATOSES

Many chronic skin diseases are morphologically recognizable and may occur on other areas of the body as well as the vulva. There are several different types of chronic vulvar diseases—some common, and others more rare. Some examples of common vulvar diseases that can become chronic are lichen simplex chronicus/neurodermatitis, psoriasis, vulvovaginal candidiasis, genital herpes, contact dermatitis, intertrigo, and persistent bacterial vaginal infections (2). It is much more difficult to manage and treat patients with more debilitating vulvar diseases such as vulvodynia and all of its subsets, including dysesthetic vulvodynia, cyclic vulvitis, and vulvar vestibulitis syndrome. Other, less common vulvar diseases include chronic vulvovaginal *Candida albicans* and *non-albicans* vulvovaginitis, desquamative vulvo-vaginitis/lichen planus, and lichen sclerosus (2). Symptoms are quite variable among the vulvar dermatoses and may be altered by previous therapy (3).

Vulvodynia

The term vulvodynia refers to symptoms of constant or intermittent vulvar burning and pain, of uncertain etiology, not explained by clinical findings. Until recently, vulvodynia was thought to represent an uncommon manifestation of depression, anxiety, or psychosexual dysfunction (4). Physical examination may reveal a normal-appearing vulva or some degree of erythema. Although psychological factors do play a role in some patients, this condition has finally achieved recognition in the medical literature and is thought to be a manifestation of any inflammation or neuropathy. The pain associated with vulvodynia often has a "burning quality" and is usually chronic and recalcitrant to treatment (5). Vulvodynia is quite different from pruritus vulvae, for the patient with vulvar burning seldom has the abnormal physical findings that one may see with continuous scratching or rubbing (6).

Vulvar Vestibulitis

Vulvar vestibulitis presents with severe localized pain around the introitus, dyspareunia, and at times inflammation of the vestibular glands around the introitus and urethral opening, respectively. It is a subcategory of vulvodynia thought to be related to pelvic floor dysfunction, pudendal neuralgia, and reflex sympathetic dystrophy (7). It encompasses a constellation of symptoms and findings limited to the vulvar vestibule that consists of (1) severe pain to vestibular touch on attempted vaginal entry, (2) tenderness to pressure localized around the vulvar vestibule and (3) physical findings confined to vulvar erythema of the vestibule (7,8).

Lichen Sclerosus

Lichen sclerosus is a relatively common hypopigmented skin disorder which has a predilection for genital skin. Clinically, it presents with severe pruritus and well-demarcated white plaques of thin, fragile skin. Excoriations may often be superinfected with yeast and bacteria. Patients may develop purpuric macules, blisters, and, eventually, obliteration of the normal vulvar architecture due to scarring (9).

Lichen Planus

Lichen planus is a relatively uncommon mucocutaneous disease that sometimes affects the genitalia. The classic lesions clinically appear as violaceous, flat-topped papules as well as reticulate annular white papules. Vulvar lichen planus may also be erosive with a desquamative vulvovaginitis, profuse vaginal discharge, and ulceration. Advanced disease results in progressive scarring, vaginal adhesions, and even obliteration of the vaginal space (10).

Lichen Simplex Chronicus

Lichen simplex chronicus, also known as neurodermatitis, is a chronic condition of severe pruritus of the vulva or scrotum. Clinical examination reveals lichenification and thickening of genital skin with hyperpigmentation, excoriations, and erythema. Habitual scratching and rubbing may even occur at night, and an "itch-scratch cycle" is invariably present (6,11).

STUDY OBJECTIVE

The objective of the study was to measure the quality of life and the impact that chronic vulvar dermatoses and their associated symptoms have on a group of 43 women patients. Since chronic vulvar diseases tend to be progressive, they can cause severe intractable symptoms, which affect each patient differently. This chapter will attempt to describe the distress caused by these patient's chronic symptoms and how their chronic vulvar disease affected their interpersonal and sexual relationships, activities of daily living, and emotional well-being.

METHODS

Forty-three patients with chronic vulvar disorders ages 13 to 73 (with a mean age of 44) were evaluated between November of 1994 and September of 1996 in a private dermatology office in Miami, Florida. Forty-one (95%) of these patients were referred by another physician for chronic vulvar symptoms. Demographics as to the patient's race, marital status, and age were recorded. Also included were questions about the specific vulvar symptoms, their duration, and if their symptoms were constant or intermittent. In addition, other questions investigated all patients' prior treatments, medical history, history of sexually transmitted diseases, frequency of coitus, and whether they experienced any pain during or after coitus. Questions were asked regarding how their vulvar condition affected their quality of life, their activities of daily living, their emotional well-being, and their interpersonal and sexual relationships. All patients were asked what they thought could be causing their vulvar problem, what fears and concerns they had regarding their condition, and if anything in particular brought on their symptoms or made them worse or better. Areas evaluated by these patient's chronic symptoms included activities of daily living, exercise, sexual activity, and emotional well-being. All patients were thoroughly evaluated by a careful history and physical and given an appropriate diagnosis.

RESULTS/FINDINGS

Of the 43 patients, 11 (26%) were single, 30 (70%) were married, and 2 (5%) were widowed. The majority of patients, (40, or 93%) were Caucasian, and only 3 (7%) were Hispanic. The most common chronic vulvar disease was vulvodynia, which was diagnosed in 17 (40%) of the patients evaluated. The second most common problem was vulvovaginal candidiasis, which occurred in 11 (26%) patients, 3 of which had atypical nonalbicans yeasts. Many patients had tolerated variable degrees of symptoms for a long time, such as pain, burning, itching, irritation, and swelling. The majority of patients reported that their complaints were not acknowledged by other physicians they had seen. Table 1 shows the diseases as well as the number of patients diagnosed. Some patients had more than one diagnosis.

Symptoms (Table 2)

The patient's symptoms ranged from 2 months to 40 years (mean symptom duration of 48 months). It was difficult for many patients to describe or quantitate their symptoms and their level of discomfort. The term "burning" was used by the majority of the patients when they were asked to describe the quality of the pain. Other symptoms included rawness, irritation, soreness, stinging, swelling, and chronic vaginal discharge. The majority of patients stated that topically applied medications burned and actually worsened their symptoms. Most patients developed their own ways of handling the symptoms including bed rest, prolonged bathtub soaks, ice packs, and resigning themselves to accepting their pain and suffering. It was

Table 1 Final Diagnoses of Study Patients

Vulvar disease	No. and percentage of patients
Vulvovaginal candidiasis	8/43 (19%)
Vulvodynia	17/43 (40%)
Lichen sclerosis	2/43 (5%)
Lichen planus	3/43 (7%)
Atrophic vulvovaginitis	5/43 (12%)
Lichen simplex chronicus	2/43 (5%)
Hidradenitis suppurativa	1/43 (2%)
Contact dermatitis	1/43 (2%)
Vulvar vestibulitis	2/43 (5%)
Staphylococcal furunculosis	1/43 (2%)
Vulvar intraepithelial neoplasia	1/43 (2%)
Vulvar varices	1/43 (2%)
Bacterial vaginosis	2/43 (5%)
Postherpetic neuralgia	1/43 (2%)
Chronic nonalbicans vulvovaginitis	3/43 (7%)
Molluscum contagiosum	1/43 (2%)
Condyloma acuminatum	4/43 (9%)

not uncommon to hear patients report unexplained symptom-free periods lasting for hours to days. In many cases the patients indicated a strong degree of preoccupation with the pain during waking hours. Twenty-four patients (56%) had intermittent symptoms, while 17 (40%) had constant

Table 2 Multiple Vulvar Symptoms and Complaints of Study Patients

Symptoms	No. and percentage of patients
Pain	13/43 (30%)
Pruritus	22/43 (51%)
Irritation	13/43 (30%)
Vulvar swelling	6/43 (14%)
Burning	18/43 (42%)
Vaginal discharge	8/43 (19%)
Frequency of urination	3/43 (7%)
Urgency of urination	3/43 (7%)
Hesitancy of urination	3/43 (7%)
Burning worse with urination	4/43 (9%)
Vulvar fissures	4/43 (9%)
Dysuria	1/43 (2%)

vulvar symptoms. Only 5% (2 patients) had intermittent symptoms, which became constant. Three patients complained of "rawness," and two had perianal itching and burning associated with their vulvar symptoms. Some patients complained of a great deal of discomfort and pain from the motion of their pubic hairs. One patient had been treated previously with a vestibulectomy, and two patients had CO_2 vaporization of their entire genital tracts.

Activities of Daily Living (Table 3)

Normal daily activities which may be taken for granted, such as physical exercise, sitting, walking, and wearing slacks, may be affected by chronic vulvovaginal symptoms. Many patients avoided common daily activities such as recreational activities, hobbies, and household chores. To lessen their discomfort, many patients did not wear undergarments or pantyhose and could wear only dresses or skirts to decrease any excess pressure on the vulva. Many patients complained about having to cancel dinner plans that would involve sitting for several hours, alienating friends or relatives, canceling a golf or tennis tournament, and generally feeling that they did not have a sense of control over their lives. One patient was upset because she could not participate in the bridge games that she had faithfully attended for the past 10 years. Another patient gave up gardening, which she greatly enjoyed. Many patients were upset that their symptoms interfered with exercise and keeping active and fit. The pain was worse with walking long distances, damp clothing, perspiration, heat, friction, and any type of pressure on the genital area. Pain was ameliorated by keeping one's legs apart

Table 3 Activities of Daily Living Adversely Affected by Chronic Vulvar Dermatoses in Study Patients

Activities of daily living affected	No. and percentage of patients
Symptoms awaken patient from sleep	5/43 (12%)
Difficulty wearing jeans or underwear	8/43 (19%)
Discomfort during exercise	10/43 (23%)
Discomfort during ambulation	3/43 (7%)
Interference with social activities	8/43 (19%)
Interference with hobbies (e.g., yardwork)	3/43 (7%)
Inability to sit for long periods of time	6/43 (14%)
Interference with travel plans	2/43 (5%)
Difficulty riding a bike	5/43 (12%)

as much as possible and allowing air to circulate in the area. One patient's burning was much worse after urinating, and she would need to rinse her vulvar after each voiding. This proved to be very inconvenient in public restrooms and limited her activities outside her home. For the majority of patients, their discomfort was exacerbated by sitting for long periods of time.

Human Sexuality (Table 4)

Patients with chronic vulvar disease often suffer symptoms that continue for many months or years. This can cause significant marital discord, feelings of guilt, and a decreased libido. Vulvar pain can cause a marked decrease in the frequency of coitus in that it is frequently provoked by intercourse. Five (12%) patients abstained from sexual intercourse completely, nine (21%) never had comfortable sex, and four (9%) were not sexually active. The majority of the patients expressed a decrease in libido and considerable anxiety about having sexual relations due to the pain they would likely experience. Most sexually active women experienced decreased lubrication during foreplay, which exacerbated their dyspareunia and decreased the frequency of intercourse. Lubricants were helpful, yet did not always relieve the dyspareunia. More than 50% of patients complained of burning pain with penetration during sexual intercourse. After sex, many patients complained of discomfort which would last for hours or even days. Three patients (7%) stated that coitus would cause fissures or small cuts

Table 4 How Disease Affected Sexual Activity of Study Patients

Sexual problem	No. and percentage of patients
Abstinence from sexual intercourse	5/43 (12%)
No pain with sexual intercourse	8/43 (19%)
Decreased libido	20/43 (47%)
Never had comfortable intercourse	4/43 (9%)
Pain with intromission (dyspareunia)	22/43 (51%)
Coitus caused cuts and fissures	3/43 (7%)
Pain and symptoms worse after intercourse	10/43 (23%)
Discharge worse after intercourse	3/43 (7%)
Pain and symptoms worse during coitus	8/43 (19%)
Decreased frequency of coitus	10/43 (23%)
Avoids intercourse during symptom flare	5/43 (12%)
Decreased lubrication	18/43 (42%)

along the vaginal opening, which were painful and took several days to heal. One patient was told that her symptoms were due to a "lack of sexual activity" and therefore she engaged in more frequent intercourse, which only exacerbated her pain. Many patients feared that their problem would ruin their sexual enjoyment and that they would never be able to have sexual pleasure again. One patient described feeling like she had "brush burns on her vulva after sex." Patients who suffered from chronic vaginal discharge state that vaginal discharge worsened after coitus. Many patients with dyspareunia sought relief after intercourse with cool sitz baths, topical creams, and ice packs.

Emotional Well-Being and Interpersonal Relationships

During the interviews, many patients were tearful and expressed anger and frustration about their previous medical care and the difficulty they experienced finding a doctor who could evaluate their symptoms and diagnose and treat their problem. Many of these patients are told that nothing is wrong with them and that "it is all in their heads." This may lead to a patient feeling that his symptoms are not being acknowledged and, subsequently, may lead to feelings of depression, anger, frustration, and anxiety. Many patients became preoccupied with their pain and were aware of it constantly. Only a handful of patients were undergoing psychotherapy to cope with their disease and emotional pain. In most cases, the spouse or partner was described as supportive, helpful, and understanding. However, in several instances, a few husbands grew impatient and expressed unhappiness about the decreased frequency of sexual intercourse. One patient stated that she was "depressed about the distance that occurred between her and her husband as a result of her chronic vulvar pain over the past year." She stated that her husband told her "Can't you just find out what is wrong with you, and have it fixed?" Interestingly, only two (5%) of the partners accompanied the patients to their initial clinical evaluation.

Patient's Fears and Concerns

Some of the patients were not sure why they had their vulvar disease and felt that it was making their life miserable. They stated that they could not function the way they wanted to in life. "It affects everything in my life, I fear that I am not normal and will never be the same," one patient stated. Many patients stated that they were concerned about the decreased intimacy and sexual intercourse. A few patients scrubbed their vulvas several times a day because they thought they were "dirty." A common fear in over 50% of the patients was that the cause of their vulvar pain would never be determined and that it would worsen and never be cured. Three patients

(7%) feared having a malignancy, and one patient was concerned about developing a vulvar deformity. Two patients feared that their husbands had some abnormality that may be contributed to their problem, such as a sexually transmitted disease. Two patients believed that their vulvar condition was a punishment for sexual promiscuity.

CONCLUSION

Patients with chronic disease define their quality of life primarily in terms of positive relationships, recreational activities, a sense of security and meaning in life, and the ability to function independently (12). An individual's quality of life is constantly changing and is very difficult to measure. It encompasses the capacity to perform activities of daily living, be free from pain and suffering, preserve our senses and sensuality, and have a social support system. It also allows one to have a purpose outside of oneself and some degree of happiness and morale (13). These basic elements are affected by one's personality characteristics and how they adapt to stress and physical pain. Women are especially affected physically, psychologically, emotionally, and sexually by chronic vulvar diseases. Basic human functions such as urination, ambulation, physical exercise, and sexual relations may be affected. Emotionally, many patients felt alone and in despair about their private condition. The majority of patients felt that few individuals could truly empathize with their pain. Some of the patients belonged to support groups and networks.

The anxiety and depression that long-standing genital pain produces can potentially cause psychological injury to a woman's self-esteem and devastate her sensuality and sexual enjoyment. Relationships may also suffer, since a partner or spouse may not understand the fact that many chronic vulvar diseases have no cure. Since intercourse may not be possible, counseling is often very beneficial to patients and their sexual partners, especially when neither the patient nor the physician fully understands what is causing the pain. Joint counseling can help both partners cope with their frustrations and guilt over their inability to always have a mutually satisfying sexual relationship. Patients with chronic vulvar disease experience a decreased libido, loss of self-esteem, and a sense of loss. Many patients emotionally distance themselves from their partners and may feel that they are not in control of what is happening to their bodies. Patients may withdraw from intimate relationships because of fear of undesirability, discovery, disapproval, and rejection, leading to increasing isolation and withdrawal (14).

Often patients are labeled as neurotic, crazy, depressed, and hypochondriacal. In patients with pain co-existing with depression, it is often unclear which came first, i.e., whether the pain is a somatic symptom of a primary depression or a reactive depression that developed from being in chronic pain (15). It has been suggested that even when depression is not obvious in a patient with chronic painful symptoms, it is often present, but subclinical, the theory being that the pain may be an expression of depression (16). Patients may naturally develop anxiety and depression due to the chronicity of their disease and the hopelessness of finding a cure. Stress of any kind can worsen the symptoms these patients experience. Patients who are predisposed to psychological problems may have a prior history of depression and/or anxiety, which may exacerbate and/or contribute to their coping mechanisms of dealing with a chronic disease. Certain personality characteristics can be adaptive or transcend the most physical and mental pathology (13). Emotionally, patients have different perceptions about their capabilities of healing, their level of motivation, their thought patterns and their emotional reactions to various stimuli (17).

Chronic vulvar dermatoses can also affect activities of daily living. As one patient stated in her own essay, "I could no longer wear tight jeans or panty hose, use tampons, exercise freely, lift a child, sit in any position, or ride a bicycle without experiencing extreme pain" (18). Patients often give up many aspects of their usual lifestyle with obvious detriment to their social interactions, interpersonal relationships, psychological well-being, and overall quality of life. Activities such as household chores, travel plans, hobbies, and entertainment may be particularly restricted by chronic symptoms of vulvar itching, burning, pain, and irritation.

In particular, patients with chronic vulvar pain are traumatized and often devastated by their condition. Chronic vulvar disease is not only physically painful, but emotionally debilitating. Despite this, many women with chronic vulvar diseases do not seek help for their condition due to embarrassment or do so only after years of suffering and private misery. Simple screening methods to detect patients suffering from chronic vulvar symptoms who have not yet been properly diagnosed and treated include taking a thorough medical history and including gynecological symptoms on standardized office medical history questionnaires.

Physicians need to understand that although a patient may have a paucity of clinical findings, their pain is real and may cause significant emotional morbidity even though its etiology is unknown or physical examination reveals a paucity of clinical findings. Clinicians do not always automatically assume that sexuality is important to older women patients, and as a result may fail to evaluate and explore its existence and expression (13). A striking feature in this study was the patients' gratitude and appreciation that their disease was taken seriously and treated in a sympathetic manner after struggling with their chronic vulvar disease day after day. It is important for physicians to understand the many sensitive concerns that these patients may have and their many hopes, fears, and frustrations that need to be explored. The impact of a patient's disease on activities of daily living may be more important than the actual diagnosis itself.

A thorough literature search from 1966 to the present day showed no appreciable research literature on QOL for chronic vulvar dermatoses. Standard quantitative measures and existing QOL instruments which currently exist for various dermatological conditions, such as the Dermatology Life Quality Index (DLQI) (19), are not sufficient to measure the sensitive features inherant in chronic vulvar diseases. Disease-specific health-related quality of life (HRQOL) (20) instruments in combination with generic QOL instruments need to be designed to measure the impact that chronic vulvar diseases have on affected patients (21). Dimensions should explore physical functioning, emotional well-being, social interaction, sexual functioning, interpersonal relationships, psychological functioning, and overall quality of life. Clinicians and patients would benefit a great deal if more utility measures assessed the value placed on chronic vulvar diseases and the measurement of the QOL. There is a definite need for descriptive and clinical trials that include QOL outcomes and QOL instruments specific and sensitive to chronic vulvar dermatoses. A disease-specific HRQOL could provide useful information about the impact of the vulvar disease on a patient's life experiences as well as the biological and physical functioning of human behavior.

REFERENCES

1. Kelleher CJ, Cardozo LD, Toozs-Hobson PM. Quality of life and urinary incontinence. Curr Opin Obstet Gynecol 1995; 7:404–408.
2. Lynch PJ, Edwards L. Genital Dermatology. New York: Churchill-Livingstone, 1994.
3. McKay M. Vulvodynia. Arch Dermatol 1989; 125:256–262.
4. Dodson MD, Friedrich EG. Psychosomatic vulvovaginitis. Obstet Gynecol 1978; 51(suppl):23s.
5. Lynch PJ. Vulvodynia: a syndrome of unexplained vulvar pain, psychologic disability and sexual dysfunction. J Reprod Med 1986; 31:773–780.
6. McKay M. Vulvodynia vs. Pruritus vulvae. Clin Obstet Gynecol 1985; 28:123–133.
7. Marinoff SC, Turner MLC. Vulvar vestibulitis syndrome: an overview. Am J Obstet Gynecol 1991; 165:1228–1233.
8. Baggish MS, Miklos JR. Vulvar pain syndrome: a review. Obstet Gynecol Surv 1995; 50:618–627.
9. Ridley CM. Lichen sclerosus. Dermatol Clin 1992; 10:309.
10. Edwards L. Vulvar lichen planus. Arch Dermatol 1989; 125:1677–1680.
11. Sherertz EF. Clinical pearl: Symptomatic dermatographism as a cause of genital pruritus. J Am Acad Dermatol 31:1040–1041.

12. Burckhardt CS, Woods SL, Schultz AA, Ziebarth DM. Quality of life of adults with chronic illness: a psychometric study. Res Nurs Health 1989; 12:347–354.
13. Butler RN. Quality of life: can it be an endpoint? How can it be measured? Am J Clin Nutr 1992; 55:1267S–1270S.
14. Vanderplate C, Aral SO. Psychosocial aspects of genital herpes virus infection. Health Psychol 1987; 6:57–72.
15. Block B. Antidepressants in the treatment of pain. Res Staff Phys 1993; 39:49–52.
16. Blumer D, Heilbronn M. Chronic pain as a variant of depressive disease: the pain-prone disorder. J Nerv Ment Dis 1982; 170:381–406.
17. Headley BJ. Self-efficacy and chronic pain. Clin Manage 1990; 10:47–50.
18. Smith H, Pomerantz E. Getting back to normal: one woman's experience with vulvodynia. J Obstet Gynecol 1996; 20:10–13.
19. Finlay AY, Khan GK. Dermatology Life Quality Index (DLQI): a simple practical measure for routine clinical use. Clin Exp Dermatol 1994; 19:210–216.
20. Revicki DA. Health-related quality of life in the evaluation of medical therapy for chronic illness. J Fam Pract 1989; 29:377–380.
21. McKenna KE, Stern RS. The outcomes movement and new measures of the severity of psoriasis. J Am Acad Dermatol 1996; 34:534–538.

19

Aging Skin and Quality of Life

Madhulika A. Gupta *University of Western Ontario, London, Ontario, Canada*

INTRODUCTION

Some of the clinical sequelae of cutaneous aging and/or photodamage include wrinkling, pigmentary changes, roughness, laxity, and telangiectasia, which can result in the aging of the overall appearance (1). This in turn can have a negative impact on various aspects of quality of life (1–3), including (1) social interactions, most commonly manifesting as uneasiness and anxiety during interpersonal interactions, (2) occupational functioning, in that a youthful appearance may be associated with better employment opportunities, and (3) the psychological state of the individual, resulting in decreased self-esteem, body image problems, and, in some instances, an adjustment disorder. Among some individuals, concerns about an aging appearance can culminate in an excessive preoccupation with dieting, exercise, and thinness. The perceived negative appraisal of the appearance resulting from cutaneous aging and photodamage culminates in significant expense for cosmetic treatments. Studies (4–7) have shown that a reduction in the cutaneous signs of photodamage and/or aging with topical tretinoin or cosmetic makeovers is associated with an improvement in these dimensions of quality of life.

It should be emphasized that the cutaneous stigmata of aging are an ubiquitous experience and therefore do not represent a physical disorder like many other dermatoses that affect the quality of life. However, with the aging of the population at large and the relatively high value placed by society on the maintenance of a youthful appearance, the impact of photo-damaged and/or aging skin on the quality of life cannot be ignored by dermatologists (1). This chapter reviews some of the literature on the impact of aging and/or photodamaged skin on the quality of life.

REVIEW OF THE LITERATURE

Cutaneous Aging and Social Interactions

The skin as an organ of communication represents various socially important attributes such as age, social status, wealth, and sexuality (1–3). Physical appearance, especially the appearance of the face, plays a major role in human transactions (4), and youthful skin contributes significantly to an individual's physical attractiveness. In one study (5), 20 observers representing both sexes rated photographs of 48 white women (age range 54–96 years) for physical attractiveness. Two essentially nonoverlapping groups of 16 women each who were on the opposite ends of the attractiveness spectrum were selected from the 48 subjects (5). The attractiveness ratings were strongly affected by physical stigmata typically associated with aging, i.e., wrinkling, sagging, sallowing, etc., by both the male and female judges. Second, the group of women rated as good-looking by the judges also reported greater satisfaction with their lives and described themselves as more socially outgoing (4,5), further supporting the positive influence of an attractive appearance upon social functioning. In one study of 20 patients with clinically mild to moderately aged skin secondary to photodamage (6), who had entered a study to evaluate the efficacy of topical tretinoin for the treatment of photodamaged skin, the study volunteers had high scores on Interpersonal Sensitivity and Phobic Anxiety subscales of the Brief Symptom Inventory (BSI) (8) prior to starting the study. High scores on these subscales indicate that these subjects were experiencing uneasiness during their interpersonal interactions. The Interpersonal Sensitivity (8) subscale measures a lack of ease during interpersonal interactions and the Phobic Anxiety (8) subscale provides an index of a persistent fear response to certain situations, including social situations, that leads to avoidance of the anxiety-providing situations. After 24 weeks of therapy both the Interpersonal Sensitivity and Phobic Anxiety scores decreased significantly ($p < 0.05$) in the tretinoin but not in the control group (receiving the inactive vehicle) (6). These findings were confirmed in another study (7) involving 40 additional subjects with moderate to severe photodamage among whom a significant decrease in Phobic Anxiety (8) ($p < 0.05$) was observed after 24 weeks of therapy with topical tretinoin, with an increase ($p < 0.05$) in this symptom dimension in the group receiving the inactive vehicle (7). These findings indicate that photodamage causes increased social anxiety in some subjects, and this anxiety decreases with treatment of some of the cutaneous changes of photodamage.

Aging Skin and Physical and Occupational Functioning

Aging skin does not generally have a direct impact on the physical functioning of an individual. However, when the individual depends on others to carry out their physical activities, an aging appearance can have an important effect on the type of care the individual receives (1). For example, it has been observed that caregivers in nursing homes and hospitals sometimes emotionally disengage from a patient when their grooming habits and hygiene and/or appearance begins to deteriorate or when the patient appears aged (9). Alternately, an improved appearance secondary to improved hair care and cosmetics has been associated with increased interest by the caregiver and even taken as evidence that the patient's physical state is improving (9). It is likely that the older individual in the community, who uses community resources to be able to maintain an independent lifestyle, also experiences similar reactions.

Physical appearance plays an important role in the business world, and professional image consultants help both men and women project confidence and authority through their appearance and their clothing (9). Society tends to equate both beauty and productivity with youth (10), a factor contributing to the age discrimination faced by older individuals, especially women (10), since the "double standard of aging" (11) continues to be an important factor in the workplace. It has been observed, however, that an increasing number of men are also seeking a youthful appearance with the use of hair coloring, topical skin exfoliators, and cosmetic surgery (10). In contrast to older men, older women tend to face these problems to a greater degree and at an earlier age (10,12). In a study involving 8 women (ranging in age from the late twenties to the sixties), photographs taken "before" and "after" cosmetic makeovers were attached to resumés and submitted to personnel interviewers in 120 major private employment agencies and large corporations (9). The variable of physical appearance was observed to play an important role in the hiring process in all skill levels with greatest differences noted for jobs requiring the lowest skill level where a better appearance (i.e., associated with the photograph "after" the cosmetic makeover) yielded a 8–20% higher salary for the applicant.

Aging Skin and the Psychological State

An aging appearance can have a significant psychological impact on the individual. Pearlman (13) describes a transitional developmental stage sometimes reaching the proportions of a developmental crisis, which she has termed "late mid-life astonishment" (13). She describes a psychological reaction to a sudden awareness of the acceleration and stigmatization of aging, which may manifest as amazement, despair, a disruption of one's sense of self or identity, feelings of heightened vulnerability, shame, depression, and severe loss of self-esteem (13). Other cofactors such as declining health and menopause can further lead to a sense of diminished physical and/or sexual attractiveness (13). Pearlman observes that in late midlife, it is no longer possible to "pass" as younger than one's chronological age, and this factor makes the psychological adjustment to aging more difficult. This may be one reason why studies involving topical treatment of photodamaged skin with topical tretinoin (6,7) and cosmetic makeovers to cover the cutaneous stigmata of aging (4,5) have been shown to be associated with an increased sense of well-being (4,5), increased ease during interpersonal interactions (4–7), and decreased anxiety (6,7).

The impact of aging skin on body image or mental representation of the body and its organs may generalize to concerns about overall body image not related directly to the skin (1). In a study of 71 men and 102 women, all of whom were non clinical subjects attending a shopping mall (14), it was observed that concerns about the effect of aging on the appearance correlated directly ($r \geq 0.4$; $p < 0.05$) with the Drive for Thinness subscale of the Eating Disorder Inventory (EDI) (15) even after the possible effects of body mass index (weight in kilograms divided by height in meters squared) and chronological age were partialled out statistically. This correlation was significant among both men and women. The Drive for Thinness subscale of the EDI measures an excessive preoccupation with dieting and exercise and an ardent desire to lose weight (15). Furthermore, among the women the belief that having young-looking skin is a prerequisite to good looks correlated directly with Drive for Thinness, (15) ($r = 0.3$; $p < 0.01$) and Body Dissatisfaction (15) ($r = 0.4$; $p < 0.01$), after the effects of age and body mass index were partialled out statistically. The Body Dissatisfaction subscale of the EDI (15) measures dissatisfaction with body shape and weight and measures the concern that certain body regions such as the abdomen, hips, and thighs are too fat. This finding was replicated among another randomly selected sample of nonclinical subjects (16). Furthermore, in a prospective, controlled study (16) of patients undergoing treatment for photodamaged skin with topical tretinoin or the inactive vehicle (the control group), it was observed that patients receiving the active treatment with topical tretinoin and not the control group, reported a significant decline ($p < 0.01$) in both Drive for Thinness and Body Dissatisfaction after 24 weeks (16). These findings highlight the significant impact of photodamaged skin on overall body image including aspects of body image that are not necessarily related to aging, in the population at large (3). A youthful look is typically associated with a slim and well-toned physique, and some individuals may become obsessively preoccupied with diet and exercise as they develop the cutaneous stigmata of aging (3). In the small subgroup of individuals who have other risk factors for the development of an eating disorder, the fear of aging precipitated by the cutaneous stigmata of aging can culminate in anorexia nervosa (3,17).

A psychological dimension that plays a critical role in the degree to which an individual is affected by cutaneous aging is the individual's internal locus of control or the degree to which an individual sees life's outcomes as being dependent upon their own abilities and efforts (1). It has been observed that patients who were concerned about their photodamaged skin and volunteered for studies (7) evaluating the efficacy of topical tretinoin also had obsessive-compulsive traits as measured by high obsessive-compulsiveness on the Brief Symptom Inventory (8). Obsessive-compulsiveness is associated with perfectionistic personality traits, a tendency to be excessively self-critical, and an inordinate need to be in control of one's life (8). These personality traits probably predisposed these subjects to seek treatment for their wrinkles (7). After 24 weeks of therapy with topical tretinoin, the subjects reported a decrease in obsessive-compulsiveness, however, those receiving the inactive vehicle reported an increase in this symptom dimension (7). These findings also suggest that life events that adversely affect an individual's internal locus of control may heighten their concern about their aging appearance and predispose them to seek treatment for their aging skin (3). Patients with severely narcissistic personalities may develop a major adjustment disorder in reaction to the cutaneous stigmata of aging (1,3). Among such patients who have a desperate need to be admired, having a youthful appearance is often a precondition for self-acceptance and trusting that they will be accepted by others, and aging appearance can result in a significant emotional crisis (1,3).

SUMMARY

A review of the literature (1–3) suggests that cutaneous aging can affect many aspects of quality of life. The review further suggests that when assessing the patient who is requesting therapies for cutaneous photodamage, it is important for the clinician to address the psychosocial dimension. The busy dermatologist may wish to screen for whether or not psychosocial factors are important in any particular patient by, for example, enquiring why the patient had decided to seek treatments for cutaneous aging and/or photodamage at that particular time. The role of psychosocial issues, if important, is likely to emerge in the response to such a question. Some patients may also have unrealistic expectations of what treatment has to offer and should be counseled, since otherwise they are likely to be dissatisfied with treatment outcome.

In contrast to most dermatological conditions, aging and/or photodamaged skin lies within the spectrum of normal human experience, since everyone (if lucky enough to have a long life) is likely to experience some cutaneous changes related to aging and/or photodamage. Therefore there is most likely a wide variation in the degree to which an individual will consider cutaneous aging and/or photodamage to be a dermatological problem. This is most likely the reason why some preliminary studies (6,7) indicate a wide variance in the responses of individuals to typical questions addressing quality of life and aging and/or photodamaged skin. Further research is required to develop more sensitive instruments that can reliably measure the impact of cutaneous aging and/or photodamage on quality of life.

REFERENCES

1. Gupta MA, Gupta AK. Photodamaged skin and quality of life: reasons for therapy. J Dermatol Treat 1996; 7(4): 261–264.
2. Kligman AM. Psychological aspects of skin disorders in the elderly. Cutis 1989; 43: 489–501.
3. Gupta MA. The aging face: a psychocutaneous perspective. Facial Plast Surg 1995; 11: 86–90.
4. Kligman AM, Graham JA. The psychology of appearance in the elderly. Dermatol Clin 1986; 4: 501–507.
5. Graham JA, Kligman AM. Physical attractiveness, cosmetic use and self-perception in the elderly. Int J Cosmet Sci 1985; 7: 85–97.
6. Gupta MA, Goldfarb MT, Schork NJ, Weiss JS, Gupta AK, Ellis CN, Voorhees JJ. Treatment of mildly to moderately photoaged skin with topical tretinoin has a favorable psychosocial effect: a prospective study. J Am Acad Dermatol 1991; 24: 780–781.
7. Gupta MA, Schork NJ, Ellis CN. Psychosocial correlates of the treatment of photodamaged skin with topical retinoic acid: a prospective controlled study. J Am Acad Dermatol 1994; 30: 969–972.
8. Derogatis LR, Spencer PM. The Brief Symptom Inventory (BSI), Administration, Scoring and Procedures manual—I. Baltimore: Clinical Psychometric Research, Johns Hopkins University, 1982.
9. Waters J. Cosmetics and the job market. In: Graham JA, Kligman AM, eds. The psychology of cosmetic treatments. New York: Praeger, 1986: 113–124.

10. Rodeheaver D. Labor market progeria. Gender Aging, Generations 1990; (Summer): 53–58.
11. Sontag S. The double standard of aging. In: Williams J, ed. Psychology of Women. New York: Academic Press, 1979: 462–478.
12. Hutchens RM. "Do job opportunities decline with age?" Ind Labor Relat Rev 1988; 42: 89–99.
13. Pearlman SF. Late mid-life astonishment: disruptions to identify and self-esteem. Women Ther 1993; 14: 1–12.
14. Gupta MA, Schork NJ. Aging-related concerns and body image: possible future implications for eating disorders. Int J Eating Disord 1993; 14: 481–486.
15. Garner DM, Olmstead MP. Eating Disorder Inventory Manual. Lutz, FL: Psychological Assessment Resources, 1984.
16. Gupta MA. Concern about aging and a drive for thinness: a factor in the biopsychosocial model of eating disorders? Int J Eating Disord 1995; 18: 351–357.
17. Gupta MA. Fear of aging: a precipitating factor in late onset anorexia nervosa. Int J Eating Disord 1990; 9: 221–224.

20

Measuring Quality of Life in Recurrent Genital Herpes

Stephen P. McKenna and Lynda C. Doward Galen Research, Manchester, England

OVERVIEW

Genital herpes is an episodic viral infection that affects millions of people throughout the world. The adverse effects of recurrent genital herpes on quality of life relate not only to the clinical manifestations of the illness but also to the social stigma surrounding it. For some individuals the psychological impact of recurrent genital herpes can result in anger, depression, anxiety, decreased libido, diminished self-esteem, and fear of rejection or discovery. It is becoming relatively common to demonstrate the impact of pharmaceutical and other treatments on the quality of life of patients, but there has been little use of standardized measures of health status to assess the impact of recurrent genital herpes on nonclinical aspects of patients' lives.

A new measure to assess quality of life in patients with recurrent genital herpes (the RGHQoL) has been developed for use in clinical trials in the United Kingdom. It is based on the hypothesis that quality of life relates to the ability and capacity of an individual to satisfy his or her human needs.

Quality of life is at its highest when these needs are fulfilled and at its lowest when few needs are satisfied.

While the initial development work was undertaken in the United Kingdom conceptually equivalent versions were required for five European countries and the United States. The present chapter describes the initial development work and the production of the U.K. version of the instrument. The content of the RGHQoL was derived from interviews with individuals in the United Kingdom who experience recurrent genital herpes. The items are expressed, as far as possible, in the words of the patients, and consequently respondents find the measure comprehensive and highly relevant to their condition. The RGHQoL is shown to be reliable and valid.

INTRODUCTION

Genital herpes is an episodic viral infection that affects millions of people worldwide (1). For most people who contract it, genital herpes is an inconvenient but benign self-limiting infection (2). However, a number of factors influence the impact of the disease. These include the unpredictability of the timing of outbreaks, the area affected by the lesions, its association with sexual behavior, and misleading and sensational media coverage.

A large psychological burden falls on those who are infected (2). Recurrent genital herpes (RGH) can have a major negative effect on the emotional well-being of sufferers (3). For some individuals the psychological impact of the disease can result in reactions such as anger, depression, anxiety, decreased libido, and diminished self-esteem (4). These responses may be serious enough to require clinical attention (1).

Because the condition is incurable, feelings of lack of control over life and helplessness can develop together with frustration over the inadequacy of commonly used treatments, fears of the effects on sexual behavior, and anxiety about future recurrences and nonsymptomatic contagion (2). Some patients view the illness as a punishment, as a sign of personal weakness, as an enemy, and, occasionally, as a challenge (5,6).

In a survey of 3000 members of self-help groups in California, a majority of respondents reported that recurrent genital herpes had a profound effect on their sexual functioning (2). British studies have reported male impotence following initial diagnosis, although this improves over time (3,7). Fear of forming relationships and of rejection may affect the capacity for physical warmth and intimacy and the enjoyment of sex. The disorder may also lead to a loss of sexual confidence and adversely affect feelings of sexual desirability (7). Several studies have shown that at least half of those surveyed experience a reduction in the frequency of sex (2,4). Approximately 10% of patients with genital herpes adopt a celibate lifestyle (3).

Coverage of the illness in the media has made it more difficult for individuals both to admit to having herpes and to disguise the fact. Infected individuals often believe that they will not be sexually or socially acceptable once their secret is known (1,6). Herpes has been called the "new sexual leprosy" (*Time*, July 28, 1980) and the "new scarlet letter" (*Time*, August 2, 1982). Telling a partner can lead to arguments or to the breakdown of the relationship. Consequently, the adverse effects of genital herpes on quality of life result from both the disorder itself and the condemnatory climate that surrounds it.

It is clear that recurrent genital herpes has a profound psychological impact on patients and, consequently, a major effect on their quality of life.

Measuring the Impact of Recurrent Genital Herpes

There has been little use of standardized measures to assess the impact of genital herpes on non-clinical aspects of patients' lives. Goldmeier et al. (8) employed the General Health Questionnaire (GHQ) and the Eysenck Personality Inventory (EPI) in a comparison of patients with primary attacks and those experiencing recurrent episodes. However, neither measure is particularly suitable for assessing the illness. The GHQ is designed to identify psychiatric cases, and the EPI is of questionable value in health research.

Carney (9) used the Hospital Anxiety and Depression scale (HAD) and the GHQ to assess the effectiveness of oral acyclovir in the treatment of genital herpes. Results from the GHQ were inconclusive, but the HAD showed a reduction in anxiety with treatment.

Three herpes-specific questionnaires have been developed. The Genital Herpes Questionnaire, covering sexual functioning, interpersonal relationships, emotional reactions, self-concept, and effects on work or school, was developed by Drob in the United States (6). A second questionnaire was produced at the Herpes Research Center in the United States and contains 183 items exploring social relationships, self-image, sexual attitudes and behavior, psychological reactions, and effects on work performance and enjoyment (4). The length of this measure makes it impractical for use in a clinical setting.

A scale assessing knowledge and attitudes towards genital herpes has also been produced (10). This was intended to explore myths and fears about the illness, rather than its impact on patients.

Quality of Life

It is becoming increasingly common to investigate the impact of pharmaceutical and other interventions on the quality of life of patients. However, rather than present a theory or model of the construct, test authors tend to define "quality of life" in terms of a varying number of components, all of which require measurement. These differ between instruments but commonly include physical, social, and emotional well-being and functioning. Without a theoretical basis it is not possible to establish that such measures have construct validity, a fundamental requirement of all measurement (11). Unlike clinical indicators and measures of symptoms, if an instrument is intended to assess quality of life, the questions must derive directly from relevant patients. Many generic instruments that have been referred to as measures of quality of life, such as the SF-36 (12) and the EuroQOL (13), are unsuitable for assessing the health status of patients with recurrent genital herpes because much of their content is inappropriate to this patient group.

Recently, a model of quality of life has been proposed that postulates that life gains its quality from the ability and capacity of the individual to satisfy his or her human needs (14). Quality of life is at its highest when these needs are fulfilled and at its lowest when few needs are satisfied. Different illnesses interfere with the fulfillment of different needs. Consequently it is possible to develop condition-specific measures that are able to determine the impact of the illness and its treatment on the quality of life of the patient.

Such an approach has a number of positive features. As the instrument focuses on needs rather than functioning, questions that are irrelevant to certain respondents are avoided. For example, many patients with recurrent genital herpes do not currently have a sexual partner. Rather than ask directly about sexual behavior, it is possible to look at the needs satisfied by such behavior that may be satisfied in other ways. Thus, questions about sharing, intimacy, and touch are relevant to all respondents, whether or not they are in a sexual relationship.

A second advantage of the needs approach is that measures based on this model can cope with adaptation to chronic illness. Patients with recurrent genital herpes will adapt their lifestyle to allow for the limitations imposed by their illness. For example, such a patient may avoid spending time away from home, making new sexual relationships, or taking part in sports that involve communal washing and dressing facilities. Such activities may be replaced by others, which can be equally satisfying. A measure of the satisfaction of needs will avoid questions about particular functions and activities, which may have been replaced.

The remainder of this chapter will discuss the development of a new measure of quality of life specific to patients with recurrent genital herpes, which is based on the conceptual model of needs fulfillment. The measure was required for use in a clinical trial to be conducted in five European countries and the United States. While the initial development work was undertaken in the United Kingdom, conceptually equivalent versions were required for each country. The present chapter describes the initial development work and the production of the U.K. version of the instrument.

DEVELOPING THE RECURRENT GENITAL HERPES QUALITY-OF-LIFE QUESTIONNAIRE

Patient Interviews

Two genito-urinary consultants in northern England were approached and agreed to assist the researchers in the recruitment of patients for interview. All patients with recurrent genital herpes attending outpatient clinics were asked whether they would be willing to meet an interviewer. In this way it was possible to recruit patients who had a range of severity of illness. If the patient agreed to be interviewed, he or she was given the telephone number and address of the researcher to arrange a convenient appointment. When a patient called, the purpose of the interviews was explained and, if the patient was still willing to participate, an appointment was made for the interview.

Interviews took place either at the home of the patient or, if preferred, at the researcher's base. Interviewees were assured of the confidential nature of the interviews and were told that they could terminate the meeting at any time.

Participants were interviewed individually by a researcher of the same sex. Interviewees were encouraged to discuss the effects of herpes on their daily life and to raise any aspect of their experience of herpes that they considered important. While the interviews were unstructured, the interviewer had a list of topics to be raised if they had not arisen spontaneously. These topics included personal relationships, occupational difficulties, social activity, leisure pursuits, emotional reactions, and self-confidence. This list had been derived from a review of the work of the major theorists in the field of motivation and had been employed in the development of a previous quality-of-life measure (14).

With the consent of the interviewee, the conversations were audio-recorded. One of the participants preferred not to be recorded, and in that case comprehensive notes were taken by the interviewer and written up as soon as possible after the interview.

The recordings were transcribed and all clues to the identity of the interviewee were removed. After transcription, the tapes were wiped clean, thus ensuring the anonymity of the written transcripts.

Twenty-six patients (12 men and 14 women) between 23 and 54 years of age were interviewed. The interviews lasted between three quarters of an hour and 3 hours. None were prematurely terminated. Many of the participants reported that the interview had been of value in allowing them a rare opportunity to discuss, with a sympathetic outsider, their problems with and attitudes towards genital herpes.

Findings from the Interviews

This section reports comments commonly made during the interviews, with isolated events and experiences excluded. It is important to note that the reported impact of the illness on the interviewees varied considerably. While some claimed that their lives were severely affected, others reported that it was a minor inconvenience that did not concern them greatly. However, all interviewees had sought treatment for their genital herpes, and such a decision was likely to have been influenced by the extent to which their quality of life had been adversely affected.

For most respondents, having herpes had profoundly affected their quality of life. Some of the issues raised were related to how they had contracted the infection and whether or not a partner had been unfaithful or untruthful. Thus, where individuals were in a sexual partnership at the time they contracted herpes, suspicion and doubt entered their relationship. Partnerships became strained, leading to feelings of insecurity.

Sometimes it appeared that a "pact of ignorance" had been agreed upon, whereby both partners knew that one or both of them had herpes but neither referred to it. This resulted in a reduction in feelings of intimacy. Moreover, because of the perceived problems associated with forming new partnerships, some interviewees felt trapped in their current (sometimes unsatisfactory) relationship. Some participants went to considerable lengths to conceal the fact that they had herpes. These included making excuses for not having sex and hiding medication.

Almost all interviewees felt that there was a stigma attached to having herpes and were afraid of friends and family finding out. Genital herpes was associated in most people's minds with promiscuity, even when they knew that this did not apply to them personally. Most interviewees reported having had only two or three sexual partners. Individuals described themselves as feeling dirty and contaminated, feeling like a "leper," feeling ashamed, and having suffered a blow to their self-esteem. Some felt anger towards the person (known or unknown) who had infected them.

Many people lived in dread of their next attack. Consequently, they felt that they could never forget that they had herpes. Some individuals reported bouts of depression and self-blame. There was a fear of rejection if others should find out or of becoming the object of gossip.

Some people had strategies that they believed could stave off an outbreak. These included taking frequent baths, putting on lotion, and avoiding tight clothes, sexual intercourse, and "stress." In some cases it was believed that worry could initiate an outbreak. Consequently, worrying about the next outbreak became a vicious circle.

The uncertainty associated with when an outbreak would occur meant that it was difficult to plan for outings and other social occasions. There was a reluctance to stay in other people's homes because of fears of contaminating towels or toilets.

The respondents' major fear was of passing on the infection to others, and this led some interviewees to give up all sexual relationships. Even where this was not the case, sex was often accompanied by the anxiety that the infection would be passed on, even though precautions were taken. In some instances, people had developed a fear of physical contact and were reluctant to touch others or to be touched. Respondents with children were particularly afraid of infecting them and sometimes took elaborate precautions to prevent it happening. Moreover, the possibility that the children would find out caused respondents a great deal of anxiety.

A small number of the interviewees did not regard having herpes as a serious problem and treated it much like any other infection, as a minor inconvenience.

Many people complained about the length of time it had taken for them to have the condition correctly diagnosed. In particular, general practitioners had been found to be unwilling or unable to diagnose genital herpes, and patients had been told that they had a "cold sore" or a fungal infection. One interviewee had waited 2 years before receiving a correct diagnosis. Naturally, during the interval between presenting with the symptoms and receiving a correct diagnosis, some individuals had, unwittingly, passed on the infection. This caused them feelings of guilt and, in some cases, anger towards their doctor.

General practitioners were reported to be generally unsympathetic, in some cases apparently sharing the common stereotype of genital herpes as a sign of promiscuous sexual behavior. There was a lack of support for herpes sufferers and insufficient counseling available. Possibly as a consequence, there was considerable confusion about the facts. Interviewees were unsure about when they were infectious and for how long, in how many ways and by what routes the infection could be passed to others, and if there were long-term adverse effects of medication. Some women wanted to know more about the implications of becoming pregnant and if, and how, the infection might be transmitted to the baby.

Drug costs largely fall on the national health service in the United Kingdom, and problems associated with the cost of suppression therapy arose. Conflict between hospital consultants and general practitioners was reported. Where the clinic had recommended suppression, general practitioners (particularly those who had responsibility for their own budgets) were often reluctant or unwilling to prescribe the medication.

Constructing the Draft Questionnaire

The interviews were transcribed and then content analyzed to identify potential questionnaire items. Items were chosen for the measure using the following criteria:

They were commonly reported by interviewees.
They were short and expressed a single idea.
They used the respondents' own words, as far as possible.
They were applicable to all potential respondents.
They were consonant with the needs-based quality-of-life model (14).
They appeared suitable for translation into other European languages.

This last criterion was important because of the need to develop other language versions. The decision on the suitability of items for translation was based on the extensive experience of the authors in adapting patient-completed measures for use in other languages (see for example, Ref. 15). A pool of 54 potential items (some of which were alternative wordings for the same concept) was created, which was considered large enough to allow for rejection of items at later stages in the developmental process.

An international panel was then convened to consider the suitability of the 54 items for translation. The panel consisted of researchers from each of the countries in which the Recurrent Genital Herpes Quality-of-Life scale (RGHQoL) was required: the United Kingdom, the United States, France, Spain, Italy, Germany, and Denmark. The meeting lasted 2 days, and the participants considered the most appropriate response format and questionnaire instructions in addition to the cultural relevance and translatability of the individual items. Following the meeting, 27 items remained and were used in the first draft of the questionnaire.

It was decided that the content of the measure should be in the form of personal statements, in the original words of the interviewees where possible. Previous work has suggested that such a format has the greatest immediacy and appeal to respondents (16). A dichotomous response system ("yes"/"no") was considered most suitable for the different language versions. The RGHQoL items were scored 1 for a response that indicated that a need was not being met and 0 where the need was fulfilled. Item scores were then summed to give an overall score on the measure, with a high score indicating poor quality of life.

TESTING THE PSYCHOMETRIC PROPERTIES OF THE RGHQoL

Selecting the right questions is the most important stage in the development of any health status or quality of life instrument. However, it is also essential to establish that the instrument has adequate psychometric properties, in particular, that it is reliable and valid.

Field-Testing for Face and Content Validity

A new sample of 20 patients with recurrent genital herpes was recruited from the same clinics as the interviewees and two further clinics in northern England. The respondents were asked to complete the RGHQoL in the presence of an interviewer. Note was taken of any difficulties observed by the interviewer or reported by the respondent. After completing the measure, patients were asked to comment on the items and response system. In particular, they were asked whether they thought any of the items were irrelevant and whether any important aspects of their experience had been omitted. Overall, the respondents found the instrument acceptable, understandable, and relevant. Minor changes to the wording of items were made as a result of the field-test interviews. None of the respondents suggested additional areas for inclusion in the measure. Scores ranged from 1 to 23, with a median score of 13.

As a result of field-testing in other countries, four items were removed from the draft questionnaire. The item "I have to tell lies about my illness" was thought to be unacceptable to respondents in the United States. Two items, "I worry about the future" and "I have to be careful what I wear," were considered too ambiguous by respondents in several countries, particularly in the United States. The item "Herpes puts a strain on my personal relationships" was rejected because it was seen as ambiguous by many respondents with partners and considered irrelevant by others without partners.

The field-testing in different countries suggested that there were some differences in the perception of the impact of recurrent genital herpes. In particular, it was found that genital herpes was considered a less severe illness by patients in the United States and Denmark than in the United Kingdom. Consequently, a new response format was produced which consisted of four alternative responses for each item. It was intended that such a response format would minimize ceiling and basement effects in the different countries. With the new format, items are scored from 0 to 3, with, as before, 0 indicating that the need is met.

A second field test was undertaken with seven patients recruited from one of the clinics in northern England to test the acceptability of the new response format. Again the measure was found to be acceptable to the respondents whose scores ranged from 19 to 55. Examples of the items in the measure and the new response categories are shown in Figure 1.

Testing the Reliability and Construct Validity of the U.K. Version of the RGHQoL

A new sample of 39 patients with recurrent genital herpes was recruited from the same clinics as before. Patients were sent the quality-of-life instrument, a demographic questionnaire, and a reply-paid envelope. They were

1. HERPES MAKES IT DIFFICULT FOR ME TO PLAN AHEAD

Yes, very difficult ☐

Yes, quite difficult ☐

Yes, a little difficult ☐

No, not at all difficult ☐

2. I WORRY THAT SEX WILL TRIGGER AN OUTBREAK

Yes, I worry a great deal ☐

Yes, I worry quite a lot ☐

Yes, I worry about it a little ☐

No, I don't worry about it at all ☐

Figure 1 Sample items on the RGHQoL.

asked to complete the two questionnaires and return them in the envelope provided. If they had a herpes attack at the time they received the package, they were asked to delay completing the questionnaires. Thirty-six patients returned completed questionnaires. These patients were sent a similar package (excluding the demographic questionnaire) to arrive 2 weeks after they completed the first set of questionnaires.

Thirty-four of those approached on the second occasion (12 men and 22 women) returned a completed questionnaire. The high overall response rate (87%) is very good considering the intimate nature of the items and reflects the acceptability of the measure to patients. Furthermore, none of the returned questionnaires contained missing data. The respondents were aged between 20 and 49 years. A majority (21) of the patients reported that they had had genital herpes for between 1 and 5 years. Three respondents had had the condition for less than a year, and one reported having had herpes for more than 10 years. Less than half of the sample (46%) were living with a partner at the time of the study. Twenty-four (71%) of the respondents had experienced four or more herpes outbreaks in the previous year.

Internal Consistency

This statistic indicates the extent to which items in a scale are interrelated. A Cronbach's alpha value of 0.85 or above is required to indicate adequate consistency (16). The alpha values for the RGHQoL were 0.95 at Time 1 and 0.94 at Time 2. Although this showed that the new measure had adequate consistency, three of the items were found to have low correlations with the total score on the measure. These items were "I enjoy mixing with other people," "I am satisfied with my sex life," and "I enjoy being cuddled." It is interesting to note that these were the only positive items in the scale. It would appear that the respondents treated these items differently from the negative items, finding it difficult to admit to dissatisfaction in these areas. Consequently, the three positive items were removed from the measure. Statistical analyses were then conducted on the remaining 20 items.

Reliability

Any measure designed for use in clinical trials must be shown to be reliable. This is because scores obtained from an unreliable measure will be made up of the true score plus high levels of random measurement error. Such error can mask changes in score associated with treatment and reduce the sensitivity of the measure. If a measure is reliable, patients will obtain the same score each time they complete it, assuming that their health status does not change between administrations of the instrument. However, health status is rarely stable and no measure is perfectly reliable. The best method of assessing reliability is the "test-retest" method, in which a group of relevant patients is asked to complete the instrument twice and scores on the two applications are correlated. Where an instrument is intended to show change over time or to compare alternative interventions, a correlation coefficient of 0.85 or above is desirable (17).

Scores on the measure for the group as a whole were stable (the mean was 29.9 on the first administration and 31.2 on the second). The Spearman rank test-retest correlation coefficient was 0.90 ($p < 0.001$).

Construct Validity

A valid instrument is one that measures what it is intended to, without any systematic bias. Various methods of assessing the validity of a measure are available. The most appropriate for testing the validity of the RGHQoL would be to compare scores with some other index of quality of life (a gold standard). This was not possible given that no other such measure was available. Therefore, construct (discriminate) validity was assessed by comparing scores on the quality-of-life measure with the severity of the condition, as perceived by the patient. The demographic questionnaire employed in the study included a question that asked the respondents to rate the severity of their typical herpes outbreaks as mild, moderate, or severe.

It was hypothesized that patients who perceived themselves to have severe outbreaks of herpes would have worse quality-of-life scores. Thirty-three patients answered the question on severity of their outbreaks. Mean scores for patients rating their outbreaks mild, moderate, or severe are shown in Table 1 (for the 20-item measure, scores can range from 0 to 60). On both administrations of the measure there were statistically significant differences in mean quality-of-life score for the three levels of perceived severity.

Further tests of the RGHQoL's validity will be conducted. For example, it is necessary to show that the instrument can detect improve-

Table 1 Quality of Life by Patient-Rated Severity of Condition

Rated severity of condition	Time 1 (*n*)	Time 2 (*n*)
Mild	43.4 (5)	46.6 (5)
Moderate	30.8 (18)	32.0 (17)
Severe	21.4 (10)	22.9 (11)
Probability	0.03	0.01

ments in quality of life associated with effective suppression of herpes outbreaks. However, given the care taken in the generation of the items, it is reasonable to assume that the measure is valid.

CONCLUSIONS

The RGHQoL is based on a clear, conceptual model of quality of life that has been successfully employed in the development of a number of disease-specific quality-of-life instruments (18–23). The content of the measure is derived from individuals who experience recurrent genital herpes. The items are expressed, as far as possible, in the words of the patients, and, consequently, respondents find the measure comprehensive and highly relevant to their condition. The RGHQoL is quick and easy to administer and complete, making it suitable for use in clinical trials. The RGHQoL has been shown to be reliable and valid. As a result, confidence can be placed in the scores obtained by respondents.

Tests of the psychometric properties of the other language versions of the RGHQoL have recently been completed with satisfactory results (see, e.g., Ref. 24), and the instrument has been included in a multinational clinical trial. Data from the trial will provide further evidence of the validity of the RGHQoL and will demonstrate whether or not the instrument is responsive to changes in quality of life associated with effective suppression of herpes outbreaks.

ACKNOWLEDGMENTS

The authors wish to acknowledge the Wellcome Foundation for funding this research, as well as Dr. P. Woolley, Dr. G. Kinghorn, Dr. T. Chatterjee, Dr. B. Ghosh, Dr. M. Moola, Dr. G. Adhya, Sandra Herman, Sue Evans, and Janet Ford for their help in recruiting patients. The contributions of Sonja Hunt, Judy Tyrrell, and Diane Whalley to the project are also acknowledged. Not least, we would like to thank the many interviewees and respondents for their help in the development and testing of the new measure.

REFERENCES

1. Hunt SM, Kovachich P, McKenna SP. Genital herpes and quality of life. Br J Sex Med 1993; (January/February): 12–15.
2. Bierman S. Recurrent genital herpes simplex infection: a trivial disorder. Arch Dermatol 1985; 121: 513–517.
3. Woolley P, Kinghorn GR. Psychological aspects of genital herpes. Stress Med 1986; 2: 193–195.

4. Luby ED, Klinge V. Genital herpes. A pervasive psychosocial disorder. Arch Dermatol 1985; 121: 494–497.
5. Liponsky P. Physical illness, the individual and the coping process. Psychiatr Med 1970; 1: 91–102.
6. Drob S, Loemer M, Lifshutz H. Genital herpes. The psychological consequences. Br J Med Psychol 1985; 58: 307–315.
7. Mindel A, Carney O. Herpes: What It Is and How to Cope. London: Positive Health Guides, MacDonald Optima, 1991.
8. Goldmeier D, Johnson A, Byrne M, Barton S. Psychological implications of recurrent genital herpes. Genitourin Med 1988; 64: 327–330.
9. Carney O. Psychosocial/Psychosexual aspects of genital herpes. Recurrent Genital Herpes. A Management Focus. Paris: The Wellcome Foundation, 1991.
10. Bruce KEM, McLaughlin J. The development of scales to assess knowledge and attitudes about genital herpes. J Sex Res 1986; 22: 73–84.
11. Streiner D, Norman G. Health Measurement Scales. Oxford: Oxford University Press, 1989.
12. Brazier JE, Harper R, Jones NMB, O'Cathain A, Thomas KJ, Usherwood T, Westlake L. Validating the SF-36 health survey questionnaire: new outcome measure for primary care. Br Med J 1992; 305: 160–164.
13. EuroQOL Group. EuroQOL—a new facility for the measurement of health related quality of life. Health Policy 1990; 16: 199–208.
14. Hunt SM, McKenna SP. The QLDS. A scale for the measurement of quality of life in depression. Health Policy 1992; 22: 307–319.
15. Hunt SM, Alonso J, Bucquet D, Niero M, Wiklund I, McKenna SP. Cross-cultural adaptation of health measures. Health Policy 1991; 19: 33–44.
16. McDowell I, Newell C. Measuring Health: A Guide to Rating Scales and Questionnaires. Oxford: Oxford University Press, 1987.
17. Weiner E, Stewart B. Assessing Individuals. Boston: Little Brown, 1984.
18. McKenna SP, Hunt SM. A new measure of quality of life in depression: testing the reliability and construct validity of the QLDS. Health Policy 1992; 22: 321–330.
19. Holmes SJ, McKenna SP, Doward LC, Shalet SM. Development of a questionnaire to assess the quality of life of adults with growth hormone deficiency. Endocrinol Metab 1995; 2: 63–69.
20. McKenna SP, Patrick D. The development of a migraine-specific quality of life measure for multi-national clinical trials. Cephalalgia 1995; 15(suppl 14): 280.
21. Wagner TH, Patrick DL, McKenna SP, Froese MA. Cross-cultural development of a quality of life measure for men with erection difficulties. Qual Life Res 1996; 5: 443–449.
22. Whalley D, McKenna SP, de Jong Z, van der Heijde D. Quality of life in rheumatoid arthritis. Br J Rheumatol 1997; 36: 884–888.
23. de Jong Z, van der Heijde D, McKenna SP, Whalley D. The reliability and construct validity of the RAQoL: a rheumatoid arthritis-specific quality of life instrument. Br J Rheumatol 1997; 36: 878–883.

24. Wild D, Patrick DL, Johnson E. Measuring health-related quality of life in persons with genital herpes. Qual Life Res 1995; 4:532–539.

21

Comparative Cost-Effectiveness of Different Treatments for Psoriasis

Gary C. Lee and Gerald D. Weinstein *University of California, Irvine, Irvine, California*

INTRODUCTION

Psoriasis is a chronic, inflammatory disorder that affects about 2–3% of the U.S. population (1–3% of the world's population), which translates to approximately 6.4 million individuals (1). The annual cost of caring for these patients is enormous. In a 1984 survey (2), 2.3 million patients with psoriasis spent an average of $650 each year on medication costs, laboratory tests, and physician charges. The estimated cost for treating outpatients with psoriasis in 1984 was $1.5 billion per year. A more recent report discloses that the average annual cost of psoriasis care using systemic therapies ranges from $1130 to $6650 (3). Assuming that 20% of all psoriatic patients require some form of systemic therapy (4), the estimated average annual cost of caring for these patients alone is at least $1.5 billion!

The recent introduction of calcipotriene and cyclosporine (not approved in the United States) for the treatment of psoriasis adds further complexity to the already existing options. Physicians need to become familiarized with the therapeutic index of each available treatment modality and—especially in the current managed care climate—the pharmacoeconomics of these treatment options. This will facilitate the choice of the best or most appropriate treatment for our patients as well as the most economical one.

There are many subtypes of psoriasis, including the guttate, erythrodermic, pustular, and arthritic variants. The present discussion is limited to the most common type: chronic plaque psoriasis. The available treatment modalities for psoriasis can be divided into two main categories: topical and photo-/systemic (systemic) therapies. The great majority of patients—approximately 80%—are candidates for topical therapy, with limited or mild psoriasis affecting less than 20% of their body surface area (BSA). The advantages of topical therapy are that these medications are easy to use and side effects are usually localized to the site of application. The most effective topical therapies—topical corticosteroids, calcipotriene, and tazarotene—are discussed in detail later. However, if the disease is more severe and/or affects more than approximately 20% of BSA, topical therapy becomes impractical because of a lower therapeutic index, inconvenience, and expense. Systemic therapy (including phototherapies) should be considered for moderate to severe disease in patients with physically, socially extensive, or economically disabling psoriasis that has not responded to topical treatment. The five most effective systemic therapies are UVB, PUVA, etretinate, methotrexate, and cyclosporin, and they are discussed later.

COSTS OF THERAPY

The cost of each treatment modality is based on the:

Expense of medications
Frequency of administration
Medication dosage
Maintenance requirements
Extent (percentage) of BSA involvement (for topical therapies)
Frequency and type of laboratory tests
Physicians' fees

Certain caveats must be considered in developing these estimates. The cost of medications varies by the source of availability to the patient—local pharmacy, managed care organization, etc. The drug costs used here are the wholesale prices quoted in the 1996 Drug Topics Red Book. Larger purchasing organizations are able to get discounts of these prices, while smaller pharmacies may mark up these prices perhaps 30% or more. Evaluating the price list of a mail order pharmacy working in collaboration with the National Psoriasis Foundation, we found that their retail prices seem to closely match those of the Red Book prices quoted in this chapter. The information herein is presented with relative consistency based on the Red Book prices. The final price to the patient may be higher or lower across the board based on the pharmacy arrangements.

Since doctors' fees vary depending on health care systems and geographical and other factors, they are *not* included in the present analysis. The cost of anticipated treatments over one year are extrapolated and compared. Hopefully, analysis of the costs of available therapies together with their therapeutic indices will allow practitioners to choose the most cost-effective treatments.

TOPICAL THERAPIES

Topical Corticosteroids

Currently, topical corticosteroids are the most widely used treatment for psoriasis in North America. In 1990, about $90 million was spent on various strengths of topical corticosteroids in the treatment of psoriasis (Table 1). Although they do not cure the condition and are associated with a number of side effects (infra vide), potent topical corticosteroids are consistently effective, with action at least as fast as that of other recognized methods of topical treatments (e.g., coal tar, anthralin). Moreover, topical corticosteroids are available in a wide range of potency and formulations, none of which causes irritation or staining of skin or clothing, and they can be easily applied by patients at home. All these factors encourage compliance.

Although serious side effects are rare in the short term (5), chronic topical corticosteroid use causes local cutaneous atrophy, striae (which can occur at the application site or elsewhere secondary to steroid absorption), telangiectasia, folliculitis, perioral dermatitis, and other infrequent

Table 1 Use of Topical Corticosteroid by Class for Psoriasis in the United States (1990)

Strength	Total scripts (in millions $)	% Psoriasis	Spending on psoriasis (in millions $)
Superpotent	51	58	30
High/medium	197	29	57
Low	26	16	4
Total steroid for psoriasis	274	33	91

problems. Serious systemic side effects, including adrenal suppression and Cushing's syndrome, are well established but fortunately rare as long as the corticosteroids are not used on large body surface areas. The availability of more systemic therapies has limited extensive topical steroid usage (6,7). Fortunately, when topical corticosteroids are prescribed appropriately and patients are monitored carefully, side effects can usually be avoided.

The most difficult problem with topical corticosteroids is the induction of tolerance or resistance (tachyphylaxis) to the pharmacological action of this family of drugs (8). The maintenance of response with or without continued use of steroids is lost in 3–6 months (4). Limited responsiveness is usually regained after steroid-free rest periods.

For the majority of patients with plaque type psoriasis, potent corticosteroids (class 1 or 2) or less potent products with occlusion using hydrocolloid dressing (9) or plastic wrap (Saran®) (at the expense of increased local and systemic side effects) are needed to maximize improvement and potentially longer remissions. A recent study indeed shows that 62% of dermatologists surveyed choose potent to superpotent topical corticosteroids as their initial topical treatment for plaque-type psoriasis (4).

It is difficult to select the best or most appropriate topical corticosteroid from the multitude of products and studies that differ in efficacy. In a double-blind comparison of 0.5% betamethasone dipropionate, 0.5% diflorasone diacetate, and a vehicle alone in which all were applied as ointment once daily for 3 weeks by 139 patients with psoriasis, the condition improved of 57, 37, and 21% of patients respectively (5). The study also suggested that once-daily treatment with a topical corticosteroid may be as effective as the more conventional twice-daily regimen. It has been suggested that the most effective time to apply a single dose of topical corticosteroid is in the late afternoon (10).

There is still much debate about the equivalency of generic to brand-name topical corticosteroids (11–13). Generic and brand-name products may be chemically equivalent (in terms of the amount of the corticosteroid moiety) and biologically equivalent (in terms of their activity in vasoconstrictor assay) but not therapeutically equivalent (i.e., same safety and efficacy data derived from actual clinical trials in patients with plaque-type psoriasis vulgaris) (13).

The schedule of maintenance therapy, after the initial control with potent topical corticosteroid, is yet another unsettled issue. The majority of clinical trials on topical corticosteroids dosing are short-term only, and are designed to measure improvement rather than complete resolution of signs and symptoms of the disease (11). Thus, an appropriate dosing is crucial if topical corticosteroid is to be used solely for maintenance therapy and to

Table 2 Average Wholesale Cost[a] ($/g) of class 1, 2, and 3 Corticosteroids

	Cost of ointment	Cost of cream	Average cost of ointment/ cream	Relative cost
Class 1[b]				
Brand-name	0.86–1.09	0.86–1.09	1.01	1.17
Generic	0.82–1.13	0.82–0.85	0.86	1.0
Class 2[c]				
Brand-name	0.58–0.95	0.58–0.95	0.72	2.0
Generic	0.17–0.70	0.16–0.52	0.36	1.0
Class 3[d]				
Brand-name	0.46–0.87	0.7–0.95	0.69	17.3
Generic	0.03–0.10	0.03–0.12	0.04	1.0

[a] Wholesale prices based on 1996 Drug Topics Red Book.
[b] Class 1: halobetasol propionate, clobetasol propionate, betamethasone dipropionate augmented, diflorasone diacetate.
[c] Class 2: amcinonide, betamethasone dipropionate, mometasone furoate, diflorasone diacetate, fluocinonide, desoximeta.
[d] Class 3: triamcinolone acetonide (ointment), halcinonide, betamethasone dipropionate, fluticasone propionate, diflorasone diacetate, fluocinonide.
Source: Ref. 19.

avoid side effects. Several dosing regimens have been proposed, but most of them suffer from short remissions (11). Hradil et al. (14) found that eight of 12 patients given 0.05% clobestasol propionate ointment once a week (three times a day) were kept in remission for an average of 5 months. Svartholm et al. (15), using a similar regimen of once- or twice-weekly 0.05% clobetasol, achieved an average remission of 4 weeks. Katz et al. (16) developed the "weekend therapy" (three consecutive doses at 12-hour intervals applied over the weekend) using betamethasone dipropionate 0.05% and achieved remission for 12 weeks. A recent survey supports the growing popularity of intermittent (pulse) dosing schedules for psoriasis patients treated with topical steroids (4).

Topical corticosteroids are best for limited to isolated or relatively small BSA involvement. The elderly and children with mild to moderate psoriasis affecting >10% BSA have greater susceptibility to both the systemic and localized adverse reactions associated with the use of topical corticosteroid (11). Adjunctive treatment of topical corticosteroid with emollients or keratolytics is frequently used, depending on environmental conditions. "Combination" therapies utilizing topical corticosteroids with other topical drugs or systemic therapies are often used, but there are minimal supportive data for effectiveness (17,18).

Table 2 summarizes the retail price of selected examples of both brand-name and generic potent (class 2 and 3) and superpotent (class 1) topical corticosteroids. For both brand-name and generic products, the costs of ointment and cream are roughly the same (19), except for generic fluocinonide, the ointment form of which costs twice as much as the cream ($0.60/g vs. $0.30/g). The cost difference between brand-name and generic products is obvious. Thus, brand-name class 1, 2, and 3 corticosteroids cost 1.2 times, 2.0 times, and 17.3 times more, respectively, than the corresponding generic products.

The cost difference becomes an important issue when one considers a large percentage of BSA involved, the length of treatment required, and class of corticosteroid to be used. Table 3 summarizes the monthly cost—calculated based on the assumption that 45 g of ointment/cream is needed for a total body topical application (20)—of various classes of brand-name or generic corticosteroids in the treatment of psoriasis (5–20% BSA). It illustrates clearly the aforementioned cost issue.

The extrapolation to the annual cost of therapy requires consideration of potential usage patterns, several of which have been proposed in the literature (Table 4), over the course of 12 months. Table 5 summarizes the extrapolated annual cost of treating psoriasis (5–20% BSA) using different treatment and maintenance regimens (Table 4), assuming that a 4-week course of once-daily superpotent corticosteroid is required for controlling a flare that, on the average, occurs once every 4 months. Regimens 3, 4, and 5 in Table 4 have been proposed by Hradil et al. (14), Svartholm et al (15) and

Table 3 Monthly Cost[a] ($/month) of Psoriasis Treatment (5–20% BSA)[b] Using Classes 1–3 Corticosteroids[c]

	Class 1		Class 2		Class 3	
% BSA	Brand-name	Generic	Brand-name	Generic[d]	Brand-name	Generic
5	68	59	97	49	93	5
10	136	118	194	98	186	10
15	204	177	291	147	279	15
20	272	236	388	196	372	20

[a] Wholesale prices based on 1996 Drug Topics Red Book.
[b] Assuming 45 g of ointment or cream is needed for total body topical application.
[c] Class 1 steroid applied once daily; class 2 or 3 steroid applied twice daily.
[d] Calculation based on average cost of $0.28/g.

Table 4 Regimens for Treating Psoriasis (5–20% BSA) Using Topical Corticosteroid for 1 Year

Regimen	No. of flares year	Clearing schedule	Duration of remission (months)	Maintenance schedule
1	3	Class 1 steroid q.d. × 4 weeks	4	Class 2 steroid b.i.d. × 40 weeks
2	3	Class 1 steroid q.d. × 4 weeks	4	Class 3 steroid b.i.d. × 40 weeks
3[a]	3	Class 1 steroid t.i.d. × 9 d in 2 weeks	5	Class 1 steroid t.i.d. once/week × 46 weeks
4[b]	3	Class 1 steroid b.i.d. × 2 weeks	4	Class 1 steroid twice/ week × 46 weeks
5[c]	4	Class 1 steroid b.i.d. × 4 weeks	3	Class 1 steroid q 12 h × 3/weekend × 36 weeks

[a] Hradil et al. (14).
[b] Svartholm et al. (15).
[c] Katz et al. (16).

Katz et al. (16), respectively. Regimens 1 and 2 are hypothetical ones, involving a 4-week course of class 1 corticosteroid for controlling flare-up followed by class 2 or 3 corticosteroids twice daily for maintenance. Of the five regimens listed in Table 5, the ones proposed by Hiradil et al. (regimen 3, using three-times-a-day once-weekly class 1 corticosteroid as maintenance therapy) and Svartholm et al (regimen 4, using once daily for 2 days weekly class 1 corticosteroid as maintenance therapy) are comparable in terms of the cost involved. However, regimen 3 utilizes the smallest total amount of corticosteroid (hence fewer side effects), an important consideration when treating chronic diseases such as psoriasis.

Calcipotriene

Calcipotriene, a synthetic analog of 1,25-dihydroxyvitamin D_3, is the latest (1993) FDA-approved topical treatment for mild to moderate plaque-type psoriasis. Calcipotriene is an analog of vitamin D that has minimal effects on calcium metabolism. The efficacy of calcipotriene ointment (0.005%, 50 μg/g) in patients with plaque psoriasis is similar to that of a medium-

Table 5 Extrapolated Annual Cost ($/yr)[a] of Psoriasis Treatment (5–20% BSA) Using Topical Corticosteroids in Different Regimens

Regimen	5% BSA	10% BSA	15% BSA	20% BSA
1	1089 (616)	2178 (1232)	3267 (1848)	4392 (2464)
2	1089 (213)	2120 (426)	3180 (639)	4240 (852)
3	498 (424)	996 (848)	1494 (1272)	1992 (1696)
4	400 (341)	800 (682)	1200 (1023)	1600 (1364)
5	754 (642)	1508 (1284)	2262 (1926)	3016 (2568)

[a] Costs are calculated based on brand-name products; those in parentheses are based on generic products. All are wholesale prices based on the 1996 Drug Topics Red Book.

potency corticosteroid ointment such as 0.1% betamethasone valerate (21,22). Twice-daily treatment with calcipotriene ointment (0.005%) was shown to cause moderate improvement in 60% of patients with chronic plaque psoriasis over an 8-week period (21). Subsequent multicenter, double-blind, placebo-controlled right-left comparison studies confirmed the efficacy and safety of calcipotriene (23). In a randomized, double-blind, paired comparison of calcipotriene ointment (0.005%) with betamethasone 17-valerate ointment (0.1%) in 345 patients, the improvement was 68% in the calcipotriene group and 61% in the betamethasone group (22). As for corticosteroid, occlusion with hydrocolloid dressing enhances the efficacy of calcipotriene in clearing persistent plaques of psoriasis (24). For patients with extensive lesions, combination therapy of calcipotriene with halobetasol ointment (25), UVB (26), PUVA (27), or cyclosporine (28) has been advocated.

Long-term efficacy of calcipotriene in the treatment of plaque-type psoriasis has been confirmed in a large multicenter study, providing a 60% response over 12 months (29). A major advantage of calcipotriene over corticosteroid is that it may not induce skin atrophy in long-term treatment (30). The disadvantages are mild irritation, particularly to the face, and limitation of total dosage to 100 mg/week.

Following the guideline of using a maximum of 100 g/week of calcipotriene, both short- and long-term trials have not shown a significant change in bone and calcium metabolism (31–33). In those who used more than 100 g calcipotriene/week, serum calcium level normalized after stopping the medication (31,34,35). In the United States, calcipotriene ointment 0.005% is approved for use in a twice-daily regimen for 8 weeks. If one follows the guideline of using a maximum of 100 g calcipotriene/week, the patient must have no more than approximately 15% BSA of psoriasis.

Table 6 compares the costs of treating plaque psoriasis using calcipotriene, a class 2 steroid, a class 3 steroid, or a combination of class 1 and class 2 or 3 steroid twice a day for 8 weeks. It is obvious that treatment with calcipotriene is expensive, especially when dealing with larger BSAs. Calcipotriene costs at least twice as much as a medium-potency corticosteroid (class 3) having similar efficacy in treating psoriasis. The comparison is even more unfavorable when generic corticosteroids are considered. Combination treatment with class 1 and class 2 or 3 steroid, which is more effective than calcipotriene, is also much less expensive. The high cost of calcipotriene argues against its long-term use unless its effectiveness as an alternative or maintenance therapy is useful for the individual patient. However, the side effects commonly associated with topical corticosteroid use—localized atrophy, tachyphylaxis, and rebound—have not been reported with calcipotriene.

Topical therapy of psoriasis also includes some secondary or supplementary modalities. There is a wide assortment of emollients, including lotions, creams, and ointments. There are also several keratolytic agents, e.g., salicylic acid, lactic acid, and urea preparations, that help in the hydration and descaling of the skin surface that has a compromised barrier layer. Tar preparations and anthralin products are rarely used by themselves in

Table 6 Comparing the Costs of Calcipotriene and Class 2 and 3 Corticosteroids[a] in the Treatment of Psoriasis (5–15% BSA) for 8 Weeks Using b.i.d. Dosing Regimen

	5% BSA	10% BSA	15% BSA
1. Calcipotriene	307	614	921
2. Class 2 steroid	181 (91)	362 (182)	543 (273)
3. Class 3 Steroid	174 (10)	348 (20)	513 (30)
4. Class 1 steroid × 4 weeks, class 2 steroid × 4 weeks	154 (100)	308 (200)	462 (300)
5. Class 1 steroid × 4 weeks, class 3 steroid × 4 weeks	151 (59)	302 (118)	453 (177)

[a] Costs are calculated based on brand-name products; those in parentheses are based on generic products. All are wholesale prices based on the 1996 Drug Topics Red Book.

the United States because of lack of effectiveness and poorly tolerated cosmetic effects of smell and/or staining. While the costs of emollients are significant, they are hard to estimate for psoriasis alone and are certainly much lower than those of the FDA-approved topical medications.

SYSTEMIC THERAPY

Ultraviolet B

Ultraviolet B (280–320 nm), alone or in combination with crude coal tar (use of the latter is also known as the Goeckerman procedure), is the oldest treatment modality for patients with moderate to severe psoriasis. A retrospective study showed that, on the average, 95% improvement of the disease can be achieved within 2 to 3 weeks of treatment (36). Most patients dislike the crude coal tar, which is extremely messy to apply and stains the skin and clothing. To achieve optimal therapeutic results, patients have historically been hospitalized to ensure compliance with the treatment regimen and perhaps to provide psychological support in a protected environment. Special facilities and staff are also available in outpatient phototherapy centers.

Currently, UVB treatment of psoriatic patients is administered either with coal tar and suberythemogenic amounts of UVB or with only erythemogenic UVB and emollients (37). Both therapies are effective, but there are no data to indicate whether either approach has greater benefit, or whether the increased amount of UVB used in erythemogenic treatment has long-term toxicity.

Importantly, long-term remission can be achieved by intermittent maintenance therapy. In a four-center study, patients began a tapering maintenance schedule twice weekly for 4 to 8 weeks and weekly for up to 4 months (38). Table 7 summarizes the cost of UVB treatment, including maintenance therapy (a total of 62 treatments), on a schedule adapted from Ref. 38. The cost of emollient is not included.

As mentioned earlier, treatment with the Goeckerman regimen requires hospitalization for an average of 2–3 weeks. From the patient's perspective, it is less expensive, and for many it is desirable and convenient. Outpatient physician visits and topical medications are usually not covered expenses in most insurance policies (39), while months of outpatient therapy demands patients' compliance and tolerance to the inconvenience. Over the years, as hospital costs have soared, this traditional approach has been partially replaced by the ambulatory psoriasis treatment center (APTC) (40,41). The ATPC represents an intermediate alternative between outpatient care and hospitalization. It is designed for the select group of patients whose disease is too extensive to be treated effectively on a regular outpatient basis, yet is

Table 7 The cost[a] of UVB in Office Outpatient Treatment of Psoriasis for Approximately 1 Year

	Schedule	No. of treatments	Cost ($) per treatment	Total cost ($)
Clearing phase	3 × /week × 10 wk	30	30	900
Maintenance phase	2 × /week for 4–8 weeks, then weekly × 16 weeks	32	30	960
Grand total		62	60	1860

[a] The cost of emollient or tar is not included. Wholesale prices based on 1996 Drug Topics Red Book. The cost of inpatient therapy per clearing course is $6300–14700 (Ref. 43). The cost of outpatient ambulatory center per clearing course is $1680–5040 (Ref. 43).

not severe enough to warrant hospitalization. As a result, patients with severe psoriasis are treated effectively during the day and allowed to leave the center in the afternoon, with equal efficacy of the regimen but at a substantially reduced cost—about 1/15 of the cost of treatment in a hospital ward (42). Moreover, patients also benefit from periodic patient discussion groups, an activity designed to enhance their understanding of their disease. A recent article on the cost-effectiveness of UVB/tar treatment concluded that the cost per clearing course using a daycare center ($1680–5040) is 3.5 times that for outpatient UVB/emollient ($480–1200), while the cost of inpatient clearing ($6300–14700) is more than 13 times than that for outpatient UVB with emollient (43). One must also consider that the additional modes of therapy—PUVA, MTX, etretinate, and cyclosporine—have decreased the need for inpatient UVB therapy of severe patients. The prohibitive cost of inpatient Goeckerman therapy has made infeasible the most rapid form of therapy, and probably the safest.

PUVA

PUVA, unlike UVB/emollient phototherapy, is a form of photochemotherapy involving UVA (340–400 nm) and a photosensitizing compound, methoxypsoralen—most commonly used is 8-methoxypsoralen (8-MOP) (44). The FDA approved PUVA for the treatment of extensive psoriasis in 1982. It is generally believed that the mechanism of action of PUVA includes intercalation of methoxypsoralen into DNA, producing an interstrand cross-link of the double helix, via a bifunctional adduct (45), that interferes with DNA synthesis and blocks cell proliferation. More recent studies also suggest an immunomodualtory effect.

PUVA treatments are divided into two phases: the clearing and the maintenance phases (44,46). The clearing phase begins with the commencement of therapy and ends with the clearing of approximately 80–90% of treatable lesions in an average of 20–30 treatments. The maintenance phase, however, is subject to considerable variations in frequency and duration as well as dose adjustment.

The treatment frequency during the clearing phase varies between two or three times a week regardless of the skin type. Once the psoriatic lesions are 80–90% improved, the maintenance phase is started. The most frequently recommended maintenance program is a sequential downgrading schedule in every four treatments, starting at once a week down to once a month and eventually discontinued, as long as the patient remains relatively clear of lesions. On the average, the maintenance phase requires 30 treatments (47). For patients who remain in remission after 2 months of maintenance PUVA therapy, the likelihood of remaining in remission for 6–12 months is excellent (48).

The most worrisome side effects of long-term treatment are an increased risk of photodamage to the skin (including wrinkles, irregular pigmentation, lentigines, and premalignant keratoses) and an increased incidence of squamous cell cancer (49). To minimize the above two risks (photodamage and squamous cell skin cancer), it is recommended that the total number of PUVA treatments be less than 160 (50). For patients receiving high doses of PUVA (>250 treatments), there is an increasing risk of developing squamous cell skin cancer and even metastatic skin cancer (51).

Table 8 summarizes the cost of PUVA therapy, based on the assumption that the patient (70 kg) is taking 40 mg 8-MOP per session and the clearing phase requires 25 treatments while the maintenance phase requires 30 treatments. The only recommended pretreatment evaluation is an eye examination for cataracts. Other laboratory evaluations, including CBC, SMA12, and ANA level, are controversial (46).

Etretinate

About 40 years ago, vitamin A in the form of retinol or retinyl esters was introduced in the treatment of psoriasis (52). Unfortunately, only minimal improvement was observed, at the expense of intolerable side effects (53). Subsequently, other retinoids with better therapeutic indices were synthesized and tested. All-*trans* retinoic acid (tretinoin) used topically for the treatment of plaque psoriasis showed modest effectiveness but unacceptable irritation (54). Oral 13-*cis* retinoic acid (isotretinoin) demonstrates beneficial

Table 8 The Cost of PUVA in the Treatment of Psoriasis for Approximately 1 Year

	Schedule	No. of treatments	Cost ($) per treatment	Drug cost ($)[a] per treatment	Total cost ($)
Clearing phase	2–3 × /week	25	40	18	1450
Maintenance phase	Sequential downgrading q 4 treatments	30	40	18	1740
Laboratory tests[b]	Pretreatment cataract exam	—	90	—	—
Grand total	—	55	2200	990	3280

[a] 0.6 mg/kg of 8-MOP for a 70-kg patient. Wholesale prices based on 1996 Drug Topics Red Book.
[b] Pretreatment SMA20, CBC, and ANA titers evaluation are controversial.

effects in generalized pustular psoriasis but only minimal effects in plaque psoriasis; however, its main efficacy lies in disorders of keratinization and especially in cystic acne. Retinoid specificity became apparent with the development of etretinate (Tegison), a synthetic aromatic retinoid (55), which demonstrates good efficacy and tolerability in psoriatic patients and was approved by the FDA in 1986. The main drawback of etretinate is its long serum half-life (about 100 days) and hence slow elimination from the body (56). Acetretin, the principal metabolite of etretinate, is now being introduced in the United States. It has a much shorter half-life (about 2 days) but its use will still be limited in women of childbearing age.

Etretinate has been shown to be effective in treating different types of psoriasis (57). It is the drug of choice in the treatment of generalized pustular psoriasis and erythrodermic and acral localized psoriasis for men and nonfertile women (58). In fertile women with pustular psoriasis, isotretinoin is equally effective. Approximately half of the patients with extensive plaque psoriasis have moderate improvement (59); thus, as monotherapy the efficacy of etretinate in patients with psoriasis is limited (60). It is generally considered a less effective monotherapy than methotrexate, cyclosporine, and the phototherapies. Combination therapy, especially with PUVA, increases the efficacy of this treatment (infra vide) (61–63).

Side effects, which occur in almost all patients on systemic retinoids, resemble those of hypervitaminosis A (64). Significant ones include teratogenicity, elevation of liver enzymes and triglycerides, bony and ligament calcification and hyperostosis, premature epiphyseal closure, and hypercalcemia. Continuous therapy in responsive patients is limited to 1–2 years at a time because of cumulative side effects.

Weinstein et al. (65) recommended that the initial dose of etretinate be relatively small (0.3–0.4 mg/kg/day), and titrated upward as needed to minimize inflammatory flare of the disease. Lowe et al. (64), however, recommended an initial dose of 0.5–0.75 mg/kg/day. Once the disease is under control, titration to a lower dosage for maintenance is required. Etretinate has the shortcoming of not usually inducing remissions; thus, relapse is frequently seen as the dosage is reduced or eliminated.

The costs of using different dosages of etretinate in the treatment of plaque-type psoriasis are summarized in Table 9. Etretinate comes in only two dosage forms, 10- and 25-mg capsules, which limits a cost-effectiveness basis for exact dosing. For a 70-kg patient, it is interesting to note that the cost of using 0.4 mg/kg/day (about 30 mg/day) of etretinate is similar to that of 0.7 mg/kg/day (about 50 mg/day), and the most expensive dosage would be 0.6 mg/kg/day (40 mg/day)—two 10-mg capsules ($4.10) is more expensive than one 25-mg capsule ($3.20). Thus, dosage flexibility must be kept in mind when prescribing etretinate. For this reason, we try to average doses over 2 consecutive days, by using 25- and 50-mg doses (or 50- and 75-mg) on alternate days (10-mg capsules are rarely used except in a small patient). This permits a reasonable, adequate, and cost-effective schedule for intermediate dosages. Table 10 shows a projected annual cost of etretinate therapy. The cost of 3 months' treatment using 50 mg/day, followed by 25 mg/day alternating with 50 mg/day for 9 months as maintenance therapy

Table 9 Monthly cost ($) of Etretinate for the Treatment of Psoriasis with Various Dosing Regimens in a 70-kg Patient

Dosing (mg/kg/day)	mg/day	$/month[a]
0.3	20	123
0.35	25	96
0.5	37.5 (2 days)[b]	144
0.7	50	192
0.9	62.5 (2 days)	240

[a] Etretinate costs $2.05/10-mg capsule and $3.20/25-mg capsule.

[b] 25 mg and 50 mg on alternate days, i.e., about 37.5 mg/day (intermediate dosing), permits more economical dosing.

Table 10 Extrapolated Annual Cost of Etretinate for Treatment of Psoriasis

	Clearing phase	Maintenance phase	Total cost[a] ($)
Dosing schedule	50 mg/day × 3 months	25 mg/day alternate with 50 mg/day × 9 months	—
Cost of etretinate	576	1296	1872
Laboratory tests[b,c]:			
CBC, SMA 20	679	388	1067
Grand total	1255	1684	2939

[a] Wholesale price based on 1996 Drug Topics Red Book.
Recommended guidelines for laboratory evaluation before and during etretinate treatment (Ref. 64):
[b] Pretreatment evaluation; repeat q 2 weeks during the first 6 weeks of clearing phase; repeat q 8 weeks when on a low-maintenance dose.
[c] Etretinate rarely used in women capable of becoming pregnant.

($1872), does not differ significantly from that of using 40 mg/day for 3 months followed by 20 mg/day for 9 months ($1845). The table also summarizes the cost of currently recommended tests for patients on systemic retinoid (64). The total laboratory fees involved differ significantly from those reported earlier (3). However, neither the type nor frequency of the tests done was discussed in that report.

Methotrexate

For the 25 years since it was approved by the FDA, the folic acid antagonist methotrexate (MTX) has proven to be one of the most effective and reliable medications in the treatment of moderate to severe psoriasis unresponsive to conventional therapies (65–67). MTX is useful in patients with extensive plaque-type psoriasis as well in those with other severe forms, including acute von Zumbusch pustular psoriasis, localized pustular psoriasis, and psoriatic arthritis. The exact mode of action of MTX is unknown; however, cumulative evidence suggests that it may affect the systemic and local immune responses (68), as well as the proliferation and activation of keratinocytes, as part of its therapeutic action on psoriasis.

Studies showed that the maximum efficacy of MTX in psoriasis therapy appears similar regardless of how aggressively it is used (69). Aggressively dosed MTX improves 80% of psoriatic patients by greater than 50%, while 30–50% of patients have 90% clearing. Of the various drug schedules studied, the triple-dose regimen (70) has the best benefit-to-risk ratio. A survey of dermatologists indicates that 74% utilize the triple-dose regimen over alternative regimens involving a single weekly oral or parenteral dose (10–25 mg each week) (71).

The recurrence of psoriasis after stopping MTX has been studied in a small group of patients. Nyfors and Brodthagan (72) reported that after MTX was stopped, psoriasis recurred in nine of 19 patients (47%) at 3 months, three of 19 (16%) at 6 months, and another three of 19 (16%) at 9 months. In other words, approximately 80% had relapsed by 1 year after discontinuing MTX treatment. Thus, maintenance therapy will frequently be required after stopping MTX. The relapse rate, however, does not seem as severe or rapid as that occurring after etretinate and cyclosporine.

In general, moderate to severe psoriatic patients are treated with UVB or PUVA prior to using MTX. When using MTX, one should follow the available guidelines closely (67) to avoid unnecessary complications. Well-documented side effects of MTX on blood counts and liver-function tests call for periodic testing to avoid toxicity. To minimize the side effects of MTX, it is advisable to keep the dosage to a minimum while achieving acceptable clinical improvement. One concern associated with long-term MTX therapy is liver cirrhosis, which seems to be related to the cumulative dosages of MTX and liver damage, usually caused by excessive alcohol intake. Thus, a liver biopsy is recommended for approximately every cumulative 1.5 g of MTX in the absence of abnormal liver enzymes (67). With abnormal liver-function tests, consideration of a liver biopsy is more important, although it is expensive and not without complication. A recent retrospective study (73) on liver biopsies during long-term MTX treatment questioned the value of such a routine approach. It is still perplexing that the large number of patients receiving MTX for rheumatoid arthritis appear to have a lower incidence of liver abnormalities.

Table 11 summarizes the cost of various dosing schedules of MTX for the treatment of psoriasis (BSA >20%) for up to 1 month. The cost of using generic tablets and injectable MTX in an oral form is included for comparison. Brand-name MTX tablets are about 1.4 times more expensive than the corresponding generic product, but 5.6 times more expensive than the injection form used orally. The cost-effectiveness of using MTX solution orally in the treatment of rheumatoid arthritis was recently addressed by McLaughlin (74) and Hanson (75). Liquid MTX is available as a 50 mg/2 ml (2.5 mg/0.1 ml) solution. 0.3 ml diluted in water or juice would be the equivalent of three tablets in a single dose. The clinical effectiveness of the tablet and oral liquid forms have not yet been compared, but, as water-

Table 11 Monthly Cost ($) of Treatment of Psoriasis Using Different Dosing Schedules of Methotrexate (MTX)

Dosing schedule per week[b]	Brand-name MTX[a]	Generic MTX[a]	Injectable MTX[a]
1-1-1	51	37	9
2-1-1	68	49	12
2-2-1	85	61	15
2-2-2	102	73	18

[a] Costs of brand-name, generic, and injectable MTX are $4.25/2.5 mg, $3.06/2.5 mg, and $0.75/2.5 mg, respectively. Wholesale prices based on 1996 Drug Topics Red Book.
[b] 1-1-1 refers to a triple dosing of 2.5 mg MTX given at 12-hour intervals for three doses each week. 2-1-1 refers to triple dosing of 5 mg-2.5 mg-2.5 mg MTX. 2-2-2 refers to triple dosing of 5 mg MTX.

soluble preparations, a higher relative equivalence would be anticipated. The dosage per week in Table 11 represents either the triple-dose regimen (or a single weekly dose) ranging from three 2.5-mg MTX tablets (1-1-1) to six 2.5-mg tablets (2-2-2) per week. The annual cost of MTX treatment with these doses, excluding liver biopsy, ranges from $864 to $2153 (Table 12), which is in agreement with an earlier report (3). The table also summarizes the recommended laboratory evaluation before and during treatment with MTX (67). Considering the effectiveness of MTX for extensive psoriasis, MTX is a very economical, if not the most economical, modality for long-term treatment of extensive psoriasis (Table 14). In a recent survey, over 50% of dermatologists said they use methotrexate (4).

Cyclosporine

Cyclosporine (CSA) is the latest addition to our potential armamentarium in the treatment of severe and extensive psoriasis. Currently it is approved as treatment for psoriasis in Europe but not in the United States. Numerous clinical studies have recently demonstrated the efficacy of CSA in the treatment of extensive psoriasis vulgaris (76), psoriatic erythroderma, generalized von Zumbusch pustular psoriasis, acrodermatitis continua of Hallepeau, and a wide variety of other cutaneous diseases. However, like other treatment modalities for psoriasis. CSA is not curative. Unlike PUVA and MTX, the disease usually relapses within days or weeks after CSA treatment has been discontinued.

Table 12 Extrapolated Annual Costs ($) of Different Dosing Regimens of Brand-Name MTX for the Treatment of Psoriasis

	Dosing schedule	
	1-1-1	2-2-2
Cost of MTX[a]	663	1326
Laboratory tests		
CBC[b]	442	442
SMA 18[c]	385	385
Liver biopsy[d]	—	—
Total cost	1490	2153
Generic MTX tablets	1304	1782
Injectable liquid MTX	944	1061

[a] Wholesale price based on 1996 Drug Topics Red Book.
Recommended guidelines for laboratory evaluation before and during MTX therapy (Ref. 88):
[b] Before therapy and q month thereafter.
[c] Before therapy and q 2 months thereafter.
[d] Every 1.5 g of accumulated dose of MTX; estimated cost of liver biopsy is $700 (not included).

The mechanism of action of CSA in the treatment of psoriasis has brought major new insights into the pathophysiology of the disease, suggesting that immunological components underlie psoriasis (77).

For dermatological purposes (cyclosporine is not approved by the FDA for use in psoriasis), the recommended dose for CSA (Sandimmune®) is 4 mg/kg/day, usually administered once or twice a day. The results of a large multicenter study demonstrated that, after 1 to 3 months of treatment with CSA (3–5 mg/kg/day), 60% of patients with psoriasis showed substantial improvement (76). Once optimal improvement is reached, the dosage should be titrated downward by 0.5 to 1 mg/kg/day until the lowest effective dose is reached for maintenance therapy (78). Then, if possible, CSA should be discontinued altogether and replaced by another systemic or topical treatment modality. CSA is potentially toxic, and the most troublesome side effects include nephrotoxicity, hypertension, and a possible increased risk of malignant neoplasm. Patients receiving CSA must be carefully monitored on a periodic basis to minimize the risks of kidney and liver disease (79,80). The development of hypertension fortunately is generally reversible by adjusting the dose. The long-term use of CSA in dermatology has been addressed (81,82), and it is recommended that it not be used for more than 1 year at a time. A new formulation of CSA, Neoral (currently under FDA review), was recently introduced. It is known to have significantly better absorption and a more consistent serum level than the currently available formulation of CSA. Whether this will translate into a better safety profile for long-term usage remains to be established.

The projected annual cost (assuming dosage of 3 mg/kg/day for 3 months and 2 mg/kg/day for 9 months of maintenance) of CSA in psoriasis treatment is summarized in Table 13. The table also lists the costs of all the recommended laboratory tests (78). The projected annual costs are in close agreement with those in previous report (3). It is obvious that CSA is the most expensive drug among the currently available treatment modalities for psoriasis. However, it is extremely effective in "crisis management" of acute and severely inflamed psoriasis, especially the erythrodermic or exfoliative forms, which previously required hospitalization for control. For some of these very severe patients, if otherwise healthy, therapy may be effective on an outpatient basis. In the current managed care climate, in which cost-effectiveness is an important consideration, the use of CSA as an alternative

Table 13 Extrapolated Annual Cost of Cyclosporine for the treatment of Psoriasis in a 70-kg Patient

Dosing schedule	Clearing phase (3 mg/kg/d × 3 months)	Maintenance phase (2 mg/kg/d × 9 months)	Total cost ($)
Cost of CSA (Neoral)	1002	2004	3006
Laboratory tests[a]			
CBC, SMA 18, UA[b]	540	980	1520
Creatinine clearance[c]	96	144	240
Grand total	1638	3128	4766

Recommended guidelines for laboratory evaluation before and during CSA treatment (78):

[a] CXR, HIV tests if indicated.

[b] Pretreatment and q 2–4 weeks for the first 3 months; then q month thereafter.

[c] Pretreatment and q 3 months.

to hospitalization may be valuable for selected patients. Another advantage of using CSA rather than oral corticosteroids (not generally recommended for psoriasis) for such crisis therapy is that rebound flares or pustular conversion after the discontinuation of CSA are extremely rare. Such side effects are periodically seen on discontinuing oral corticosteroids. Following crisis management, the options remain to either continue the patient on lower maintenance doses of CSA or gradually switch to one of the other modalities for moderate to severe psorasis. In summary, CSA is not generally considered the first drug of choice. However, its rapid efficacy in the treatment of severely inflamed psoriasis, which may decrease the need for hospitalization, is certainly a major advance in the treatment of psoriasis. The significant toxicity and high cost will probably restrict its use to only severe patients and limited durations of treatment.

Rotational and Combination Treatment

A major concern in the treatment of chronic diseases such as psoriasis is the cumulative toxicity of the various treatment modalities, each of which has its own unique profile of toxicity. To maximize therapeutic benefits while minimizing both short- and long-term side effects, two general approaches—rotational therapy (83) and combination therapies—have been advocated (84). Rotational therapy, recently proposed by Weinstein et al. (83), is the rotation on and off the various available therapeutic modalities in order to minimize long-term cumulative toxicities by long periods off each treatment. Combination therapies, on the other hand, use two treatment modalities in tandem. The Goeckerman procedure (UVB and coal tar) was the first such approach. Many combination treatments have been devised and tested (104). It is beyond the scope of this chapter to discuss these treatments individually; suffice it to say that most of the combination therapies do result in a certain degree of dosage reduction of the individual treatment modality.

Combination therapy is difficult to evaluate in terms of efficacy, safety, quality of improvement, complexity, and pharmacoeconomics. Very little information exists on this subject. All combinations will inherently be more costly for at least the first half of the therapeutic regimen. If the secondary or additional therapy is indeed synergistic rather than simply additive, then there may be a cost saving. However, speed of improvement is generally in the range of 25% faster or 25% less of the therapeutic modality. The physician must evaluate on an individual-patient basis whether the advantages of specific combinations outweigh those of monotherapy. The best example of combination therapy has been the addition of systemic retinoids to PUVA therapy (RePUVA). The number of PUVA treatments is reduced

Table 14 Extrapolated Annual Cost of RePUVA for Treatment of Psoriasis (BSA > 20%)

	Clearing phase	Maintenance phase	Total cost ($)
Etretinate	50 mg/d 2 weeks prior to starting PUVA until clearing (7 weeks)	—	—
Cost	314	—	314
PUVA	15 treatments	30 treatments, sequential downgrading to q 4 week treatment	—
Cost[a]	600	1200	1800
8-MOP	40 mg/treatment	40 mg/treatment	—
Cost[b]	270	540	810
Laboratory tests (CBC, SMA 20)[c]	388	—	388
Pregnancy[d]	69	—	69
Cataract exam[e]	90	—	90
Grand total	1731	1740	3471

[a] $40/treatment.
[b] $18/treatment.
Recommended guidelines for laboratory evaluation before and during etretinate treatment (88):
[c] Pretreatment evaluation; repeat q 2 weeks during the first 6 weeks of clearing phase; repeat q 8 weeks when on a low maintenance dose.
[d] Before therapy and q month during therapy. Use 13-cis retinoic acid (accutane) in women of childbearing age.
[e] Pre- or early treatment, then q 1–2 years.

from an average of 20 in U.S. studies to approximately 15 treatments, based on a 25% reduction seen in European trials (85). In Europe, the combination approach is primarily used, while monotherapy is generally used in the United States. Nonetheless, on neither continent is there a study to show whether monotherapy or combination therapy with RePUVA is safer with respect to skin cancer. There are some poorly responsive patients in which the combination of RePUVA or another combination is required. In our experience, in patients who have had limited response after 10–15

PUVA treatments, the addition of oral retinoid facilitates satisfactory improvements. In general, we find that monotherapy will adequately care for the great majority of moderate to severe patients.

Table 14 summarizes the cost of RePUVA therapy based on the 70-kg patient taking etretinate (50 mg/day) or 13-*cis*-retinoic acid (40 mg/day) 2 weeks prior to PUVA therapy and continued until clearing. The clearing phase requires 15 treatments, which represents a 25% reduction of the typical 20 treatments when PUVA is employed as a monotherapy. RePUVA is about $450 more expensive than PUVA in our postulated treatment schedule (Tables 8 and 14). The cost saving from fewer PUVA sessions required in RePUVA is eradicated by the cost of etretinate and extra laboratory tests. Whether this extra cost in RePUVA (compared to PUVA) translates into a lower risk of skin cancer remains to be established, but it could be a justifying consideration.

SUMMARY

For patients with limited plaque-type psoriasis, BSA $<20\%$, topical corticosteroids are the initial drug of choice at this time based on their efficacy, economy, and reasonable safety profiles. Long-term response or maintenance therapy remains the greatest difficulty with corticosteroid usage. Dosing regimens for long-term maintenance therapy have been tested, and the one proposed by Hiradil et al. (using a class 1 corticosteroid three times a day once each week as maintenance therapy) is especially attractive. Treatment of plaque psoriasis with calcipotriene alone is less cost-effective than corticosteroids. However, it is an attractive potential alternative in responding patients who generally require long-term therapy. Combination therapy with other modalities (e.g., potent topical corticosteroid, UV light) will increase short-term efficacy, but cost-effectiveness of combination therapy remains an open question. Sequential combinations, e.g., steroid followed by calcipotriene, may eventually be useful.

Of all the therapeutic modalities available for moderate to severe psoriasis, UVB treatment has the best therapeutic index under optimal therapeutic conditions. The risk of inducing skin cancers is small compared to that in the other form of phototherapy, PUVA. No routine laboratory work-up is required throughout the course of treatment. Unless the patient is on topical or systemic drugs that may increase the risk of photosensitivity or has a history of photosensitivity or lupus erythematosus, outpatient UVB phototherapy is considered a good therapy for patients with extensive plaque-type or guttate psoriasis. UVB phototherapy can also be used in a home situation. Anecdotally, however, many psoriatic “experts” (including the authors) believe that PUVA is more effective and requires fewer treatments.

With respect to cost, PUVA is competitive with outpatient UVB/emollient or etretinate (Table 15). It is more expensive than methotrexate but far less expensive than intermittent hospitalization (conservatively estimated to be a minimum of $750/day for 2–3 weeks) or cyclosporine. The charges for a typical hospitalization for psoriasis are approximately 10 times greater than those for a clearing course of PUVA (86). Moreover, the duration of remission after PUVA therapy is similar to that after inpatient UVB therapy (87). With regard to the duration of remission, PUVA appears to induce a longer remission than the UVB/emollient treatment (87).

Etretinate is not usually chosen as first-line monotherapy for extensive plaque-type psoriasis; its limited efficacy does not justify the high cost, as analyzed above (Table 10). One should consider the more cost-effective treatment modalities, such as PUVA or methotrexate, if no contraindications exist. Since etretinate is only moderately effective for plaque psoriasis, it is usually used as a second- or third-line therapy. However, it plays an important role in the treatment of generalized pustular or erythrodermic psoriasis, or when used in combination therapy such as with PUVA

Table 15 Average Annual Cost[a] (Including Laboratory Fees) of Psoriasis Care

	Cost ($)	Comments
Topical therapy (BSA < 20%)		
Topical corticosteroid	500–2000	Hradil regimen, 5–20% BSA; brand-name products
Dovonex	2000–8000	5–20% BSA
Photo-/systemic therapy (BSA > 20%)		
UVB/emollient	1850	62 treatments in 34 weeks
PUV	3300	55 treatments
Etretinate	2950	50 mg/d × 3 months, then 25 mg/d and 50 mg/d on alternate days × 9 months
Methotrexate	1500–2150	2.5 mg to 15 mg per week
Cyclosporine	4800	3 mg/kg/d × 3 months; 2 mg/kg/d × 9 months

[a] Calculation based on wholesale prices of brand-name products quoted in 1996 Drug Topics Red Book. Values rounded off to nearest $50.

(RePUVA). As mentioned earlier, whether the extra cost of RePUVA translates into lower skin-cancer risks remains to be seen.

Methotrexate remains the most effective and economical means of treating extensive psoriasis. Forty-five years of generally favorable experience with this drug for psoriasis, and more recently for rheumatoid arthritis, makes this the gold standard for psoriasis therapy. In a new update of the MTX guidelines (88), a modest decrease in the MTX liver problem will be analyzed.

CSA is not generally considered the first drug of choice. However, its great efficacy in the treatment of acute extensive or severely inflamed psoriasis, which may decrease the need for hospitalization, is certainly a major advance in the treatment opportunities for severe psoriasis.

The pharmacoeconomics of the management of psoriasis reflect several variables, including the extent of disease involvement, the severity and location of lesions, the past treatments, possible cumulative toxicity, and the therapeutic options available. Thus, patients with limited disease—arbitrarily defined as affecting less than 15–20% BSA—will generally use topical therapies, and the costs of those few drugs available will vary depending on the amount of surface area involved and the number of times per day the patient is instructed to use that medication. Another hidden variable here is how the patient applies the drug: sparingly, spread thinly, or smeared on in thick globs, wasting significant amounts of drug and requiring the purchase of more medication. The sum of all these factors in topical therapy can cause the drug cost alone to range from $500 to over $6000 per year.

For patients with moderate to severe psoriasis, several more therapeutic options are available, most of which seem to work better (4) and have longer maintenance potential than the topical therapies. The cost of these photo-/systemic treatments, regardless of the extent of BSA involved, is either lower than or competitive with that of the topical therapies, assuming similar effectiveness. With this background, it is not unusual to see patients with limited disease who are unresponsive to topical treatment be switched to the more aggressive modalities.

The discussion of pharmacoeconomics has dealt mainly with the price of the medications and the necessary tests associated with these treatments. Physician costs have been left out because of the variables in fees regionally, the type of health provider, and the frequency with which a patient might be seen by the doctor. Two other significant cost factors are involved, albeit indirectly, in the management of psoriatic patients. One is patients' loss of income if unemployable or the cost of time needed to care for their skin and visit physicians. While psoriasis very rarely causes total incapacitation, job opportunities may be limited by patients cosmetic appearance or inability to work on the schedule needed by the employer. The other, more difficult economic factor to judge is the psychological distress of many patients and the possible financial burdens stemming from this difficult-to-quantitate part of the psoriasis picture.

REFERENCES

1. Koo J. Population-based epidemiologic study of psoriasis with emphasis on quality of life assessment. In: Koo J, ed. Dermatologic Clinics. Philadelphia: Saunders, 1995:485–496.
2. Krueger GG, Bergstressen PR, Lowe NJ, Voorhees JJ, Weinstein GD. Psoriasis. J Am Acad Dermatol 1984; 11:937–947.
3. Sander HM, Morris LF, Phillips CM, Harrison PE, Menter A. The annual cost of psoriasis. J Am Acad Dermatol 1993; 28:422–425.
4. Liem WH, McCullough JL, Weinstein GD. Effectiveness of topical therapy for psoriasis, results of a national survey. Cutis 1995; 55:306–310.
5. Lane AV, Wachs GN, Weston WL. Once-daily treatment of psoriasis with glucocorticoid ointments. J Am Acad Dermatol 1983; 8:523–525.
6. Nilsson JE, Gips LS. Systemic effects of local treatment with high doses of potent corticosteroids in psoriatics. Acta Derm Venereol (Stockh) 1979; 59:246–248.
7. May P, Stein ES, Ryter RJ, Hirsh FS, Michel B, Levy RP. Cushing's syndrome from percutaneous absorption of triamcinolone cream. Arch Intern Med 1976; 136:612–613.
8. Du Vivier A. Tachyphylaxis to topically applied steroids. Arch Dermatol 1976; 112:1245–1248.
9. Volden G. Successful treatment of chronic skin disease with clobetasol propionate and a hydrocolloid occlusive dressing. Acta Derm Venereol (Stockh) 1992; 72:69–71.
10. Pershing LK, Corlett JL, Lambert LD, Poncelet CE. Circadian activity of topical 0.05% betamethasone dipropionate in human skin in vivo. J Invest Dermatol 1994; 102:734–739.
11. Katz HI. Topical corticosteroids. In: Lebwohl M, Zanolli M, eds. Dermatologic Clinics. Philadelphia: Saunders, 1995:805–815.
12. Stoughton RB. Are genetic formulations equivalent to trade name topical glucocorticoids? Arch Dermatol 1987; 123:1312–1314.
13. Storm BL. Generic drug substitution revisited. N Engl J Med 1987; 316:1456–1462.
14. Hradil E, Lindstrom C, Moller H. Intermittent treatment of psoriasis with clobetasol propionate. Acta Dermatol Venereol SR 1978; 58:375–377.
15. Svartholm H, Larsson L, Fredereiksen B. Intermittent topical treatment of psoriasis with clobetasol propionate (Dermovate). Curr Med Res Opin 1982; 8:154–157.
16. Katz HI, Hien NT, Prawer SE, Scott JC, Grivna EM. Betamethasone dipropionate in optimized vehicle: intermittent pulse dosing for extended maintenance treatment of psoriasis. Arch Dermatol 1987; 123:1308–1311.

17. Trozak DJ. Topical corticosteroid therapy in psoriasis vulgaris. Cutis 1990; 46:341–350.
18. Meola T Jr, Sote NA, Lim HW. Are topical corticosteroid useful adjunctive therapy for the treatment of psoriasis with ultraviolent radiation? A review of the literature. Arch Dermatol 1991; 127:1708–1713.
19. 1996 Drug Topics Red Book. Montvale, NJ: Medical Economics Data, 1996.
20. Schlagel CA, Sanborn EM. Weights of topical preparations required for topical and partial body inuction. J Invest Dermatol 1964; 42:253–256.
21. Kragballe K. Treatment of psoriasis by the topical application of the novel cholecalciferol analog calcipotriol (MC 903). Arch Dermatol 1989; 125:1647–1652.
22. Kragballe K, Gjertsen BT, De Hoop D, Karlsmark T, van De Kerkhof PCM, Larko O, Nieboer C, Roed-Peterson J, Strand A, Tikjob G. Double-blind, right-left comparison of calcipotriol and betamethasone valerate in treatment of psoriasis vulgaris. Lancet 1991; 337:193–196 (erratum, Lancet 1991; 337:988).
23. Dubertret L, Wallace D, Souteyrand P, Perussel M, Kalis B, Meynadier J, Chevranti-Breton J, Beylot C, Bazex JA, Jurgensen HJ. Efficacy and safety of calcipotriol (MC 903) ointment in psoriasis vulgaris. J Am Acad Dermatol 1992; 27:983–988.
24. Gamborg NP. Calcipotriol of clobetasol propionate occluded with a hydrocolloid dressing for treatment of nummular psoriasis. Acta Derm Venereol (Stockh) 1993; 73:394.
25. Lebwohl M, Siskin SB, Epinette W, Breneman D, Funicella T, Kalb R, Moore J. A multicenter trial of calcipotriene ointment and halobetasol ointment compared with either agent alone for the treatment of psoriasis. J Am Acad Dermatol 1996; 35:268–269.
26. Kragballe K. Combination of topical calcipotriol (MC 903) and UVB radiation for psoriasis vulgaris. Dermatology 1990; 181:211–214.
27. Speight EL, Farr PM. Calcipotriol improves the response of psoriasis to PUVA. Br J Dermatol 1994; 130:79–82.
28. Grossman RM, Thivolet J, Claudy A, Souteyrand P, Guilhou JJ, Thomas P, Amblard P, Belaich S, de Belilovsky C, de la Brassinne M, Martinet C, Bazex JA, Beylot C, Combemale P, Lambert D, Ostojic A, Denoeux JP, Lauret PH, Vaillant L, Weber M, Pamphile R, Dubertret L. A novel therapeutic approach to psoriasis with combination calcipotriol ointment and very low-dose cyclosporin: results of a multicenter placebo-controlled study. J Am Acad Dermatol 1994; 31:68–74.
29. Ramsey CA, Berth-Jones J, Brandin G, Cunlife WJ, Dubertret L, van de Kerkhof PCM, Menne T, Wegmann E. Long term use of topical calcipotriol in chronic plaque psoriasis. Dermatology 1994; 189:260–264.
30. Kragballe K, Fogh K, Sogaard H. Long term efficacy and tolerance of topical calcipotriol in psoriasis. Arch Derm Venereol (Stockh) 1991; 71:475–478.
31. Kragballe K. Vitamin D_3 analogues. In: Lebwohl M, Zanolli M, eds. Dermatologic Clinics. Philadelphia: Saunders, 1995:835–839.

32. Mortensen L, Kragballe K, Wegmann E, Schifter S, Risteli J, Charles P. Treatment of psoriasis vulgaris with topical calcipotriol has no short-term effect on calcium or bone metabolism. Acta Derm Venereol (Stockh) 1993; 73:300–304.
33. Gumowski SD, Rizzoli R, Saurat JH. Effects of topical calcipotriol on calcium metabolism in psoriatic patients: comparison with oral calcitriol. Dermatologica 1991; 183:275–279.
34. Cunliff WJ, Claudy A, Fairiss G, Goldin D, Gratton D, Henderson CA, Holden CA, Maddin WS, Ortonne JP, Young M. A multicenter comparative study of calcipotriol and betamethasone 17-valerate in patients with psoriasis vulgaris. J Am Acad Dermatol 1992; 26:736–743.
35. Dwyer C, Chapman RS. Calcipotriol and hypercalcemia. Lancet 1991; 338:364–365.
36. Perry HO, Soderstrom CW, Schulze RW. The Goeckerman treatment of psoriasis. Arch Dermatol 1968; 98:178–182.
37. Adrian RM, Parrish JA, Momtaz TK, Karlin MJ. Outpatient phototherapy for psoriasis. Arch Dermatol 1981; 117:623–626.
38. Stern RS, Armstrong RB, Anderson TF, Bickers DR, Lowe NJ, Harber L, Voorhees J, Parrish JA. Effect of continued ultraviolet B phototherapy on the duration of remission of psoriasis: a randomized study. J Am Acad Dermatol 1986; 15:546–552.
39. Bohm M, Voorhees JJ. White paper on hospitalization for psoriasis care. J Am Acad Dermatol 1984; 10:842–851.
40. Cram DL, King RI. Psoriasis day care center. JAMA 1976; 235:177–178.
41. Bohm M, Voorhees JJ, Armstrong KB, Bickers DR, Cram DL, Farber EM, Harber LC, Menter A, Roenigk HH. The role of the ambulatory psoriasis treatment center as a cost-effective program for severe psoriasis. J Am Acad Dermatol 1985; 12:740–747.
42. Larko O, Swanbeck G. Acta Derm Venereol (Stockh) 1982; 62:413–418.
43. Stern RS. The benefits, costs and risks of topical tar preparation in the treatment of psoriasis: consideration of cost effectiveness. Ann Acad Med (Singapore) 1988; 17:473–476.
44. Melski JW, Tannenbaum L, Parrish JA, Fitzpatrick TB, Bleich HL. Oral methoxsalen photochemotherapy for the treatment of psoriasis: a cooperative clinical trial. J Invest Dermatol 1977; 68:328–335.
45. Pathak MA, Fitzpatrick TB, Parrish JA. Pharmacologic and moelcular aspects of psoralen photochemotherapy. In: Ferber E, Cox AJ, Jacobs PH, Nall ML, eds. Psoriasis: Proceedings of the Second International Symposium. New York: Yorke Medical Books, 1977:262–271.
46. Gonzales E. PUVA for psoriasis. In: Lebwohl M, Zanolli M, eds. Dermatologic Clinics. Philadelphia: Saunders, 1995:851–866.
47. Melski JW, Stern RS. Annual rate of psoralen and ultraviolet—A treatment of psoriasis after initial clearing. Arch Dermatol 1982; 118:404–408.
48. Stern RS, Fitzpatrick TB, Parrish AJ, Honigsmann H, Wolff K. Oral psoralen photochemotherapy. In: Roenigk HH Jr, Maibach HI, eds. Psoriasis. 2nd ed. New York: Marcel Dekker, 1991:603–623.

49. Stern RS, Laird N, Melski J, Parrish JA, Fitzpatrick TB, Bleich HL. Cutaneous squamous-cell carcinoma in patients treated with PUVA. N Engl J Med 1984; 310:1156–1161.
50. Stern RS, Lange R. Non-melanoma skin cancer occurring in patients treated with PUVA five to ten years after first treatment. J Invest Dermatol 1988; 91:120–124 (erratum, J Invest Dermatol 1989; 92:300).
51. Stern RS, Laird, N. The carcinogenic risks of treatments for severe psoriasis: photochemotherapy follow-up study. Cancer 1994; 73:2759–2764.
52. Frey JR, Schoch MA. Therapeutische versuche bei psoriasis mit vitamin A, zugliech ein beitrag zur A-hypervitaminose. Dermatologica 1952; 104:80–86.
53. Saurat JH. How do retinoids work on human epidermis? A breakthrough and its implications. Clin Exp Dermatol 1988; 13:350–364.
54. Frost P, Weinstein GD. Topical administration of vitamin A acid for ichthyosiform dermatoses and psoriasis. JAMA 1969; 207:1863–1868.
55. Bollag W. The development of retinoids in experimental and clinical oncology and dermatology. J Am Acad Dermatol 1983; 9:797–805.
56. Paravicini U. On the metabolism and pharmacokinetics of an oral aromatic retinoid. Ann NY Acad Sci 1981; 359:54–67.
57. Dubertret L, Chastang C, Beylot C, Bazex J, Rognin C, Touraine R. Maintenance treatment of psoriasis by tigason: a double-blind randomized clinical trial. Br J Dermatol 1985; 113:323–330.
58. Moy R, Kingston TP, Lowe NJ. Isotretinoin vs. etretinate therapy in generalized pustular and chronic psoriasis. Arch Dermatol 1985; 121:1297–1301.
59. Gollnick HPM, Orfanos CE. Clinical efficacy of etretinate and acitretin, European experience. In: Roenigk HH Jr, Maibach HI, eds. Psoriasis. 2nd ed. New York: Marcel Dekker, 1991:725–748.
60. Ellis CN, Hermann RC, Gorsulowsky DC, Goldfarb MT, Voorhees JJ. Etretinate therapy reduces inpatient treatment of psoriasis. J Am Acad Dermatol 1987; 17:787–791.
61. Momtaz-T K, Fitzpatrick TB. Modification of PUVA. In: Lebwohl M, Zanolli M, eds. Dermatologic Clinics. Philadelphia: Saunders, 1995:867–873.
62. Parker S, Coburn P, Lawrence C, Marks J, Shuster S. A randomized double-blind comparison of PUVA-etretinate and PUVA-placebo in the treatment of chronic plaque psoriasis. Br J Dermatol 1984; 110:215–220.
63. Saurat JH, Geiger JM, Amblard P, Beani JC, Boulanger A, Claudy A, Frenk E, Guilhou JJ, Grosshans E, Merot Y, Meynadier J, Tapernoux B. Randomized double-blind multicenter study comparing acitretin-PUVA, etretinate-PUVA and placebo-PUVA in the treatment of severe psoriasis. Dermatologica 1988; 177:218–224.
64. Wieder JM, Lowe NJ. Systemic retinoids for psoriasis. In: Lebwohl M, Zanolli M, eds. Dermatologic Clinics. Philadelphia: Saunders, 1995:891–896.
65. Greaves MW, Weinstein GD. The treatment of psoriasis. N Engl J Med 1995; 332:581–588.
66. Bukaty L, Weinstein G. The therapy of moderate-to-severe psoriasis with methotrexate. In: Weinsten G, Gottlieb A, eds. National Psoriasis Foundation: Therapy of Moderate to Severe Psoriasis. Harber and Flora, 1993:75–93.

67. Roenigk H, Auerbach R, Maibach HI, Weinstein GD. Methotrexate in psoriasis: revisted guidelines. J Am Acad Dermatol 1988; 19:145–156.
68. Jeffes EWB, McCullough JL, Pittelkow MR, McCormick A, Almanzor J, Liu G, Dang M, Voss K, Voss J, Schlotzhauer A, Weinstein GD. Methotrexate therapy of psoriasis: differential sensitivity of proliferating lymphoid and epithelial cells to the cytotoxic and growth-inhibitory effects of methotrexate. J Invest Dermatol 1995; 104:183–188.
69. Jeffes EWB, Weinstein GD. Methotrexate and other chemotherapeutic agents used to treat psoriasis. In: Lebwohl M, Zanolli M, eds. Dermatologic Clinics. Philadelphia: Saunders, 1995:875–890.
70. Weinstein G, Frost P. Methotrexate in psoriasis: a new therapeutic schedule. Arch Dermatol 1971; 103:33–38.
71. Peckham PE, Weinstein GD, McCullough JL. The treatment of severe psoriasis: a national survey. Arch Dermatol 1987; 123:1303–1307.
72. Nyfors A, Brodthagen H. Methotrexate for psoriasis in weekly oral doses without any adjunctive therapy. Dermatologica 1970; 140:345–355.
73. Boffa MJ, Chalmers RJG, Haboubi NY, Shomaf M, Mitchell DM. Sequential liver biopsies during long-term methotrexate treatment for psoriasis: a reappraisal. Br J Dermatol 1995; 133:774–778.
74. McLaughlin GE. Parental vs. oral methotrexate, a cost comparison [letter]. Arthritis Rheum 1994; 37:779.
75. Hanson DL. Cost-effectiveness of orally administered liquid methotrexate: comment on the letters by McLaughlin and by Wase [letter]. Arthritis Rheum 1994; 37:1713.
76. Ellis CN, Fradin MS, Messana JM, Brown MD, Stiegel MT, Hartley AH, Rocher LL, Wheeler S, Hamilton TA, Parish TG, Ellis-Madu M, Duell E, Annesley TM, Cooper KD, Voorhees JJ. Cyclosporin for plaque-type psoriasis: results of a multidose, double-blind trial. N Engl J Med 1991; 324:277–284.
77. Bos J. The pathomechanism of psoriasis: the skin immune system and cyclosporin. Br J Dermatol 1988; 118:141–155.
78. Koo J, Lee J. Cyclosporin: what clinicians need to know. In: Lebwohl M, Zanolli M, eds. Dermatologic Clinics. Philadelphia: Saunders, 1995:897–907.
79. Korstanje MJ, Bilo HJG, Stoof TJ. Sustained renal function loss in psoriasis patients after withdraw of low-dose cyclosporin therapy. Br J Dermatol 1992; 127:501–504.
80. Zachariae H, Hansen H, Kragballe K, Olsen S. Morphologic, renal changes during cyclosporin treatment of psoriasis. J Am Acad Dermatol 1992; 26:415–419.
81. Zachariae H. Long-term use of cyclosporin in dermatology. Arch Dermatol 1996; 132:692–694.
82. Koo J. Cyclosporin in dermatology: fear and opportunities. Arch Dermatol 1995; 131:842–845.
83. Weinstein GD, White GM. An approach to the treatment of moderate and severe psoriasis with rotational therapy. J Am Acad Dermatol 1993; 28:454–459.

84. Psoriasis. In: Lebwohl M, Zanolli M, eds. Dermatologic Clinics. Philadelphia: Saunders, 1995:717–923.
85. Grupper C, Berretti B. Treatment of psoriasis by oral PUVA therapy combined with aromatic retinoid (Ro-10-9359). Dermatologica 1981; 162:404–413.
86. Stern RS. Long-term use of psoralens and ultraviolet A for psoriasis: evidence for efficacy and cost savings. J Am Acad Derm 1986; 14:520–526.
87. Kenicer KJA, Lakshmipathi T, Addo HA. An assessment of the effect photochemotherapy (PUVA) and UV-B phototherapy in the treatment of psoriasis. Br J Dermatol 1981; 105:629–639.
88. Roenigk H, Maibach HI, Weinstein GD, et al. Methotrexate guidelines. J Am Acad Dermatol 1997. Accepted.

22

Allergic Contact Dermatitis

Cost-Effectiveness of Early Confirmed Diagnosis and Patch Testing

Rukmini Rajagopalan,[1] Roger T. Anderson,[2] Syam Sarma,[3] John Kallal,[1] Carol M. Retchin,[3] John T. Jones,[3] Joseph F. Fowler, Jr.,[4] and Elizabeth F. Sherertz[2]

[1] *Glaxo Wellcome Inc., Research Triangle Park, North Carolina*
[2] *Bowman Gray School of Medicine of Wake Forest University, Winston-Salem, North Carolina*
[3] *PharmaResearch Corporation, Wilmington, North Carolina*
[4] *University of Louisville School of Medicine, Louisville, Kentucky*

INTRODUCTION

Background

Allergic contact dermatitis (ACD) is a common allergic condition affecting the skin. It presents as an acute or subacute eruption characterized by erythema, vesicles, and scaling after exposure to the contact allergen. The diagnosis of ACD is traditionally based on a subject's history of symptoms and substance contact, physical examination, and other diagnostic methods, including patch-testing. Patch-testing is a practical tool available to the clinician for confirming the diagnosis of ACD (1) due to common substances. It is indicated as an aid in the diagnosis of ACD, but it is not a substitute for taking the subject's history or for direct physical examination (2). The overall usefulness of the patch-testing depends on the experience of the physician interpreting the results (3,4). General clinical experience in the use of patch-testing assists the physician in defining the clinical relevance of a subject's reaction to test allergen(s) (5).

In 1995, the National Center of Health Statistics survey recorded over 697 million physician visits, about 3.6% (25.0 million) of which were due to dermatology-related causes. Further, 7.6 million visits were for contact dermatitis, atopic dermatitis, and other eczema (6). In 1989, Rietschel (7) demonstrated that patch-testing is a valuable tool to provide an accurate, relatively simple means of diagnosis that allows the physician to initiate appropriate management to alleviate patients' suffering without losing precious time. In a recent retrospective study (8), data were collected on 260 subjects with suspected ACD. Results from that study indicated that patch-tested subjects experienced a shorter postdiagnosis duration of the disease than subjects who were not patch-tested. This finding was particularly noticeable in subjects who had more than 2 months' history of ACD prior to the diagnosis. Following these results from the retrospective study, and on consultation with opinion leaders in contact dermatitis, a prospective study was designed to evaluate the benefits of patch-testing in obtaining an early confirmed diagnosis in patients with a suspicion of contact allergy.

Rationale

Early identification and subsequent avoidance of the contact allergen by the patient combined with an adequate treatment of the initial skin rash should reduce the duration and intensity of the disease, its progression to a chronic form, and the aggregate cost of patient management.

Patch-testing may play a very important role in this early identification process. Comparative analysis of subject data representing quality of life, satisfaction with care, and the use of health care resources categorized by key subject characteristics may allow us to develop strategies for targeting subjects who are the most appropriate candidates for patch-testing.

OBJECTIVES

The objectives of this 12-month study are:

1. To identify appropriate populations for whom patch-testing is cost-effective as a diagnostic tool

2. To determine the cost-effectiveness of patch-testing in these populations by:
   a. Evaluating the sensitivity of the patch test
   b. Collecting data on:
      i. Cost of disease and cost of treatment
      ii. Frequency of patch-testing
      iii. Duration of disease, frequency of episodes, and number of office visits
      iv. Treatment outcomes
      v. Subjects' perception of diagnosis and treatment
      vi. Quality of life

STUDY DESIGN AND METHODS

Study Design

This was a multicenter, observational study to evaluate cost-effectiveness of patch-testing in the diagnosis and treatment of moderate to severe ACD. The study was designed to prospectively collect data on the use of the several commercially available patch-testing products as diagnostic aids in the management of ACD. No treatment plan or diagnostic method was assigned to subjects. A variety of data that represent health care resource utilization and the outcomes of care provided to ACD subjects during the 6- and 12-month follow-up periods were collected and analyzed as specified in the study protocol.

The study was planned for a period of 12 months, with evaluations at the end of 6 and 12 months after enrollment. This report provides the results of the planned analysis of the data collected at the end of 6 months.

The study was performed in 10 outpatient dermatology clinics. To obtain a representative sample of dermatologists in the United States, we recruited two investigators from the North American Contact Dermatitis Group, four dermatologists who had considerable experience in patch-testing, and four who recently started patch-testing. These 10 investigators recruited a total of 567 subjects in order to acquire data for at least 500 evaluable subjects. The sample size was chosen such that each investigator would provide evaluable data on at least 50 subjects. No hypothesis testing was planned and no power calculation for sample size was used for comparison of cost-effectiveness. Prospectively collected data for all eligible subjects were evaluated for outcomes related to ACD and patch-testing. The primary outcome measures included diagnosis, disease management, and pharmacoeconomic assessments. Secondary outcomes were the quality of life measures used to estimate the impact of ACD on the subject's quality of life. Diagnosis was assessed by the proportion of subjects with confirmed diagnosis, proportion of subjects with positively identified allergen, number of subjects advised to avoid allergenic substances, and number of subjects who were benefited by change in lifestyle. Disease management was assessed by: results of patch-testing, investigators' global evaluation, the disease management summary, and ACD severity index.

Data were collected using a pharmacoeconomic questionnaire, one component of which was a validated dermatology-specific quality of life (DSQL) instrument. Additionally, data were collected on investigators' global assessment and disease management using case report forms to extract information from subjects' medical charts, which were the source documents.

QOL Methods

The validated DSQL instrument used for collecting data on subjects' quality of life had items on the following dimensions: 1) physical symptoms, 2) activities of daily living, 3) social activities and functioning, 4) work/school, 5) self-perception, 6) mental, 7) vitality, and 8) global items under each of the above headings. The "mental" and "vitality" domains were lifted verbatim out of the SF-36 (9) instrument. Two-sample *t*-tests of mean QOL change were performed between patch-tested and non-patch-tested groups to determine 1) whether patch-testing appeared to result in better outcomes and 2) whether one subgroup characteristic (e.g., having chronic disease) appears to have a better prognostic outcome with patch-testing than another (such as chronic dermatitis of unknown etiology or recurrent dermatitis).

Statistical Methods

In order to assess the associated impact of patch-testing on the clinical, pharmacoeconomic (PE), and quality of life assessments, subjects are divided into two groups: 1) patch-tested—at screening or before or during the 6-month visit—and 2) non-patch-tested—those who do not qualify as "patch-tested."

For statistical summaries and analyses, data are presented by patch-testing status. All statistical tests are two-sided and performed at a 5% significance level. Sample size was chosen with the expectation that each investigator would provide evaluable data on at least 50 subjects.

An evaluable patch-tested subject should have been patch-tested at any time between screening and 6-month evaluation, and an evaluable non-patch-tested subject should not have been ruled out as having ACD between screening and 6-month evaluation. All evaluable subjects should have completed a PE questionnaire at the 6-month visit and a DSQL questionnaire at the screening and at the 6-month visit.

Descriptive summary statistics were provided for all PE variables. The time to confirmed diagnosis in the patch-tested and non-patch-tested groups was compared using Kaplan-Meir estimates and the unstratified log-rank test. For quantitative variables, the two groups were compared using the Cochran-Mantel-Haenszel test with modified ridit scores. Changes within the groups for severity index before and after confirmation of diagnosis were compared using the Wilcoxon signed-rank test.

Total costs per month (of prescriptions and physician visits) from the day of confirmed diagnosis were compared over the period of the study between the subjects who had confirmed diagnosis within 8 days of screening and those who were confirmed after 8 days of screening. These costs were compared to the prediagnosis costs. At the end of the study, the usefulness of early diagnosis to the managed-care organizations will be assessed and estimated from the cost of physician office visits, the number of prescriptions filled, and the improvement in quality of life after confirmation of the diagnosis.

RESULTS

Population Characteristics

Five hundred sixty-seven subjects were recruited for the study, and 124 were discontinued. Reasons for discontinuation are summarized in Table 1. A total of 136 subjects, including the 124 discontinued subjects, were excluded from the 6-month analysis. One hundred twenty-one subjects were

Table 1 Reasons for Discontinuation

Reason for discontinuation	Patch-tested (232) No. (%)	Non-patch-tested (320) No. (%)	Overall (552)[a] No. (%)
Dermatitis cleared up	1 (0)	2 (1)	3 (1)
Lost to follow-up	18 (8)	48 (15)	66 (12)
Other disease/condition that precluded continuation in study	6 (3)	23 (7)	29 (5)
Personal reasons	14 (6)	12 (4)	26 (5)

[a] Total enrolled: 567; subjects excluded due to protocol violations: 15.

Table 2 Summary of Preliminary Diagnosis by Patch-Testing

Preliminary diagnoses	Patch-tested No. (%)	Non-patch-tested No. (%)	Overall No. (%)
Number			
One	163 (70)	167 (52)	330 (60)
Two	54 (23)	103 (32)	157 (28)
Three or more	15 (6)	50 (16)	65 (12)
Categories			
Acute dermatitis with pattern of contact dermatitis-short cutoffs/pattern combined with ACDs	60 (26)	146 (47)	209 (38)
Chronic dermatitis with questionable (unknown) etiology	86 (37)	98 (31)	184 (33)
Recurring dermatitis with questionable (unknown) etiology	86 (37)	128 (40)	214 (39)
Chronic and/or recurring hand eczema	59 (25)	83 (26)	142 (26)
Chronic and/or recurring stasis eczema	2 (1)	1 (0)	3 (1)
Pruritus: chronic and/or recurrent	5 (2)	12 (4)	17 (3)
Nummular eczema	6 (3)	11 (3)	17 (3)
Patchy eczema	9 (4)	17 (5)	26 (5)
Atopic dermatitis: worsening, nonresponding chronic and/or recurrent	9 (4)	26 (8)	35 (6)
Shoe dermatitis or foot dermatitis	4 (2)	10 (3)	14 (3)

nonevaluable for such reasons as lack of QOL and/or PE data, ACD being ruled out, or failure of a 6-month visit to take place (within a 1-month window). Fifteen subjects were excluded because of extraneous protocol violations and improper administration of the QOL instrument. The remaining 431 subjects (76%) were considered evaluable: 186 patch-tested and 245 non-patch-tested.

The overall population was 71% female and 87% Caucasian. The mean age was 45.5 years. The percentage of time with bothersome signs/symptoms prior to enrollment averaged 64% and 65% for the patch-tested and non-patch-tested subject groups, respectively. The prestudy duration of dermatitis was 10 and 12 months (median), respectively. Table 2 summarizes the preliminary diagnoses of the subjects. The most common diagnoses reported were: 1) acute dermatitis with a pattern of contact dermatitis—sharp cutoffs/patterns combined with ACD, 2) chronic dermatitis of questionable (unknown) etiology, 3) recurring dermatitis of questionable (unknown) etiology, and 4) chronic and/or recurrent hand eczema.

Evaluable subjects were stratified by disease severity based on their perception of how severe their skin problem had been on average over the previous month prior to screening. In the assessment of quality of life, subjects were asked to rate the severity on a scale from 1 (very mild) to 10 (very severe). A rating from 1 to 3 was considered "mild," 4–7 was "moderate," and 8–10 "severe." Dermatitis severity as classified thus for this evaluable population is tabulated in Table 3.

The numbers of subjects enrolled were unevenly distributed across sites; the number per site ranged from 31 to 76. Some sites studied twice as many as others. Consequently, some results may vary by site.

Diagnosis

Before we review the results of the disease management, it is important to understand the differences between an observational study and a randomized controlled clinical trial. This is an observational study to perform economic evaluation in real-life situations. Clinicians who are used to randomized clinical trials often ask why subjects were not randomized to "patch-testing" and "non-patch-testing." The current design, with no randomization, is looked on as introducing bias. In an observational study to evaluate outcomes and cost-effectiveness, randomization introduces an artificial component that mars the concept of "real-life" situations. Second, with randomization, subjects would be either forced to undergo

Table 3 Subject Perception of Disease Severity for Evaluable Subjects ($n = 429^a$)

Disease severity	Patch-tested No. (%)	Non-patch-tested No. (%)	Evaluable No. (%)
Mild (1–3)	11 (6)	38 (5)	49 (11)
Moderate (4–7)	73 (40)	107 (44)	180 (42)
Severe (8–10)	100 (54)	100 (41)	200 (47)

[a] Response to the disease severity rating item in the QOL instrument was not provided by two subjects.

unwarranted patch-testing or overlooked for patch-testing when it was necessary, or both. Therefore, the decision to patch-test is left to the discretion of the clinician, based on the history and physical characteristics and the diagnosability of the condition, and to reduce the bias and reflect the reality, the investigators are chosen with various levels of practice experience with ACD. Four investigators patch-tested 15–30% of the subjects, another four patch-tested 30–60% of the subjects, and the remaining two patch-tested 90–100% of the subject (Table 4). Cost-effectiveness studies performed with as little intervention as possible best reflect the real-life scenario and produce results close to reality. Hence, this study is designed with no randomization.

There was a significant difference between the patch-tested and non-patch-tested groups in terms of the time to confirmed diagnosis* (median = 8 days and 175 days, respectively; $p < 0.001$) and, as shown in Table 5, in the ratio of subjects who had a confirmed diagnosis (88% and 69%, respectively; $p < 0.001$). These findings show the effectiveness of patch-testing as a tool to diagnose the cause of disease as quickly as possible after the enrollment of the subject so that appropriate treatment can be administered without undue delay. In the patch-tested group, the investigators advised 76% of the subjects to avoid substances based on the identification of the allergen, while only 43% in the non-patch-tested subjects received that advice. As a result of changes made in their lifestyle, 66% in the patch-tested group and 51% in the non-patch-tested group reported improvement of 75% or more in their disease symptoms.

Considering the large difference between the two groups in terms of the time to confirm the diagnosis, it is evident that there was not enough time

Table 4 Variation in Practice Style Among the Investigators

Investigator sites	Rate of patch testing (%)
Four investigators (40%)	15–30
Four investigators (40%)	30–60
Two investigators (20%)	90–100

* For non-patch-tested subjects, physicians used their customary methods to confirm diagnosis.

Table 5 The Diagnostic Effectiveness of Patch-Testing in Subjects with Suspected Allergic Contact Dermatitis

	Patch-tested	Non-patch-tested
Total number of subjects	186	245
Subjects with confirmed diagnosis	164 (88%)	168 (69%)
Median time to confirmed diagnosis	8 days	175 days
Subjects advised to avoid substances based on the identification of allergen	141 (76%)	106 (43%)
Subjects who made changes in lifestyle	125 (67%)	114 (47%)
75% or more improvement reported as a result of changes in lifestyle	66%	51%

after confirmation of diagnosis to monitor the postdiagnosis improvement and pharmacoeconomic outcomes in subjects not patch-tested for the 6-month data analysis. Highlights of the 12-month results are presented here; detailed final results will be presented at a later date.

The Value of Patch-Testing

The objective of this study is to demonstrate the usefulness of patch-testing to patients, physicians, and managed-care organizations.

Its value to the patients is demonstrated by the following facts:

89% (161 of 180) of patients felt that the patch-testing was worthwhile

88% (134 of 153) of those who felt the cost was "as expected" or "more than expected" reported that patch-testing was worthwhile

72% (13 of 18) of the patients who "did not like" or "strongly disliked" patch-testing acknowledged that it was worthwhile

Specific results demonstrating improvement in quality of life are shown in the next section.

The value of patch-testing to the physician is evident from the higher probability of a confirmed diagnosis and the shorter time to a confirmed diagnosis than when patch-testing is not employed.

The fact that patch-testing is considered worthwhile by patients and physicians alike points to the added value of the services. Early confirmation of diagnosis and education of the patient are very important aspects of disease management in ACD. Subjects who were diagnosed within 8 days of screening incurred lower expenses for prescriptions and office visits (an average of $111) in the prediagnosis period because the diagnosis process took place right after their screening. In contrast, for those whose prediagnosis period extended from 1 to 12 months, expenses ranged from $55 to

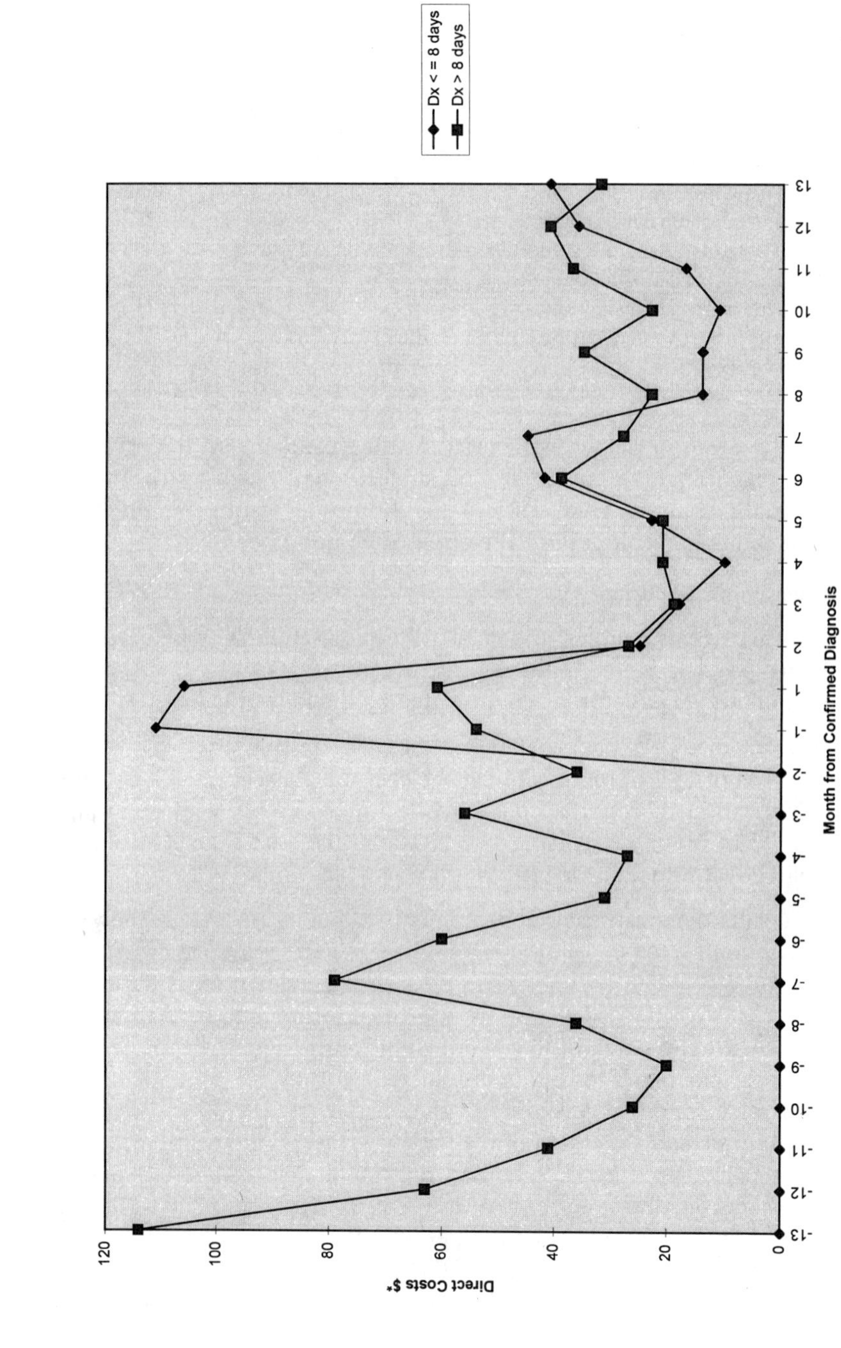

Figure 1 Pre- and post-confirmed-diagnosis cost for patients whose diagnosis was confirmed within 8 days and after 8 days. * Dollar costs represent prescription costs (without generic substitution) and visit costs.

\$622. The former group also had lower expenses for prescriptions and office visits in the postdiagnosis period compared to subjects diagnosed more than 8 days after screening (Figure 1). Further, the longer the delay in confirming the diagnosis, the longer the period during which patients were subject to symptomatic disease activity; the earlier the diagnosis was confirmed, the sooner patients could reduce disease activity by avoiding the causative substances.

Quality of Life

The changes in DSQL scales are well correlated ($0.25 < r < 0.59$; $p < 0.0001$) with changes in self-rated severity of the disease; after treatment of ACD, the 6-month QOL scores are significantly lower (indicating less impact of disease) than baseline scores. This evidence indicates that the DSQL scales reflect changes in QOL associated with improvement after the treatment of ACD (Table 6).

Use of patch-testing in patients with moderate to severe ACD who otherwise met the eligibility criteria of the protocol is associated with greater QOL benefit at 6-month evaluation than when patch-testing was not used (Table 7). This result is obtained even though those not patch-tested, as a group, have less severe ACD than those patch-tested. The greatest QOL benefit from patch-testing, relative to non-patch-testing, occurred in patients with recurrent and/or chronic ACD (Tables 8 and 9, respectively). Less benefit was found for patients with mild or moderate disease.

The results suggest that patch-testing less than one-half of patients classified as having chronic or recurrent ACD would leave many of those not

Table 6 Correlation of Change in DSQL Scores with Patient-Perceived Change in Severity

DSQL scale	*N*	Correlation coefficient (*r*)	*P*-value
Physical symptoms	414	0.592	0.0001
Activities of daily living	398	0.383	0.0001
Social functioning	412	0.468	0.0001
Mental health	409	0.307	0.0001
Vitality	404	0.246	0.0001
Work/school functioning	251	0.288	0.0001
Self-perception	410	0.545	0.0001

Table 7 Comparison of Mean Change in Score on DSQL Scales

	Non-patch-tested group			Patch-tested group			
DSQL scale	N	Mean change	SE	N	change	Mean SE	P-value
Physical symptoms	240	−0.79	0.07	180	−0.99	0.08	0.054
Activities of daily living	234	−0.20	0.05	171	−0.39	0.06	0.017
Social functioning	243	−0.37	0.06	175	−0.55	0.08	0.075
Mental health	238	−0.15	0.06	177	−0.44	0.06	0.001
Vitality	234	−0.10	0.07	177	−0.41	0.08	0.004
Work/school functioning	156	−0.09	0.04	97	−0.26	0.08	0.035
Self-perception	239	−0.51	0.07	171	−0.73	0.09	0.050

Table 8 Comparison of Mean Change in Score for DSQL Scales Between Patch-Tested and Non-Patch-Tested Groups: Recurrent ACD ($N = 169$)

DSQL scale	Non-patch-tested group			Patch-tested group			
	N	Mean change	SE	N	Mean change	SE	P-value
Physical symptoms	97	− 0.58	0.10	69	− 1.23	0.12	0.001
Activities of daily living	96	− 0.09	0.09	68	− 0.44	0.10	0.001
Social functioning	98	− 0.30	0.10	69	− 0.63	0.12	0.039
Mental health	94	− 0.18	0.09	67	− 0.45	0.10	0.052
Vitality	93	− 0.13	0.11	66	− 0.37	0.12	0.137
Work/school functioning	64	− 0.15	0.08	33	− 0.17	0.12	0.916
Self-perception	97	− 0.47	0.11	67	− 0.77	0.13	0.081
Self-perceived severity (global item)	98	− 1.85	0.33	69	− 3.59	0.36	0.001

Table 9 Comparison of Mean Change in Score for DSQL Scales Between Patch-Tested and Non-Patch-Tested Groups: Chronic ACD (N = 139)

	Non-patch-tested group			Patch-tested group			
DSQL scale	N	Mean change	SE	N	Mean change	SE	P-value
Physical symptoms	74	−0.71	0.11	62	−0.98	0.16	0.157
Activities of daily living	72	−0.18	0.10	56	−0.56	0.11	0.009
Social functioning	75	−0.19	0.10	60	−0.54	0.14	0.034
Mental health	74	−0.06	0.09	60	−0.40	0.12	0.026
Vitality	73	−0.01	0.11	63	−0.31	0.14	0.101
Work/school functioning	47	−0.01	0.05	30	−0.45	0.12	0.001
Self-perception	74	−0.21	0.12	56	−0.86	0.17	0.002
Self-perceived severity (global item)	75	−2.09	0.37	61	−3.18	0.44	0.050

Table 10 Comparison of Mean Change in Score at 12 Months for DSQL Scales Between Early and Late Patch-Tested Subjects: Chronic ACD ($N = 139$)

	Patch-tested within 7 days of screening			All others patch-tested			
DSQL scale	*N*	Mean change	SE	*N*	Mean change	SE	*P*-value
Physical symptoms	58	−0.74	0.14	36	−0.01	0.14	0.001
Activities of daily living	58	−0.43	0.13	37	−0.03	0.12	0.016
Social functioning	58	−0.75	0.14	37	−0.01	0.13	0.001
Mental health	58	−0.50	0.12	38	−0.02	0.17	0.021
Vitality	58	−0.21	0.16	38	−0.32	0.16	0.648
Work/school functioning	38	−0.55	0.15	21	0.15	0.13	0.001
Self-perception	56	−0.88	0.16	37	−0.19	0.15	0.001
Self-perceived severity (global item)	60	−3.83	0.36	37	−1.91	0.52	0.002

patch-tested with little or no QOL improvement over 6 months. Increased utilization of patch-testing may result in better QOL outcomes across patients. However, data also show that patch-testing all, or nearly all, such patients probably represents overutilization from a QOL effectiveness standpoint since a proportion of patients (less than 50%) with chronic or recurrent ACD in some dermatology practices apparently can be selected to have good prognoses without patch-testing. In summary, QOL benefits from patch-testing appear to be moderated by patient-selection processes that guide treatment allocation, and that optimal effectiveness is reached at some point between 50% and 100% utilization.

When QOL improvements were compared between chronic ACD subjects patch-tested in the first week of the study and those patch-tested much later in the study period, the former group showed improvement remarkably superior to the latter, and the differences were statistically significant (Table 10). This shows the importance of early confirmed diagnosis. This difference in QOL improvement also influences the differences in frequency of visits, number of prescriptions, and other direct and indirect costs.

When subjects are not patch-tested in the beginning of the study, delay in diagnosis and identification of the allergen contributes to the worsening of the disease and leads to chronicity. When such subjects do not respond to treatment, and are patch-tested at a later date, they cross into the patch-tested group and are liable to increase the postdiagnosis costs for the patch-tested group. Thus, the patch-tested group is defined as comprising only those subjects who were patch-tested within the first 8 days of screening.

CONCLUSION

Patch-testing is considered worthwhile by subjects in spite of the discomfort and additional cost involved. Patch-testing also helps to confirm diagnosis earlier and at a higher rate. More patch-tested subjects than non-patch-tested subjects were appropriately advised to avoid a substance to aid in management of ACD, and at the end of 6 months, a larger proportion of patch-tested subjects reported 75% or more improvement in their symptoms. By confirming the diagnosis earlier, the prediagnosis costs of prescriptions and office visits were reduced; the postdiagnosis costs of prescriptions and office visits were comparatively lower for the subjects diagnosed within the first 8 days of the screening than for those diagnosed later. Overall, the improvement in quality of life is greater in subjects who had their diagnosis confirmed earlier with patch-testing than in those with late patch-testing or none at all. On all but one of the DSQL scales, the subjects who were patch-tested in the first week had greater quality of life and economic benefits than did those patch-tested at later times. On the whole, the data demonstrated clearly the importance of early confirmation of diagnosis (and patch-testing's role in that), and thus early identification and avoidance of the causative allergens and early treatment.

ACKNOWLEDGMENTS

We acknowledge the valuable contributions of all the investigators and the clinical monitors from PharmaResearch Corporation toward the success of this study. We also appreciate Suzanne Peace for her diligent editorial services.

REFERENCES

1. Fisher AA. The use and abuse of patch testing. CUTIS 1985; 36:451.
2. Kieffer M. Nickel sensitivity: relationship between history and patch test reaction. Contact Dermatitis 1979; 5:398–401.
3. Motolese A, Seidenari S. Patch test reading: a comparison between two application methods. Contact Dermatitis 1994; 30:49–50.
4. Brasch J, Henseler T, Aberer W, Baucrle G, Frosch PJ, Fuchs T, et al. Reproducibility of patch tests: a multicenter study of synchronous left-vs.-right-sided patch tests by the German Contact Dermatitis Group. J Am Acad Dermatol 1994; 31:584–91.
5. Ruhnek-Forsbeck M, Fischer T, Meding B, Pattersson L, Stenberg B, Strand A, et al. Comparative multi-center study with TRUE Test and Finn Chamber patch test methods in eight Swedish hospitals. Acta Derm Venereol (Stockh) 1988; 68:123–28.
6. National Center for Health Statistics. Advance data, 1995.
7. Rietschel RL. Human and economic impact of allergic contact dermatitis and the role of patch-testing. J Am Acad Dermatol 1995; 21:812–815.
8. Rajagopalan R, Kallal JE, Fowler JF, Sherertz EF. A retrospective evaluation of patch-testing in patients diagnosed with allergic contact dermatitis. CUTIS 1996; 57:360–364.
9. Ware, JE Jr. SF-36 Health Survey. The Health Institute, New England Medical Center, Boston, 1993.

23

Atopic Dermatitis

Economic Evaluation of Treatments for Eczema and Atopic Dermatitis

Steven R. Arikian* *Columbia University, New York, New York*

Thomas R. Einarson *University of Toronto and Hospital for Sick Children, Toronto, Ontario, Canada*

John J. Doyle* *Columbia University, New York, New York*

OVERVIEW

In the United States, an estimated 30 million physician office visits annually are due to dermatology-related causes (1). Despite this high incidence, relatively little health economic work has been done in the field of dermatology. This is due in part to the fact that dermatological disorders are not life-threatening ailments and therefore do not occupy the health care policy spotlight in the same way that conditions such as heart disease, high blood pressure, and cancer do. Nonetheless, chronic disease of the skin presents serious quality-of-life issues for sufferers, while the complications that may arise from delayed, denied, or inappropriate medical care can raise serious economic issues for payers.

* *Current affiliation*: The Analytica Group, Scarsdale, New York.

The characteristics of atopic dermatitis, or eczema, make it an ideal model for health economic analysis in dermatology. Atopic dermatitis is marked by early onset and is often chronic in nature; it is of uncertain etiology and frequently refractory to treatment; and, finally, serious complications can result if the condition is untreated or improperly treated. Atopic dermatitis, therefore, can provide an example of the way in which quality-of-life measures in the health economic evaluation of a medical condition may have significant consequences for both patients and payers.

Few studies of the economic impact of atopic dermatitis have been conducted, despite the fact that the condition is a common and important cause of morbidity in children of all ages. Atopic dermatitis has been found to be the most frequent diagnosis made in pediatric dermatology clinics—it is the most common skin condition among children younger than 11 years old (2).

This chapter provides a detailed clinical background on atopic dermatitis and a case model for the health economic analyses of the disease that we believe may have broader application in future health economic research in the field of dermatology.

EPIDEMIOLOGY

According to Larsen et al. (3), it is estimated that 9% to 12% of children will suffer from atopic dermatitis. The disease may occur as early as at 2 months, and before age 7 in 80% to 90% of patients, with a female-to-male ratio of 1.4 : 1. There is good evidence from twin studies that genetic factors do influence the development of atopic dermatitis (3).

A personal or family history of allergic disease occurs in 75% to 80% of patients with atopic dermatitis. Even with a family history of atopy, it is difficult to predict the incidence of atopic dermatitis, but it may climb to as high as 80% when both parents have atopic dermatitis. Studies show that severe childhood dermatitis will carry forward into adulthood in about 70% of cases, whereas milder cases will persist in 60% of patients (4).

Atopic dermatitis involves a hypersensitivity reaction within the skin and is characterized by inflammation, itching, and scaling. It has a worldwide distribution and affects all races. It is estimated that 60% of atopic dermatitis cases begin within the first year of life. Ninety percent of cases are found in the first 5 years of life (3). Fewer than 2% of patients had onset after age 20. Late onset of symptoms is a significant diagnostic consideration, since this should alert the physician to rule out other possible conditions such as cutaneous lymphoma or contact dermatitis (4). Of those patients diagnosed with atopic dermatitis, it is estimated that 70% is irritant and 30% is allergic (5). The frequency of cases of atopic dermatitis has increased over the past three decades, from 3% to 10%. Patients with atopic eczema account for 10% to 20% of all referrals to dermatologists and 30% of dermatological consultations in general practice (6).

Most studies of long-term prognosis have been retrospective surveys of clinic or hospital patients. Few prospective studies relating to the epidemiology of atopic dermatitis have been published. Vickers (7), however, provided a structure upon which future prospective studies could be built. His research was based on the study of a large population of eczema patients followed for more than 20 years in Liverpool. Quielle-Roussel et al. (8) carried out a comprehensive computer-based, prospective study of atopic dermatitis in which half of the newborns with a family history of atopy were found to have developed atopic dermatitis within 20 months of birth.

HISTORY

Atopic eczema most frequently occurs in people with a family history of asthma, hay fever, or eczema. It may begin in the first few months of life, with red, crusted lesions. The tendency to scratch these lesions aggravates the condition. Although eczema is usually limited to the hands, scalp, face, neck, and back of the knees and elbows, it may become generalized and cover the entire body. This form of eczema often subsides by age 3 or 4, or in adulthood, but there is always the possibility of recurrence, especially when the patient is under stress.

Although it has been shown that atopic dermatitis has a strong genetic influence, the mode of inheritance remains unknown. Expression may depend largely on environmental factors, including chemical irritants, infection, stress, and allergens.

CLINICAL SPECTRUM OF ATOPIC DERMATITIS

Features

The primary clinical features of atopic dermatitis are:

- Pruritus (itch)—often more severe at night, attributable to the absence of distraction, capillary dilation, and increased skin temperature
- Xerosis (dry skin)—scaling, chapping, and a feeling of skin roughness, exacerbated by frequent use of detergents or defatting substances
- Eczematous lesions—polymorphic, erythematous, papulovesicular, erosive, and crusted appearance that is most prevalent in infantile atopic dermatitis
- Prurigo—a dome-shaped papule, sometimes with a tiny vesicle on top
- Lichenification—a lichenified plaque is a poorly demarcated, slightly tan to red plaque with grossly accentuated skin markings

Dennie Morgan fold—extrainfraorbital eyelid fold—a consequence of scratching of eyelids

Characteristically, atopic dermatitis presents in acute, subacute, and chronic phases with recurring remissions and relapses. The acute phase presents with intense pruritus and erythematous papules and vesicles that become excoriated and exudative with scratching. Secondary infection is common during the subacute stage, with resultant erythema, scaling, and plaque formation. Lichenification, in which the skin is thickened and marked, occurs during the chronic eczematous phase secondary to unrelenting rubbing and scratching. Table 1 describes the four phases of atopic dermatitis.

Complications

Bacterial Infection

The most common bacterial pathogen found in atopic dermatitis is *Staphylococcus aureus*, colonized on the skin in more than 95% of cases. Small superficial pustules, crusting, and weeping occur. Antistaphylococcal antibiotics have an excellent response.

Viral Infection

Infections caused by herpes simplex, vaccinia, warts, and molluscum contagiosum may complicate atopic dermatitis. Generalized spread of herpes

Table 1 The Four Phases of Atopic Dermatitis

Phase	Predominant features
Infantile phase	Lesions first appear on cheek, forehead, and scalp; may also occur on trunk, neck, hands, and feet.
Childhood phase	Eczematous lesions are replaced by lichenification. Prurigo papules occur and are extremely itchy. Commonly, there are elbow, knee, wrist, ankle, and neck flexures. Neck may display reticulate repigmentation.
Adolescent/young-adult phase	Predominant features include pruritus, lichenification, prurigo papules, scratch marks, and crusting. Localized patches of eczema may occur around the nipple or vermilion of the lip. Psychological difficulties may occur in some patients.
Adult phase	Atopic dermatitis ends in most patients after age 20. Majority of patients still have sensitive, unstable skin, and a higher tendency to develop dermatitis.

simplex may occur, causing a possibly toxic condition called eczema herpeticum and/or involvement of the nervous system. Herpes labialis infection may spread on the face to mimic herpes zoster and may involve the eye. Warts and molluscum respond poorly to the usual treatment.

Fungal Infections

Patients with atopic dermatitis are increasingly susceptible to chronic infections of the hands and feet by *Trichophyton rubrum.* This pathogen may cause flareups of dermatitis in areas not involved with fungus. Head and neck flareups respond to ketoconazole treatment.

Exfoliative Erythroderma

In patients with widespread infection of their atopic dermatitis or those in whom systemic steroids have been withdrawn, exfoliative erythroderma may occur. These people develop generalized erythema and scaling with lymphadenopathy, fever, and general systemic toxicity.

Mental and Emotional Dysfunction and Growth Retardation

Symptoms of anger, frustration, anxiety, and depression are commonly experienced in patients with atopic dermatitis. In one study, psychic stress appeared to be the aggravating factor in one-half to two-thirds of these patients (9).

Children who are severely affected by generalized atopic dermatitis may develop growth retardation secondary to being placed in a catabolic state (10). Growth is resumed, even at an accelerated rate, when the dermatitis is controlled. Adults may lose weight and become fatigued but improve when the dermatitis is controlled.

DIAGNOSIS

The diagnosis of atopic dermatitis is based on the patient's history and family history and a physical examination. A skin biopsy is generally not considered helpful. The patient's symptoms of itchiness—increasing in such areas as the folds of elbows, behind or the front of knees, or around the neck—is a key indicator. A history of asthma or hay fever and the occurrence of general dry skin within the past year are also important in a diagnosis. Kjellman (11) has detailed six factors for diagnosis:

1. *Family history of atopic disease*: immediate and/or remote
2. *Case history*: unspecified symptoms indicating a high risk of atopic allergy
3. *Eosinophils in blood*: higher in allergy as well as in certain infections

4. *Clinical finding*: unspecified indicators of possible atopic constitutions
5. Total serum IgE concentrations: high in allergy, parasitosis, and other infections
6. *Specific IgE antibodies against common allergens in blood, skin, or mucous membranes*: may be detected in the presymptomatic stage

Pathology and Laboratory Findings

Controversy exists as to whether atopic dermatitis is a primary inflammatory skin disease or the product of rubbing and scratching. There are difficulties in interpreting existing literature since biopsies are rarely performed on children with atopic dermatitis, on whom diagnostic criteria are best established. Studies in adults rarely mention the criteria used for inclusion and do not specify whether the disease was present in childhood.

The itchy erythematous papule that has been referred to as the earliest clinical lesion in atopic dermatitis is said to be characterized by slight spongiosis, papillary dermal edema, and a sparse perivascular and slightly interstitial infiltrate of lymphocytes, macrophages, and eosinophils (12). However, spongiosis can also occur beneath and to the side of ulcers produced by excoriation. One study has shown spongiosis in nonexcoriated papules from adults with authentic atopic dermatitis (13,14).

Immunohistochemical examination of the inflammatory infiltrate in atopic dermatitis has shown differing ratios of the two types of T lymphocytes present compared to normal skin (15,16). Blood eosinophilia is often noted in patients with atopic dermatitis, tending to be very high in patients with severe atopic dermatitis and respiratory atopy while being normal or moderately elevated in severe cases with no personal or family history of respiratory atopy (17). Langerhans' cells (18,19) and mast cells (14) are increased in chronic lesions of atopic dermatitis.

Serum IgE levels are elevated in more than 80% of patients with atopic dermatitis (19–22). When asthma or rhinitis is associated with atopic dermatitis, the serum IgE level may be markedly elevated (23), while mildly elevated in those patients with only skin involvement (24).

Pathogenesis

Most studies agree that some immune dysfunction exists in patients with atopic dermatitis, but it still remains to be clarified whether the dysfunction is the cause or the effect. Studies on mouse subsets of T-helper cells, named Th1 and Th2, showed the former producing interferon-γ, tumor necrosis factor-α, and other lymphokines, while the latter produce interleukin (IL-4, 5, 6, and 10), and both subsets produce IL-2. Evidence has been found for the existence of these subsets in patients with atopic dermatitis (25,26). Many factors confirm a Th1/Th2 imbalance in atopic dermatitis. The cytokines produced by Th2 cells are important for driving the IgE response in atopic dermatitis. The various interleukins affect IgE synthesis (27,28).

Monocytes are increased in atopic skin lesions. Peripheral blood monocytes in atopic dermatitis produce elevated levels of prostaglandin E2 which affect secretions of Th1 cells. The Langerhans' cells have increased autologous T-cell reactivity, affecting resting CD4-positive T cells without any antigenic stimulation.

Food allergens, aeroallergens such as trees and grass pollens, and house dust mites may also play an important role in the exacerbation of atopic dermatitis (29–33).

Staphylococcus aureus has also been known to flare atopic dermatitis, possibly because of secretion of enterotoxin B.

TREATMENT

Restoration of proper hydration to the affected skin, identification and elimination of triggering factors, and decrease of pruritus and inflammation of the skin are the goals of treatment in atopic dermatitis. Table 2 describes the features of each stage of inflammation, and lists the corresponding treatment (34).

Hydration

Hydration is an important factor in the successful treatment of both acute and chronic stages of atopic dermatitis. During the acute stage the inflamed area may be soaked for 15 to 20 minutes in tepid water two or three times daily.

Besides providing hydration, this process will remove crusts and reduce exudates. A compress of 1:40 dilution of Burow's solution applied for a short time provides astringent and antibacterial effects for localized weeping lesions. Sodium bicarbonate or colloid substances such as oatmeal (Aveeno) or starch can produce a soothing effect if added to bathwater. After bathing, skin should be dried with a soft towel, followed by the application of the appropriate topical medication. Evaporation, which could lead to excessive drying of the skin, should be avoided by occluding the skin within 3 to 5 minutes. Uninvolved skin should be treated with white petrolatum or a moisturizing cream. When the inflammation is controlled, bathing may be reduced to one or two times a day. Use of moisturizers on a regular basis is encouraged.

Table 2 Eczema Treatment Plan Based on Stage of Inflammation

Stage	Morphology of lesions	Symptoms	Examples	Treatment
Acute	Vesicles, blisters, intense red	Intense itch, stinging, burning	Acute contact dermatitis, acute nummular eczema, stasis dermatitis pompholyx	Cold wet compress, steroid, antihistamine, antibiotics
Subacute	Red, scale, fissuring, parched or scalded appearance	Slight to moderate itch, stinging, burning	Contact allergy, irritation, atopic dermatitis, stasis dermatitis, nummular eczema, asteatotic eczema	Topical steroid, emollients, antihistamine, antibiotics
Chronic	Thickening skin, lichenified, excoriation, fissuring	Moderate to intense itch	Atopic dermatitis, lichen simplex chronicus, fingertip eczema, hyperkeratotic eczema	Topical steroid, antihistamine, antibiotics, emollients

Source: Ref. 34.

Trigger Factors

Irritants

Patients with atopic dermatitis have dry, sensitive skin easily irritated by soaps, solvents, and fabrics such as those made of wool and nylon. Drying of the skin may be prevented by using soaps with a neutral pH and minimal defatting, for example, Dove, Tone, Alpha Keri, Basis, Lowila, and Neutrogena. Soapless cleansers such as Cetaphil and Aquinil may be used. To avoid the irritation caused by laundry detergent, extra rinsing of the clothes may be necessary. If the hands are involved in atopic dermatitis, jobs that require frequent washing or exposure to chemical irritants should be avoided if possible. Activities should be modified to minimize sweating, which may cause itching. Ideally, the patient with atopic dermatitis should work and sleep in an environment of controlled temperature and humidity.

Allergies

Atopic dermatitis may be exacerbated by various foods and aeroallergens. Electrostatic air purifiers may be of benefit, and, for mite-sensitive patients, plastic encasement of mattresses and pillows may be helpful. While food avoidance in cases of food sensitivities is helpful, strict compliance should be relaxed in children's diets to avoid malnutrition.

Infection

Recurrent flares of dermatitis may be caused by cutaneous infections with bacteria, viruses, or fungi, which are fairly common in atopic dermatitis. The most common of the bacterial infections is caused by *S. aureus*, which is usually resistant to penicillin. Culture sensitivities should be carried out to facilitate proper antibiotic choice. However, acute flares may be treated initially with erythromycin. In resistant cases, dicloxacillin or an oral cephalosporin may be indicated.

Antibiotic creams are prescribed to treat infected eczema. The older, sedating type of antihistamine tablets or syrups such as Aterax will reduce itching, especially at night. Antihistamine cream may sensitize the skin and thus should be avoided.

Mild herpes simplex infections require no topical or systemic medication. Acyclovir, systemically, is indicated in patients with extensive local or widespread infection and those who are immunocompromised. Burow's solution compresses may be used to dry out vesicles, and an ointment such as bacitracin applied to prevent crusting.

Topical antifungal agents should clear most dermatophyte infection; resistant infections may require systemic treatment with griseofulvin.

Antipruritic Agents

Pruritus is one of the most common symptoms in atopic dermatitis. Antihistamines have been the mainstay of therapy for pruritus, but many studies have found that antihistamines have little effect on the control of pruritus or the improvement of dermatitis (35,36). Studies of both sedating and nonsedating antihistamines show that these agents are not clinically effective in the treatment of pruritus (37). Control of environmental humidity and temperature and the wearing of loose-fitting cotton clothing may help pruritus.

Anti-Inflammatory Agents

Corticosteriods

Topical corticosteroids are effective in decreasing inflammation and pruritus in atopic dermatitis. The lowest effective potency topical corticosteroid should be used. The agent should be applied immediately after bathing to maximize penetration. The choice of potency of the corticosteroid should vary with the location of the inflammation, and it should be applied no more than twice daily. In the acute flare of atopic dermatitis, a medium-potency corticosteroid such as triamcinolone ointment 0.025% to 0.1% may be applied to all affected areas except the face, groin, and axillae, on which a low-potency preparation such as hydrocortisone 1% may be used. As the dermatitis improves, the frequency of the application as well as the strength of the corticosteroid should be decreased and a tar preparation or a moisturizer substituted. Monitor for atrophy and depigmentation.

The absorption of cortisone cream over wide areas of eczematized skin can be potentially dangerous in infants and young children (38). In that study, Feiwel and colleagues found that some children treated with topical steroids had low plasma-cortisol levels, indicating depressed adrenal function.

While these agents may cause dramatic relief, their use is highly discouraged because of the serious side effects associated with long-term use. In addition, they may promote flares when discontinued. If a short course of systemic steroids such as Kenalog IM is given, it is important to institute intensified skin care to suppress flares of dermatitis while tapering off the steroids.

Tar

The anti-inflammatory effects of tar are not as great as those of corticosteroids, but their topical use has a place, especially in subacute or chronic cases. Those commonly used are coal tars, liquor carbonis detergens (LCD), and tar gels. Tar gels such as Estar Gel and Psorigel are the most cosmetically acceptable formulations of crude coal tars, but the alcoholic content of these preparations may cause burning, especially when applied to acutely inflamed skin. A tar preparation consisting of a 2.5% to 5% solution of LCD in a base such as Aquaphor, Dermabase, or petrolatum has been found to be acceptable in patients with atopic dermatitis.

Ultraviolet Therapy

Psoralens plus ultraviolet A (PUVA) is the most effective treatment of atopic dermatitis, but combinations with ultraviolet B (UVB) have been used. UVB alone is not therapeutic unless combined with topical corticosteroids. It appears that the treatment works by modulating the immune response in the skin. The number of treatments of PUVA is high—ranging from 20 to 40, given two or three times weekly, then tapered to weekly and biweekly. Treatment with PUVA resulted in resumption of normal growth in children who were previously growing poorly (39,40). Some patients suffer flares when exposed to ultraviolet therapy, and others experience phototoxicity.

Interferon-Gamma

Patients with atopic dermatitis seem to have decreased secretion of interferon-gamma. Recombinant IFN-γ injected daily by subcutaneous injection over a 12-week period seems to be safe and effective in reducing inflammation, clinical symptoms, and eosinophilia in severe atopic dermatitis (41). However, relapse occurs once the treatment is discontinued. Side effects of the treatment include headaches, fever, myalgia, and nausea but may be avoided by pretreating with acetaminophen and taking the medication at night. The mechanism of action of recombinant IFN-γ is currently unknown.

Cyclosporine

While relatively new to dermatology, the immunosuppressive agent cyclosporine has been studied in patients with severe atopic dermatitis. Its use systematically produced a dramatic effect initially, with skin inflammation and pruritus improving within 10 days. After discontinuation of the drug, there was a rapid relapse (42,43). Careful monitoring is essential, since the drug is associated with serious side effects such as hypertension, elevated serum creatinine, and paresthesias. Cyclosporine gel 10% applied topically was efficacious compared with placebo. Local side effects in the form of irritation and burning were transient (44). Further studies are needed with better excipients.

Thymopentin

Thymopentin is a synthetic pentapeptide that mimics thymopoetin, a thymic hormone that influences the immune system by promoting the differentiation of thymocytes and, perhaps more importantly, by affecting the function of mature T cells. Studies utilizing thymopentin have shown moderate improvement in the dermatitis of patients after 6 weeks of treatment, but with some relapses after 7 weeks. Further studies are needed to determine whether thymopentin acts by correcting the various immune abnormalities in atopic dermatitis (45,46).

Traditional Chinese Medicine

Sheehan and Atherton (47) conducted a controlled trial of traditional Chinese medicinal plants in widespread nonexudative atopic dermatitis. Patients received daily oral decoctions of a mixture of these plants over an 8-week period with effective clinical results. Palatability was a problem, but efforts are being made to develop forms with a less unpleasant taste. This is certainly a treatment to be pursued, considering some of the hazards of conventional therapeutic measures.

ECONOMIC CONSIDERATIONS

The factors to consider in assessing the cost of atopic dermatitis management include drug costs, physician visits, procedures, laboratory tests, and hospitalization. It is estimated that more than $300 million is spent on managing dermatitis annually (48). This cost may be partially or completely paid by the third party, government, or patient. Over-the-counter drugs and preparations may also impact these overall medical costs. For example, 1981 over-the-counter sales of hydrocortisone were estimated to be $74,300,000 and noncorticosteroid poison ivy preparations to be $31,400,000, a total of $105,700,000.

Health economic evaluations are designed to examine resource consumption and consequences of alternative therapies. The design of a particular study may be determined by the perspective adopted, since health economic and pharmacoeconomic investigations may be conducted from many viewpoints, including those of payors, providers, administrators, or patients—as well as from the perspective of society at large. But whatever the study design, the overall goal is to quantify the costs associated with care (whether tangible or intangible) and to establish objective criteria for the valuation of this investment.

Typically, health economic research can help decision makers address such questions as:

What is the best drug for treating a particular patient?

How do two clinical pharmacy services compare?
What is the cost per quality-adjusted life year extended by a particular therapy?
What are the clinical outcomes associated with various therapies?

In the care of atopic dermatitis, the research perspectives that appear to be most meaningful in the application of health economic measures are those of patients and payers, since these two groups are most heavily impacted by the condition.

Perspectives and Costs: The First Step

In designing a health economic model for the management of atopic dermatitis from the patient and payer perspectives, rigorous cost-of-illness studies must be conducted to determine the economic consequences of the disease. The cost of illness is the sum of direct medical costs, direct nonmedical costs, and indirect costs (49).

Some initial cost-of illness work has been done in atopic dermatitis in the United States and the United Kingdom. In a 1993 study of inpatient and outpatient discharge diagnosis logs and computerized ambulatory billing records from Children's Hospital of Philadelphia, Lapidus, Schwartz, and Honig (50) were able to extrapolate a total national cost of treatment for childhood atopic dermatitis of $364 million annually.

The estimates of national costs for treatment were made in four categories: ambulatory care, emergency department care, inpatient care, and pharmaceutical supplies. Ambulatory care cost utilization estimates were based on the 1989 National Ambulatory Medical Care Survey obtained from the National Center for Health Statistics, which used a representative sample of physician practices, excluding fixed-panel HMO and hospital-based providers.

Tables 3 and 4 show the major cost findings of the Philadelphia study (50). This study, however, captured only some of the direct costs of illness associated with atopic dermatitis. In a more recent analysis (51), Herd et al. of the Department of Dermatology and Public Health Sciences, University of Edinburgh, identified the expenditures of 155 patients with atopic dermatitis (eczema) over a 2-month period. The study revealed that the mean personal cost to patients was £25. The mean cost to the health service was £16.20. Among the primary group studied there were 58 lost working days and 17 lost school days. A cohort of 10 seriously affected patients attending the Royal Infirmary of Edinburgh were also studied. Each of these patients spent an average of £325 in 2 months, with a mean health service expenditure per patient of £415. When these results were extrapolated to the total U.K. population, the annual personal cost of atopic dermatitis to patients

Table 3 Projected Reimbursement for Atopic Dermatitis at Children's Hospital of Philadelphia (1990–1991)

	No. of visits	Reimbursement ($)
Hospitalizations	82	268,301
Other practice settings	672	28,900
ER visits	1144	113,229
Total		410,430

Source: Ref. 50.

was found to be £297. The health services cost was £125. The annual social cost due to lost working days was £43, making the total outlay for atopic dermatitis £465. This study targeted a semirural population of 9786 patients served by eight general practitioners, all of whom used computerized records with diagnostic coding for various forms of eczema. The use of computer-based data greatly simplified patient identification and analysis.

To assess the personal costs of the illness, patients were provided with the following instructions:

1. Keep containers of all creams or ointments, bandages, or tablets used for your skin that you buy or are prescribed by your doctor.
2. Record dates of all consultations with a doctor or nurse and expenses involved.
3. Record dates for all visits to the hospital and expenses involved.
4. Record all dates of missed work or school.
5. Record any loss of salary.

Table 4 National Costs for Atopic Dermatitis (1990)

	Cost (millions $)
Hospitalizations	49
Other practice settings	107
ER visits	87
Total	364

Source: Ref. 50.

6. Record any new clothing or bedding purchased as a result of your skin condition and extra laundry expenses.
7. Record any other expenses incurred directly or indirectly as a result of your skin condition.

This study suggests some of the complexities involved in determining the cost of illness—one of the underlying difficulties in health economic analysis is the lack of data on either the costs or the consequences of medical intervention.

Activity-Based Costing

A reliable method for determining the true costs of care comes from analytical models based on actual data collected in the practice setting. While activity-based costing (ABC) is new to health care, methodologies of this type have long been applied in the industrial sector. Some of the earliest efforts to discover the costs of manufacturing production were based on the classic time and motion studies that attempted to quantify the efforts of workers on the factory floor.

In health care, ABC can be used to develop a cost model from composite data derived—in the private practice setting—from profit-and-loss statements of the business; tax records; a detailed examination of the floor plan to determine allocations of space for treatment rooms, physician offices, storage, and other requirements; and, finally, the treatment activities themselves. By carefully tracking the clinical activities of the practitioners in observational studies, one can relate clinician time and medical resources to specific ICD-9 codes. These data can then be consolidated with reasonable "overhead" allocations for the nonmedical costs of rent, space, etc., determined in the baseline paper audit.

The financial accounting definition of "full cost" consists of consumables, labor, and facility. In determining an average cost per medical service delivered, the total accounting cost is divided by a predetermined activity base. The selected proxy for activity should correlate with the cost in the numerator. Activity-based costing is a comprehensive and functional mechanism employed to produce generalizable cost data (52).

To define the full cost of gradation of care, it is necessary to establish the type of resources provided when care is delivered at each level, the quantity of those resources, and their cost per unit. The cost-per-unit calculation accounts for both fixed and variable costs, direct and indirect costs, and specific values of activity. The cost-finding approach consists of five phases:

1. Cost center identification
2. Cost classification

3. Allocation of indirect costs
4. Allocation of full (direct and indirect) costs
5. Intensity level cost adjustment

Using this method, is it possible to determine a specific cost of illness that can be used in a more broad-based health economic analysis of atopic dermatitis.

It is important to recognize that costs are multidimensional in the health care setting. They include:

The cost of treatment
The cost of treating adverse effects
Expenses incurred in nonmedical services such as patients' transportation to provider sites
Earnings lost by patients or family members as a result of treatment

However, in atopic dermatitis, it is likely that once the initial diagnosis is made the most consistently recurring cost element will be the cost of pharmaceuticals and medical service for treatment of both the primary condition and secondary infections.

A Plan for a Prospective Cost-Effectiveness Study of Atopic Dermatitis

Once critical health economic parameters have been identified and defined for a particular illness, it is possible to begin construction of an analytical model that will provide a statistical picture of the prognosis associated with the various possible treatment arms. (See phases I, II, and III below.) An example for such a study by the authors employed an economic model that incorporated elements of both meta-analysis and pharmacoeconomic analysis (53).

Phase I

The purpose, scope, and perspectives of the analysis will be defined. A complete literature review will be conducted to identify comparators and recognized therapeutic guidelines for each comparator in the study. Primary comparators in the study will include the topical agents used to treat atopic dermatitis. Three sets of data will be evaluated: cost of the therapeutic regimen, total expected cost, and cost-effectiveness. Separate analyses will be performed for moderate–severe and mild illness because of differences in cure rates and choice of duration of treatment.

Phase II

The second phase of the research will be composed of four distinct analytical components: clinical management analysis, decision-analytical modeling, meta-analysis, and probability analysis. An expert panel of clinicians will be assembled and interviewed to identify and describe the usual treatment approaches including:

- Treatment regimens (amount, frequency, and duration of therapy)
- Routine medical care required (number and frequency of office visits and laboratory tests performed)
- Adverse-event-management medical care rendered (number and frequency of physician visits and laboratory tests performed; regimens of prescribed and over-the-counter drugs
- Hospitalization
- Other ancillary services
- Drug treatment in the event of treatment failure or disease recurrence
- Alternative choices of therapy

Patients' outcomes will then be identified, including treatment success, failure, and relapse. The failure rate for each drug product will be defined as the proportion of patients that were neither cured nor markedly improved 2 weeks after a course of therapy.

Clinical outcomes will be quantified using meta-analysis of published literature. A stepwise meta-analytic approach will then be employed to determine the relative efficacy and relapse rates of the various treatments. Profiles of adverse events will be developed for each drug.

Results will be combined using the method of Dersimonion and Laird (54) and modified for single-group analysis. This method produces a sample-sized weighted average value for each rate for each comparator along with a standard error so that a 95% confidence interval may be constructed. Two separate meta-analyses will be performed, one for each level of infection. Success rates will be set by analyzing results from published clinical drug trials. The results from this phase of the study will provide quantitative point estimates of clinical outcomes that can be used in the economic analysis.

Phase III

This study will focus on the relative cost of alternative drug regimens and their relationship to clinical outcomes. It is therefore necessary to calculate and sum expected utilities for each drug. All possible patient outcomes will be identified, valued, and classified for relevance to the analytical perspective. The pharmacoeconomic analysis will encompass cost of drug, cost of regimen, expected cost analysis, cost-effectiveness, and robustness analysis. The cost of physicians' services will be extracted from national schedule of benefits records. The cost of medical care will be calculated by multiplying the number of incidents by the unit cost of each incident indicated in the schedule of benefits.

The expected cost analysis will represent the total net cost of each treatment regimen plus the costs of additional therapy when either the regimen fails or the illness relapses.

Finally robustness analysis—a type of breakeven analysis—will be performed to evaluate the sensitivity of the model to change. Values will vary for all drivers of the model, including drug costs, medical care, and laboratory tests.

USE OF DECISION ANALYSIS

In decision analysis, the decision process can be represented diagrammatically as a "decision tree" (Figures 1 and 2). A choice node, represented by a square, indicates a point in time when one of several options or actions may be selected. In developing a decision tree for atopic dermatitis based on the clinical classifications show in Table 2—acute, subacute, and chronic—it is clear that the diagrammatic representation quickly becomes complex and somewhat cumbersome.

In the clinical management of long-term illness, the practitioner faces a series of treatment decisions as the natural history of the disease progresses. A decision tree model can effectively depict only a finite number of decision points. For example, after treatment is administered at any one of the stages of atopic dermatitis, the condition will be either controlled or not. When the long-term illness is not controlled, this pattern is likely to be repeated many times.

An alternative is to employ the Markov process to develop a decision-analytical model for atopic dermatitis (Figure 3), because, while decision-analytical formalism works well for problems involving events that occur once over a short period of time (e.g., the results of a surgical procedure), the natural history of a disease involves events that occur repeatedly or over a prolonged period of time. Under these conditions, a classic decision tree becomes "bushy" and unwieldy. The utility structure also becomes

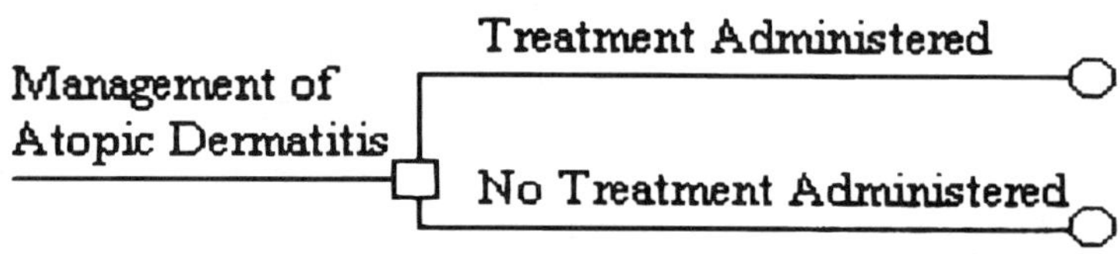

Figure 1 A decision tree for management of atopic dermatitis. The square represents a choice node, a point in time when one of several actions may be taken.

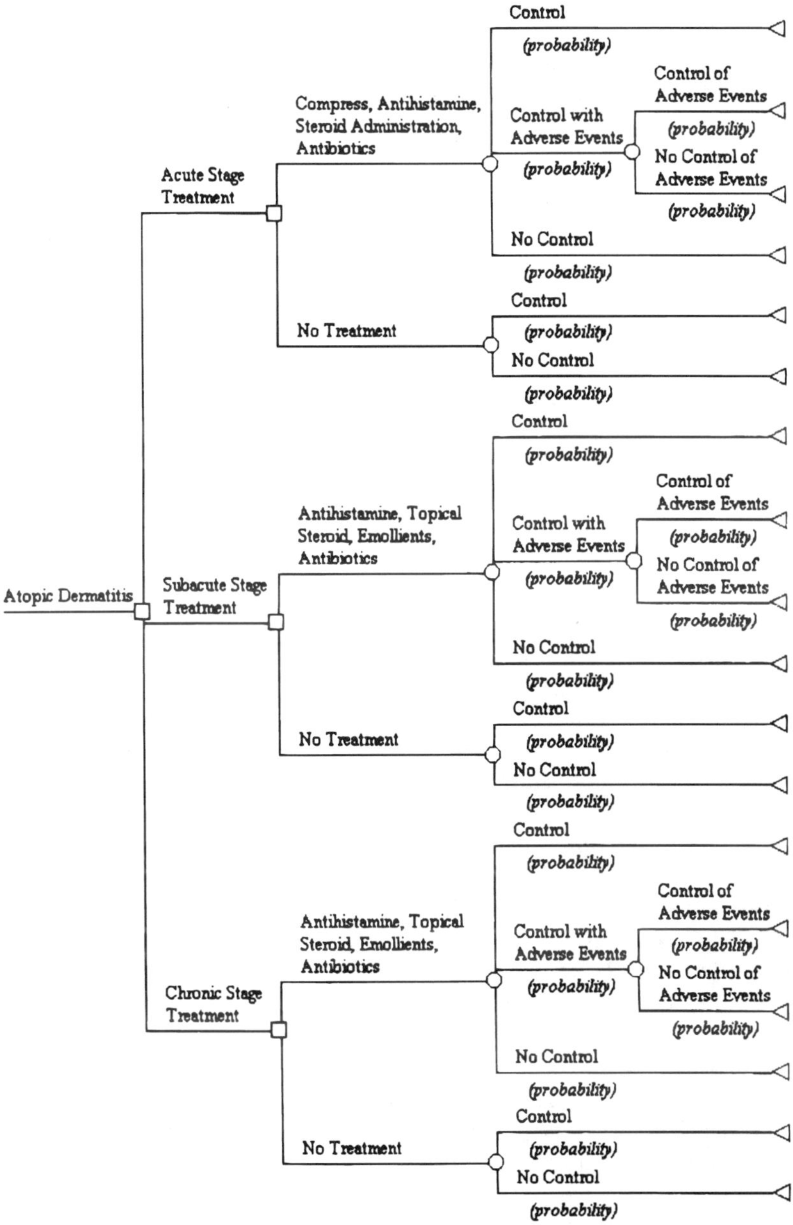

Events in this decision patterns

Figure 2 Further development of the decision tree for clinical management of atopic dermatitis. The events shown occur at probabilities dictated by clinical practice patterns.

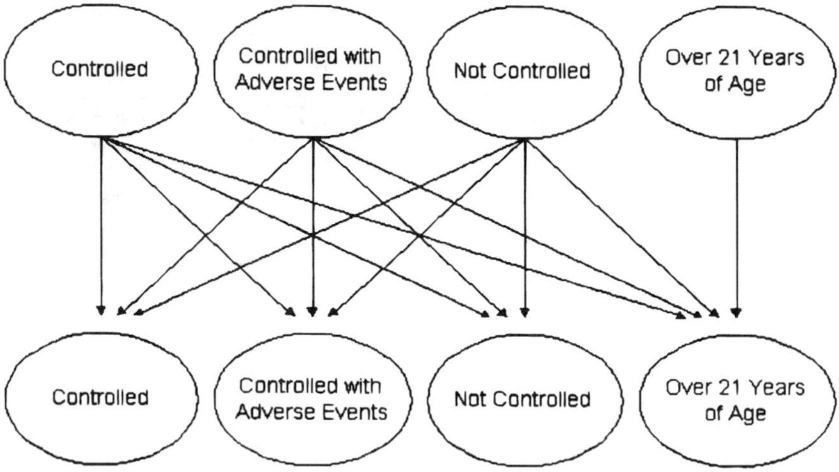

Figure 3 A Markov decision-analytical model for clinical management of atopic dermatitis.

unmanageable because utility must be related to the *time* at which positive or negative clinical events take place.

In applying the Markov model to a long-term, remitting illness such as atopic dermatitis, an individual patient is seen as passing through a sequence of particular states of health. The possible changes of state or transitions occur over the fixed time interval. In the Markov model, the passage of time is represented by cycles or "ticks" of the model's implied "clock".

For purposes of this example, the patient will be classified into one of four categories: controlled, controlled with adverse events, not controlled, and greater than 21 years of age. The reason for this final classification is that the Markov model needs what is called an "absorbing state." Once all patients have entered this state, no further transitions are possible and the process is said to have been absorbed. It is important to note that each change of state is represented by a single transition from one health status to another. The Markov process is said to have "an absence of memory." In other words, the process has no memory of prior states. "All patients in a given state at a given time have the same prognosis, no matter how they got to the present state" (55).

In creating decision-analytical models, it is possible to replace a formalized decision tree with a Markov model and to "graft" the Markov onto a standard decision tree as an equivalent to the utility structure (55).

Whether or not a hybrid approach is used, the power of decision analysis is that it forces the analyst to place the changing situation into a clearly defined structure, moving the process of medical decision making from a largely intuitive process to one that can be graphically articulated.

CONCLUSIONS

It is clear from the clinical profile and the initial cost-finding research that has already been done that the personal and health economic consequences of atopic dermatitis are significant. What is lacking in the current literature is a comprehensive economic analysis of the disease in its various stages and in different practice settings. It would seem appropriate that the condition be evaluated in both private and managed care practice, and that the impact of aggressive self-care and preventive measures such as the avoidance of triggers be measured in a controlled study.

ACKNOWLEDGEMENTS

We would like to thank John Read, Panos T. Lappas, and Thevaki Thambirajah for their help in the research and development of this project.

REFERENCES

1. Office visits to dermatologists: National Ambulatory Medical Care Survey, United States, 1990–91. In: Advanced Data, 1995. Division of Health Care Statistics, National Center for Health Statistics.
2. Hanifin JM, Rajka G. Diagnostic features of atopic dermatitis. Acta Derm Venereol (Stockh) 1980; 92:44–47.
3. Larsen FS, Holm NV, Henningsen K. Atopic dermatitis. J Am Acad Dermatol 1986; 15:487–494.
4. Hanifin, JM. Epidemiology of atopic dermatitis. Monogr Allergy. 1987; 21:116–131.
5. Lantinga H, Nater JP, Coenraads PJ. Prevalence, Incidence and course of eczema on hands and forearms in a sample of the general population. Contact Dermatitis 1984; 10:135–139.
6. Rook AR, Wilkinson DS, Ebling FJG, Champion RH, Bunton JL, eds. The Prevalence, Incidence, and Ecology of Disease of the Skin. Textbook of Dermatology. 4th ed. London: Blackwell: 1986:40.
7. Vickers CFH. The natural history of atopic eczema. Acta Derm-verner, Stockh 1980; 92(suppl):113–115.
8. Quielle-Roussel C, Raynaud R, Saurat, JH. A prospective computerized study of 500 cases of atopic dermatitis in childhood. Actaderm-vern, Stockh 1985; 114(suppl):87–92.
9. Lammintausta K, Kalimo K, Raitala R, et al. Prognosis of atopic dermatitis: a prospective study in early adulthood. Int J Dermatol 1991; 30:563–568.

10. Abrahamov A, Schifmann R, Goldstein R, et al. Growth failure due to protein loss in dermatitis. Eur J Pediatr 1986; 145:223–226.
11. Kjellman NIM, Prediction and prevention of atopic allergy. Allergy 1982; 363–473.
12. Baer RL, Atopic Dermatitis. Med Clin North Am 1959; 43:765–767.
13. Hurwitz RM, DeTrana C. The cutaneous pathology of atopic dermatitis. Am J Dermatopathol 1990; 12:544–551.
14. Mihm MC, Soter NA, Dvorak HF, et al. The structure of normal skin and morphology of atopic eczema. J Invest Dermatol 1976; 67:305–312.
15. Leung DYM, Geha RS, Schnecberger EE, et al. Characterization of the mononuclear cell infiltrate in atopic dermatitis using monoclonal antibodies. J Allergy Clin Immunol 1983; 71:47–56.
16. Lever R, Turbitt M, Sanderson A, et al. Immunophenotyping of the cutaneous infiltrating and of the mononuclear cells in the peripheral blood in patients with atopic dermatitis. J Invest Dermatol 1987; 89:4–7.
17. Uehara M, Izukura R, Sawai T. Blood cosinophilia in atopic dermatitis. Clin Exp Dermatol 1990; 15:264–266.
18. Uno H, Hanifin JM. Langerhans cells in acute and chronic epidermal lesions of atopic dermatitis, observed by L-dopa histofluorescence, glycol methacrylate thin section, and electronic microscopy. J Invest Dermatol 1980; 75:52–60.
19. Zachary CB, Allen MH, MacDonald DM. In situ quantification of T-lymphocyte subsets and Langerhans cells in the inflammatory infiltrate of atopic eczema. Br J Dermatol 1985; 112:149–156.
20. Juhlin L, Johansson SGO, Bennich H, et al. IgE in atopic dermatitis. Arch Dermatol 1971; 103:575–580.
21. Gurevitch AW, Heiner DC, Reisner R. IgE in atopic dermatitis and other common dermatoses. Arch Dermatol 1973; 107:712–715.
22. Stone SP, Muller SA, Gleich GJ. IgE levels in atopic dermatitis. Arch Dermatol 1973; 108:806–811.
23. Jones HE, Inouyc JC, McGerity LM. Atopic disease and serum immunoglobulin-E. Br J Dermatol 1975; 92:17–25.
24. Ohman S, Johansson SGO. Immunoglobulins in atopic dermatitis with special reference to IgE. Acta Derm Venereol 1974; 54:193–202.
25. Fiorentino DF, Bond MW, Mossman TR. Two types of mouse T helper cell. IV. TH2 clones secrete a factor that inhibits cytokine production by TH1 clones. J Exp Med 1989; 170:2081–2095.
26. Wierenga EA, Snoek M, deGroot C, et al. Evidence for compartmentalization of functional subsets of CD4 + T lymphocytes in atopic patients. J Immunol 1990; 144:4651–4656.
27. Pene J, Rousset F, Brier F, et al. IgE production by normal human lymphocytes is induced by interleukin-4 and suppressed by interferons gamma and alpha prostaglandin E_2. Proc Natl Acad Sci USA 1988; 85:6880.
28. Romagnani S, Maggi E, DelPrete G, et al. Regulatory mechanisms of in vitro human IgE synthesis. Allergy 1989; 44(suppl 9):9–15
29. Adinoff AD, Tellez P, Clark RAF. Atopic dermatitis and acroallergen contact sensitivity. J Allergy Clin Immunol 1988; 81:736–742.

30. Clark RAF, Adinoff AD. Acroallergen contact can exacerbate atopic dermatitis: patch tests as a diagnostic tool. J Am Acad Dermatol 1989; 21:863–869.
31. Beck HI, Korsgaard J. Atopic dermatitis and house dust mites. Br J Dermatol 1989; 120:245–251.
32. Colloff MJ. Exposure to house dust mites in homes of people with atopic dermatitis. Br J Dermatol 1992; 127:322–327.
33. Mitchell EB, Crow J, William G, et al. Basophils in allergen-induced patch test sites in atopic dermatitis. Lancet 1982; i:127–130.
34. Tang YM, Ho HF. Social hygiene handbook: eczema. Hong Kong: Social Hygiene Service Department of Health, 1994. http://www.hkma.com.hk/std/eczema.htm.
35. Frosch PJ, Schwantitz HJ, Macher E. A double-blind trial of H_1 and H_2 receptor antagonists in the treatment of atopic dermatitis. Arch Dermatol Res 1984; 276:36–40.
36. Savin JA, Dow R, Harlow BJ, Massey H, et al. The effect of a new nonsedative H_1 receptor antagonist (LN 2974) on the itching and scratching of patients with atopic eczema. Clin Exp Dermatol 1986; 11:600–602.
37. Wahlgren CF, Hagermark O, Bergatrom R. The antipruritic effect of a sedative and a nonsedative antihistamine in atopic dermatitis. Br J Dermatol 1990; 122:545–551.
38. Feiwell M., James VHT, Barnett HS. Effect of potent topical steroids on plasma—cortisol levels of infants and children with eczema. Lancet 1969; i:485.
39. Atherton DJ, Carabett F, Glover MT, et al. The role of psoralen chemotherapy (PUVA) in the treatment of severe atopic eczema in adolescence. Br J Dermatol 1988; 118:791–795.
40. Jekler J, Larko O. Combined UVA-UVB vs. UVB phototherapy for atopic dermatitis. J Am Acad Dermatol 1990; 22:49–53.
41. Hanifin JM, Schneider LC, Leung DYM, et al. Recombinant interferon gamma therapy for atopic dermatitis. J Am Acad Dermatol 1993; 28:189–197.
42. Van Joost T, Stolz E, Muele F. Efficacy of low dose cyclosporin in severe atopic disease. Arch Dermatol 1987; 123:166–167.
43. Taylor RS, Cooper KD, Headington JR, et al. Cyclosporin therapy for severe atopic dermatitis. J Am Acad Dermatol 1989; 21:580–583.
44. DeProst Y, Bodemer C, Teillac D. Randomized double-blind placebo-controlled trial of local cyclosporin in atopic dermatitis. Acta Derm Vencreol 1989; 144(suppl):136–138.
45. Kang K, Cooper KD, Hanifin JM. Thymopetin pentapeptide (TP-5) improves clinical parameters and lymphocyte subpopulations in atopic dermatitis. J Am Acad Dermatol 1983; 8:372–377.
46. Leung DYM, Hirsch RL, Schneider L, et al. Thymopetin therapy reduces the clinical severity of atopic dermatitis. J Allergy Clin Immunol 1990; 85:927–933.
47. Sheehan MP, Atherton DJ. A controlled trial of traditional Chinese medicinal plants in widespread non-exudative atopic eczema. Br J Dermatol 1992; 126:179–184.

48. Johnson M-L, Johnson KG, Engel. Prevalence, morbidity and cost of dermatologic disease. J Am Acad Derm 1984; 11:930–936.
49. Bootman JL, Townsend RJ, McGhan WF. Principles of Pharmacoeconomics. Cincinnati: Harvey Whitney Books, 1991:35.
50. Lapidus CD, Schwartz DF, Honig PJ. Atopic dermatitis in children: who cares? who pays? J Am Acad Derm 1993; 28:699–703.
51. Herd RM, Tidman MJ, Prescott RJ, Hunter JAA. The cost of atopic eczema. Br J Dermatol 1996; 135:20–23.
52. Doyle JJ, Casciano JP, Mauskopf SRJ, Paul JE. Full-cost determination of different levels of care in the intensive care unit. Pharmacoeconomics 1996; 10:395–408.
53. Shear NH, Einarson TR, Arikian SR, Doyle JJ. Pharmacoeconomic analysis of topical treatments of tinea infections. Pharmacoeconomics 1995; 7:251–267.
54. Dersimonian R, Laird N. Meta-analysis in clinical trials. Controlled Clinical Trials 1986; 7:177–188.
55. Beck JR, Pauker SG. Medical decision making: the Markov process in medical prognosis. 1983; 3(4):419–458.

24

Onychomycosis

An Economic Evaluation of Therapies

Aditya K. Gupta, Paul I. Oh, and Neil H. Shear *Sunnybrook Health Science Center and University of Toronto, Toronto, Ontario, Canada*

Thomas R. Einarson *University of Toronto and Hospital for Sick Children, Toronto, Ontario, Canada*

INTRODUCTION

Dermatophytes are a group of closely related fungi that invade keratinized tissue such as the skin, hair, and nails of humans and other animals. In the majority of cases, the infection remains in the cutaneous layer, restricted to the nonliving cornified layers because the fungus is unable to penetrate the deeper tissues in immunocompetent individuals. The dermatophytes are represented by the three genera *Trichophyton*, *Epidermophyton*, and *Microsporum* (1).

ONYCHOMYCOSIS: DEFINITION AND CLINICAL SPECTRUM

Onychomycosis is the infection of the nail by a dermatophyte. The nail bed is involved primarily, often followed by invasion of the dorsal aspect of the nail plate. Onychomycosis may be responsible for 18% to 40% of all nail diseases and 30% of cutaneous fungal infections (2). Four clinical types of onychomycosis are recognized (3). In distal and lateral subungual onychomycosis (DLSO), the fungus first invades the hyponychium, the nailbed, and the undersurface of the free edge of the nail plate (4). This is the most common presentation of onychomycosis (5). The other types of onychomycosis are superficial white (SWO), proximal subungual (PSO), and nail disease due to *Candida* species. In SWO, white, well-demarcated islands are present on the nail plate surface. As the disease progresses, the islands may coalesce to involve the entire surface of the nail plate. The PSO variety is uncommon, with white areas extending distally from under the proximal nail fold (3). The initial lesion is not on the surface but in the deeper aspect of the nail plate. In contrast to the soft and crumbly nail plate surface in SWO, the nail plate in PSO is initially smooth and intact. A subset of PSO has been described in patients with AIDS and occasionally in other conditions (6–8). *Candida* onychomycosis is typically seen in patients with chronic mucocutaneous candidiasis. The lateral and proximal nail fold may be involved. Patients with AIDS who are unable to mount an adequate T-cell response to *Candida* antigens may also exhibit a similar clinical presentation (9). *Candida* species may also cause DLSO, especially in patients whose peripheral circulation is altered, for example, those with Raynaud's phenomenon or vasculitis (10). In some cases of distal or lateral onycholysis, *Candida* species may be cultured. In such cases, the *Candida* may be either the primary pathogen or a contaminant (11). Also, there may be a variation in the incidence of *Candida* onychomycosis in different parts of the world (12). Total dystrophic onychomycosis may be regarded the endpoint of any of the above types of the condition.

INCIDENCE AND ETIOLOGY

The incidence of onychomycosis ranges from 2% to 13% (13,14). In two North American studies, the prevalence of onychomycosis was 7% (5) and 13% (15). The incidence increases with age, and it is estimated that 15–20% of the population aged 40 to 60 years may have onychomycosis (4). In one North American survey (5), the etiological organisms associated with onychomycosis were dermatophytes (90.5%), yeasts (5.5%), and nondermatophyte molds (4%). However, in other studies, dermatophytes have been implicated in as few as 23% of cases (17). Likewise, yeasts have been isolated from nail specimens in 5.5–66% of cases (16–18). Also, nondermatophyte molds have been cultured in 2–15.5% of cases (16–19). The difference in geographical locations of the studies may explain in part the range in values. Dermatophytes are more likely to cause toenail onychomycosis, and yeasts have a higher probability of causing fingernail than toenail onychomycosis, especially in women.

The nondermatophyte molds that may act as primary pathogens include *Scytalidium dimidiatum*, *Scytalidium hyalinum*, and perhaps *Scopulariopsis brevicaulis*. The other nondermatophyte molds may enter the nail when it is damaged, e.g., secondary to trauma, or abnormal, e.g., in psoriasis. Also, nondermatophyte molds have been cultured in association with a dermatophyte. If the same organisms are recultured on a repeated basis, then the diagnosis of a mixed infection is more likely (20). On the other hand, in many instances, the same nondermatophyte mold has not been cultured from two or more consecutive specimens, suggesting that it may have been a contaminant. Patients with onychomycosis often have tinea pedis; in fact, the latter may predispose to onychomycosis. Zaias et al. (21) have suggested that the DLSO caused by *Trichophyton rubrum* infection may be familial, possibly an autosomal dominant condition. Differences in progesterone and related steroids between the sexes may lead to a differential capacity to inhibit the growth of dermatophytes (22). Trauma to the nails, occlusive footwear, and the relative degree of immunosuppression can also contribute to the development of onychomycosis (5).

DIAGNOSIS

It is imperative that, whenever possible, the clinical diagnosis of onychomycosis in an abnormal-appearing nail be confirmed by mycological examination. In a survey, Gupta et al. (5) reported that in only 40% of abnormal-appearing nails could mycological confirmation of onychomycosis be obtained. When the abnormal-appearing nail is suggestive of DLSO, a nail clipper, a #15 scalpel blade, or a 1–2 mm curette can be used to collect nail material (23,24). It is important to obtain a sample from the most proximal part of the involved nail (i.e., the end closest to the nail matrix) because this is the site most likely to yield viable organisms (25). When SWO is present, the affected nail plate surface can be scraped using a #15 scalpel blade or curette. In PSO, the fungal organisms are often deep under the nail plate in the region of the nail cuticle. A nail drill is used less often. A nail micronizer allows nail clippings to be ground to a size suitable for planting a culture (26). The potassium hydroxide (KOH) examination tells the physician whether fungal filaments are present. The identity of the organism is obtained from the culture (27). When the KOH and culture fail to confirm the diagnosis, histological evaluation of nail clippings (28) or even a nail biopsy (29) should be considered.

DIFFERENTIAL DIAGNOSIS

Several conditions can mimic onychomycosis. Age-related nail changes, sometimes accompanied by nail abnormalities from recurrent trauma, can make difficult the diagnosis of onychomycosis on clinical grounds alone (5). It is important to examine all toenails and fingernails for signs of tinea pedis or other stigmata of cutaneous disease. Nail changes in psoriasis can mimic those seen in onychomycosis. However, fine pitting or the oil-drop sign in a nail suggests psoriasis. Psoriasis may be present at other sites. It is worth noting that in psoriatics nail changes may be due to coexisting psoriasis and onychomycosis; in fact, a study has shown that psoriatics have a higher incidence of onychomycosis than the general population (30). Other conditions to consider in the differential diagnosis are changes of onycholysis (especially in fingernails) due to other causes, lichen planus, contact or irritant dermatitis, nail bed tumors, eczema, acrodermatitis continua of Halopeau, pityriasis rubra pilaris, Darier's White diseases, alopecia areata, yellow nail syndrome, keratotic scabies, and acrokeratosis paraneoplastica of Bazex (8).

THERAPIES

The response of onychomycosis to therapy depends on several factors: confirmation of diagnosis, the nature of the infecting organism (dermatophyte, yeast, other nondermatophyte mold, or mixed infection), severity (e.g., <25% nail plate involvement is mild disease; 25 to 75% is moderate severity; and >75% nailplate disease with or without proximal nail plate involvement is severe disease), thickness of diseased nail plate, immune status, other concomitant illness (e.g., chronic mucocutanoeus candidiasis, HIV, or transplant), and rate of outgrowth of the nail plate following therapy. The response to antifungal therapy is proportionately less when nail plate involvement with onychomycosis approaches total nail plate dystropy (i.e., >75% nail plate disease) (31). It is also important to adopt strategies that will reduce the chances of reinfection in the event of cure following therapy: cut nails regularly and keep them short, avoid walking barefoot in areas that may have a high density of fungal spores (e.g., communal swimming pools, gymnasiums, health spas), don't share shoes and consider discarding shoes that may have the highest density of fungal spores, wear sensible shoes that have ample room at the toe and are made of material that allows the feet to "breathe," wear socks made of natural absorbent material—e.g., cotton—and use foot powders and topical antifungal agents. Family members and/or close contacts should be examined and treated for tinea pedis and/or onychomycosis, if possible. The patient should be educated about the symptoms and signs that may suggest a recurrence of onychomycosis or tinea pedis. Onychomycosis treated at an early stage of reinfection or relapse should require less treatment than more severe disease.

Topical Therapies

In North America, there is currently no approved topical treatment that is effective for onychomycosis. In Europe and elsewhere in the world, topical treatments include ciclopiroxolamine (32,33), amorolfine (34–36), and tioconazole 28% nail solution (37,38). Similarly, chemical nail avulsion (39–43) is not used on a regular basis in North America. One situation in which this therapy may be helpful is in the management of some nondermatophyte mold infection since the response of the newer antifungal agents has been variable depending on the antimycotic and the causative agent. For example, when the onychomycosis is due to *Hendersonula toruloidea* and oral therapy with the new agents has failed, then nail avulsion followed by a topical agent should be considered (44). However, such an approach has not always been successful (45).

Surgical Therapies

Before the advent of the new generation of oral antifungal agents, which are significantly more effective than griseofulvin and ketoconazole, surgical avulsion of the nail with adjunctive topical and/or oral therapy was sometimes attempted. This course was most often taken when a patient was keen on seeking a cure and only a single nail was involved. Nail avulsion tends to be performed more commonly by podiatrists, and mostly in Europe. If the diseased nail is thick and hyperkeratotic, then one approach is to curette or file down the affected nail, thereby reducing the "fungal load" that needs to be treated (48).

Traditional Therapies: Griseofulvin and Ketoconazole

Griseofulvin was the first oral agent available to treat onychomycosis (49, 50). Cure rates of 40 to 100% were reported for onychomycosis of the fingernails; however, cure rates for pedal disease were 3 to 38% (51). Furthermore, the duration of therapy for fingernail and toenail onychomycosis was 4–9 months and 9–18 months, respectively. The long duration of therapy for pedal onychomycosis and the low cure rates often led to poor compliance. Furthermore, griseofulvin has a narrow spectrum of action, not being effective against yeasts or nondermatophyte molds.

Ketoconazole was the next significant oral antifungal agent to become available. Several comparative trials were carried out looking at the efficacy of griseofulvin and ketoconazole in treating toenail onychomycosis. Hay et al. (52) treated toenail onychomycosis with ketoconazole 200 mg/day or griseofulvin 500 mg/day. The dose was doubled after 3 months if there was an inadequate clinical response. Treatment was continued until either clinical and mycological remission was achieved or a year of therapy had been completed. The cure rates for ketoconazole and griseofulvin were 21% and 17%, respectively. In the study by Svejgaard (53), when toenail onychomycosis was treated with griseofulvin, the rates of cure and marked improvement were 0% and 57%, respectively. In the ketoconazole group, the corresponding values were 11% and 89%, respectively. Ketoconazole was also found to be effective in *Candida* infections of the nails (54). Soon after the drug became available to treat onychomycosis, there were reports of symptomatic hepatitis. This appeared to be idiosyncratic rather than toxic or immunoallergic (55). There appeared to be no relationship to the duration of therapy, daily dosage, or cumulative total dose (54–56). The incidence of hepatotoxicity has been estimated to be 1:10,000 to 1:15,000 exposures (57). With the availability of the newer antifungal agents, the use of griseofulvin and ketoconazole for the treatment of onychomycosis has markedly decreased (58).

The New Generation of Oral Antifungal Agents: Terbinafine, Itraconazole, and Fluconazole

The availability of terbinafine, itraconazole, and fluconazole has resulted in the re-evaluation of our approach to the management of onychomycosis. Griseofulvin has a poor affinity for nail keratin and is able to reach the nail only via the matrix (59). In contrast, terbinafine, itraconazole, and fluconazole reach the nail plate within 1 week of starting therapy and remain there for several months following therapy (60–66). Both griseofulvin and ketoconazole are fungistatic in vitro. This is also true for itraconazole and fluconazole. Terbinafine is fungicidal in vitro; however, this may or may not have a clinical correlation.

Terbinafine was approved in Canada for the treatment of toenail onychomycosis in May 1993, and is currently the only one of the new agents approved for this indication in that country. Terbinafine was approved for the treatment of dermatophyte onchyomycosis in the United States, in May 1996. The recommended dosage regimen is continuous therapy 250 mg/day for 6 and 12 weeks to treat fingernail and toenail onychomycosis, respectively. More recently, intermittent pulse therapy (IPT) with terbinafine 250 mg twice a day for 1 week a month has been used (67). It remains to be seen whether this will ultimately become the preferred dosage regimen since exactly one-half the amount prescribed in continuous therapy is used (68). The study by Tosti et al. (67), which involved small numbers of patients, showed no significant difference in efficacy between the continuous and IPT groups. The more common side effects observed with terbinafine therapy are gastrointestinal, cutaneous, and central nervous system changes (e.g., headache) (69,70).

Itraconazole is a triazole approved for the treatment of onychomycosis in the United States in October 1995. It is currently not approved for this indication in Canada. The drug was initially used as continuous therapy 200 mg/day for 6 weeks and 12 weeks to treat fingernail and toenail onychomycosis, respectively (71). Subsequently, De Doncker and coworkers (72) demonstrated that IPT with itraconazole was a feasible and effective alternative. The dosage regimen with itraconazole IPT is 200 mg twice daily for 1 week each month. Typically, two and three pulses are sufficient for fingernail and toenail onychomycosis, respectively. The more common side effects observed with itraconazole therapy are gastrointestinal, cutaneous, and central nervous system changes (e.g., headache).

Fluconazole is the third of the newer oral agents that can be considered for the treatment of onychomycosis. Compared to both terbinafine and itraconazole, fewer studies have been reported on its use in onychomycosis. In fact, fluconazole is currently not approved in Canada or the United States for the treatment of onychomycosis. The most commonly used dosage regimen in the literature is IPT 150 mg one dose per week for 3–12 months in toenail onychomycosis (73). A dose-finding study with fluconazole IPT has been completed in the United States, and the results should be available in the near future.

ECONOMICS

Onychomycosis has an important economic impact. Scher (74) has discussed the financial implications of onychomycosis in relation to the over-65-year-old (Medicare) population. In one year alone (year not specified), there were 1,300,000 Medicare visits for onychomycosis, which affected 662,000 beneficiaries. The total cost exceeded $43,000,000. Of the elderly population (>65 years old), 2.7% were treated for onychomycosis compared with less than 1% of individuals <65 years old. Furthermore, there was an increase of onychomycosis with age, reaching over 5% of those aged 75 years and over.

In the United Kingdom, Goodfield et al. (75) carried out a retrospective chart review to determine the direct medical costs incurred in treating dermatophyte fingernail and toenail onychomycosis from a government payer perspective. The estimated cost (including drug acquisition, administration costs, physician fees, and laboratory tests) was £349 per patient treated with griseofulvin and £176 per patient treated with terbinafine.

In a Canadian study, Einarson et al. (76) calculated the expected cost of therapy with a 100% government payer perspective. For toenail onychomycosis, the cost in Canadian dollars of using terbinafine, griseofulvin, and ketoconazole was 1049.77, 1388.54 and 1936.48, respectively. Itraconazole was not considered in this analysis.

In the United States, Halpern and Palmer (77) developed a decision model to compare the costs and outcomes of itraconazole with those of griseofulvin for the treatment of onychomycosis. Cost-effectiveness was expressed as the marginal cost per additional disease-free day gained within a 2-year period starting at treatment initiation. Recorded outcomes included adherence to therapy, occurrence of adverse events and their treatment, clinical response, and the occurrence of relapse. The authors showed that itraconazole was highly cost-effective compared with griseofulvin, with a marginal cost of \$1.56 (1996 value) per additional disease-free day for fingernail infections and \$0.30 for toenail infections. Terbinafine was not considered in this analysis.

In Germany, Van Doorslaer et al. (78) performed a pharmacoeconomic evaluation of the most commonly employed treatments in toenail onychomycosis from a health care payer perspective. They demonstrated that itraconazole IPT was the most cost-effective, at DM GER 1107 (1996 value) per successful treatment, followed by oral terbinafine at DM GER 1224, ciclopirox nail varnish, and itraconazole (continuous dosing). Sensitivity analyses indicated that itraconazole IPT and terbinafine had similar cost-effectiveness ratios with no significant difference between the two agents.

In the United States, Marchetti et al. (79) evaluated the clinical and economic effects of oral griseofulvin, continuous itraconazole therapy, ketoconazole, and terbinafine in the treatment of onychomycosis from the perspective of a third-party payer. Terbinafine had the lowest cost per mycological cure after one treatment regimen for both toenail (\$791, 1996 value) and fingernail (\$454) onychomycosis. With itraconazole continuous therapy, the corresponding costs were \$1535 and \$767, respectively. For griseofulvin, the costs for toenail and fingernail onychomycosis were \$2385 and \$837, respectively. For itraconazole IPT, the cost for toenail onychomycosis was \$1159.

Patient Utility Measurements

Patient utility measurements include quality-of-life or health-status evaluations, willingness-to-pay surveys, and satisfaction surveys (80). In one survey, the quality of life of patients with onychomycosis ($n = 299$) was significantly lower than in those without onychomycosis ($n = 381$) (81).

Therapeutic Implications of Economic Analyses

Onychomycosis is more than a cosmetic issue for many patients. This is reflected by the increase in the requests for treatment for this condition. Several pharmacoeconomic analyses have looked at the most cost-effective therapy for onychomycosis. Only the study of Van Doorslaer et al. (78) has included a topical therapy, ciclopirox alamine, as a comparator. For toenail onychomycosis, when comparing itraconazole IPT and continuous terbinafine, one study found no significant difference in cost-effectiveness between the two dosage regimens (78), whereas another study comes out in favor of terbinafine (79). We are aware of three other ongoing pharmacoeconomic analyses looking at the most cost-effective agent to treat onychomycosis.

Regardless of the agent a physician prefers to use, it is important to realize that the pharmacoeconomic analyses merely provide general guidelines. For a given patient, it is likely that the choice of drug will be individualized depending on several factors, for example, status of regulatory approval of the various agents, physician preference and past experience, etiological agent, concomitant medications, previous treatments for onychomycosis, and patient preference, such as continuous dosing vs. an intermittent pulse format. In the future it is possible that a cost-effective approach to the management of onychomycosis will be the use of combined topical and oral therapies. This may be associated with high efficacy and minimal adverse effects.

REFERENCES

1. Wietzman I, Summerbell RC. The dermatophytes. Clin Microbiol Rev 1995; 8:240–259.
2. Andre J, Achten G. Onychomycosis. Int J Dermatol 1987; 26:481–490.
3. Zaias N. Onychomycosis. Arch Dermatol 1972; 105:263–274.
4. Zaias N. Onychomycosis. Dermatol Clin 1985; 3:445–464.
5. Gupta AK, Jain HC, Lynde CW, Watteel GN, Summerbell RC. Prevalence of unsuspected onychomycosis in patients visiting dermatologists' offices in Ontario, Canada: a multicenter study of 2001 patients. Submitted.
6. Noppakun N, Head ES. Proximal white subungual onychomycosis in a patient with acquired immune deficiency syndrome. Int J Dermatol 1986; 25:586–587.
7. Dompmartin D, Dompmartin A, Deluol AM, Grosshans E, Coulaud JP. Onychomycosis and AIDS, clinical and laboratory findings in 62 patients. Int J Dermatol 1990; 29:337–339.
8. Gupta AK, Scher R. Management of onychomycosis: a North American perspective. Dermatologic Therapy. 1997. In press.
9. Conant MA. The AIDS epidemic. J Am Acad Dermatol 1994; 31:s 47–s50.
10. Hay RJ, Baran R, Moore MK, Wilkinson JD. Candida onychomycosis—an evaluation of the role of Candida species in nail disease. Br J Dermatol 1988; 118:47–58.
11. Daniel CR, Elewski BE. Candida as a nail pathogen in healthy patients. Mississippi State Medical Assoc 1996; 36:2–5.
12. Al-Sogair SM, Moawad MK, Al-Humaidan YM. Fungal infection as a cause of skin disease in the eastern province of Saudi Arabia: prevailing fungi and pattern of infection. Mycoses 1991; 34:333–337.
13. Walshe MM, English MP. Fungi in nails. Br J Dermatol 1966; 78:198–207.
14. Seebacher C. Untersuchungen über die pilzflora kranker und gesunder zehennägel. Mykosen 1968; 11:893.
15. Charif M, Elewski BE. Prevalence of onychomycosis in the United States: results of a population based survey. Arch Dermatol. 1997. In press.

16. Summerbell RC, Kane J, Krajden S. Onychomycosis, tinea pedis and tinea manuum caused by non-dermatophytic filamentous fungi. Mycoses 1989; 32:609–619.
17. Greer DL. Evolving role of nondermatophytes in onychomycosis. Int J Dermatol 1995; 34:521–524.
18. Achten G, Wanet-Rouard J. Onychomycoses in the laboratory. Mykosen 1978; 21:125–127.
19. Kritische MW. Auswertung der griseofulvinbehandlung von Onychomykosen unter besonderer Berücksichtingung des Resistenzproblems. In: Gotz H, ed. Die griseofulvinbehandlung der Dermatomykosen. New York: Springer Verlag, 1962:29.
20. Piefard GE, Arrese JE, De Doncker P, Pierard-Franchimont C. Present and potential diagnostic techniques in onychomycosis. J Am Acad Dermatol 1996; 34:273–277.
21. Zaias N, Tosti A, Rebell G, Morelli R, Bardazzi F, Bieley H, Zaiac M, Glick B, Paley B, Allevato M, Baran R. Autosomal dominant pattern of distal subungual onychomycosis caused by *Trichophyton rubrum*. J Am Acad Dermatol 1996; 34:302–304.
22. Emmons CW. Dermatophytes: natural groupings based on the form of the spores and accessory organs. Arch Dermatol Syphiol 1934; 30:337–362.
23. Hull P, Gupta AK, Summerbell RC. Comparison of different methods of obtaining nail samples for mycological evaluation. Submitted.
24. Daniel CR III. The diagnosis of nail fungal infection. Arch Dermatol 1991; 127:1566–1567.
25. Daniel RC, Lawson LA. Tinea unguium. Cutis 1987; 40:326–327.
26. Daniel CR, Elewski BE, Gupta AK. Surgical pearl: nail micronizer. J Am Acad Dermatol 1996; 34:278.
27. Elewski BE. Clinical pearl: diagnosis of onychomycosis. J Am Acad Dermatol 1995; 32:500–501.
28. Suarez SM, Silvers DN, Scher RK, Pearlstein HH, Auerbach R. Histologic evaluation of nail clippings for diagnosing onychomycosis. Arch Dermatol 1991; 127:1517–1519.
29. Scher RK, Ackerman AB. Subtle clues to diagnosis from biopsies of nails. Am J Dermatopathol 1980; 2:55–56.
30. Gupta AK, Sibbald RG, Knowles SR, Lynde CW, Shear NH. Terbinafine therapy may be associated with the development of psoriasis de novo or its exacerbation: four case reports and a review of drug-induced psoriasis. J Am Acad Dermatol. 1997. In press.
31. Gupta AK, De Doncker P, Scher RK, Haneke E, Daniel CR, André J, Baran R. Itraconazole for the treatment of onychomycosis: an overview. Submitted.
32. Qadripur VSA, Horn G, Höhler T. Zur lokalwirksamkeit von ciclopiroxolamin bei nagelmykosen. Drug Res 1981; 31:1369–1372.
33. Ulbricht H, Wörz K. Therapy of onychomycosis due to moulds with ciclopirox nail lacquer. Mycoses 1994; 37:97–100.
34. Zaug M, Bergstraesser M. Amorolfine in the treatment of onychomycoses and dermatomycoses (an overview). Clin Exp Dermatol 1992; 17:61–70.

35. Reinel D, Clarke C. Comparative efficacy and safety of amorolfine nail lacquer 5% in onychomycosis, once-weekly vs. twice-weekly. Clin Exp Dermatol 1992; 17(suppl 1):44–49.
36. Gupta AK. Amorolfine: an overview. Drugs of Today 1995; 31:145–153.
37. Hay RJ, Clayton YM, Moore MK. A comparison of tioconazole 28% nail solution vs. base as an adjunct to oral griseofulvin in patients with onychomycosis. Clin Exp Dermatol 1987; 12:175–177.
38. Hay RJ, Mackie RM, Clayton YM. Tioconazole nail solution—an open study of its efficacy in onychomycosis. Clin Exp Dermatol 1985; 10:111–115.
39. South DA, Farber EM. Urea ointment in the nonsurgical avulsion of nail dystrophies—a reappraisal. Cutis 1980; 25:609–612.
40. Hay RJ, Roberts DT, Doherty VR, Richardson MD, Midgley G. The topical treatment of onychomycosis using a new combined urea/imidazole preparation. Clin Exp Dermatol 1988; 13:164–167.
41. Ishii M, Hamada T, Asai Y. Treatment of onychomycosis by ODT therapy with 20% urea ointment and 2% tolnaftate ointment. Dermatologica 1983; 167:273–279.
42. Nolting S. Non-traumatic removal of the nail and simultaneous treatment of onychomycosis. Dermatologica 1984; 169:117–120.
43. Rollman O. Treatment of onychomycosis by partial nail avulsion and topical miconazole. Dermatologica 1982; 165:54–61.
44. Rollman O, Johansson S. Hendersonula toruloidea infection: successful response of onychomycosis to nail avulsion and topical ciclopiroxolamine. Acta Derm Venereol (Stockh) 1987; 67:506–510.
45. Tosti A, Piraccini BM, Stinchi C, Lorenzi S. Onychomycosis due to *Scopulariopsis brevicaulis*: clinical features and response to systemic antifungals. Br J Dermatol 1996; 135:799–802.
46. Baden HP. Treatment of distal onychomycosis with avulsion and topical antifungal agents under occlusion. Arch Dermatol 1994; 130:558–559.
47. Baran R, Hay RJ. Partial surgical avulsion of the nail in onychomycosis. Clin Exp Dermatol 1985; 10:413–418.
48. Gupta AK, Scher RK, De Doncker P. Current management of onychomycosis. Dermatol Clin 1997; 15:121–135.
49. Gupta AK, Shear NH, Sauder DN. New antifungal agents. Curr Opin Dermatol 1993; 2:200–206.
50. Gupta AK, Sauder DN, Shear NH. Antifungal agents: an overview. Part I. J Am Acad Dermatol 1994; 30:677–698.
51. Korting HC, Schäfer-Korting M. Is tinea unguium still widely incurable? A review three decades after the introduction of griseofulvin. Arch Dermatol 1992; 128:243–248.
52. Hay RJ, Clayton YM, Griffiths WAD, Dowd PM. A comparative double blind study of ketoconazole and griseofulvin in dermatophytosis. Br J Dermatol 1985; 112:691–696.
53. Svejgaard E. Oral ketoconazole as an alternative to griseofulvin in recalcitrant dermatophyte infections and onychomycosis. Acta Derm Venereol (Stockh) 1985; 65:143–149.

54. Holub PG, Hubbard ER. Ketoconazole in the treatment of onychomycosis. Am Podiatric Med Assoc 1987; 77:338–339.
55. Knight TE, Shikuma CY, Knight J. Ketoconazole-induced fulminant hepatitis necessitating liver transplantation. J Am Acad Dermatol 1991; 25:398–400.
56. Janssen PAJ, Symoens JE. Hepatic reactions during ketoconzole treatment. Am J Med 1983; 74:80–85.
57. Hay RJ. Ketoconazole. Br Med J 1982; 285:584–585.
58. Gupta AK, Shear NH. Attitudes of dermatologists towards prescribing for onychomycosis: a Canadian perspective. Submitted.
59. Epstein WL, Shah VP, Riegelman S. Griseofulvin levels in stratum corneum. Arch Dermatol 1972; 106:344–348.
60. Schatz F, Bräutigam M, Dobrowolski E, Effendy I, Haberl H, Mensing H, Weidinger G, Stütz A. Nail incorporation kinetics of terbinafine in onychomycosis patients. Clin Exp Dermatol 1995; 20:377–383.
61. Faergemann J, Zehender H, Millerioux L. Levels of terbinafine in plasma, stratum corneum, dermis-epidermis (without stratum corneum), sebum, hair and nails during and after 250 mg terbinafine orally daily for 7 and 14 days. Clin Exp Dermatol 1994; 19:121–126.
62. Cauwenbergh G, Degreef H, Heykants J, Woestenborghs R, Van Rooy P, Haeverans K. Pharmacokinetic profile of orally administered itraconazole in human skin. J Am Acad Dermatol 1988; 18:263–268.
63. Willemsen M, De Doncker P, Willems J, Woestenborghs R, Vandevelde V, Heykants J, Van Cutsem J, Cauwenbergh G, Roseeuw R. Posttreatment itraconazole levels in the nail. J Am Acad Dermatol 1992; 26:731–735.
64. Hay RJ. Pharmacokinetic evaluation of fluconazole in skin and nails. Int J Dermatol 1992; 31:6–7.
65. Faergemann J, Laufen H. Levels of fluconazole in normal and diseased nails during and after treatment on onychomycoses in toe-nails with fluconazole 150 mg twice weekly. Acta Derm Venereol (Stockh) 1996; 76:219–221.
66. Wildfeuer A, Faergemann J, Laufen H, Pfaff G, Zimmermann T, Seidl HP, Lach P. Bioavailability of fluconazole in the skin after oral medication. Mycoses 1994; 37:127–130.
67. Tosti A, Piraccini BM, Stinchi C, Venturo N, Bardazzi F, Colombo MD. Treatment of dermatophyte nail infections: an open randomized study comparing intermittent terbinafine therapy with continuous terbinafine treatment and intermittent itraconazole therapy. J Am Acad Dermatol 1996; 34:595–600.
68. Gupta AK, Shear NH. Terbinafine: an update. Submitted.
69. Shear NH, Gupta AK. Terbinafine for the treatment of pedal onychomycosis: a foot closer to the promised land of cured nails? Arch Dermatol 1995; 131:937–942.
70. Gupta AK, Shear NH. Terbinafine in the treatment of superficial dermatomycoses. Can J Derm 1994; 6:561–565.
71. Gupta AK, Sauder DN, Shear NH. Antifungal agents: an overview. Part II. J Am Acad Dermatol 1994; 30:911–933.

72. De Doncker P, Decroix J, Pierard GE, Roelant D, Woestenborghs R, Jacqmin P, Odds F, Heremans A, Dochx P, Roseeuw D. Antifungal pulse therapy for onychomycosis. Arch Dermatol 1996; 132:34–41.
73. Montero-Gei F, Robles-Soto ME, Schlager H. Fluconazole in the treatment of severe onychomycosis. Int J Dermatol 1996; 35:587–588.
74. Scher RK. Onychomycosis is more than a cosmetic problem. Br J Dermatol 1994; 130:15.
75. Goodfield MJD, Bosanquet N, Evans EGV. Cost effective clinical management of onychomycosis. Br J Med Econ 1994; 7:15–23.
76. Einarson TR, Arikian SR, Shear NH. Cost-effectiveness analysis for onychomycosis therapy in Canada from a government perspective. Br J Dermatol 1994; 130(suppl 43):32–34.
77. Halpern MT, Palmer CS. Modeling the cost-effectiveness of oral therapy for nail fungus. Am J Man Care 1996; 2:59–66.
78. Van Doorslaer EKA, Tormans G, Gupta AK, Van Rossem K, Eggleston A, Dubois DJ, De Doncker P, Haneke E. Economic evaluation of antifungal agents in the treatment of toenail onychomycosis in Germany. Dermatology 1996; 193:239–244.
79. Marchetti A, Piech CT, McGhan WF, Neugut AI, Smith BT. Pharmacoeconomic analysis of oral therapies for onychomycosis: a US model. Clin Ther 1996; 18:757–777.
80. Einarson TR, Gupta AK, Shear NH, Arikian S. Clinical and economic factors in the treatment of onychomycosis. PharmacoEconomics 1996; 9:307–320.
81. Lubeck DP, Patrick DL, McNulty P, Fifer SK, Birnbaum J. Quality of life of persons with onychomycosis. Qual Life Res 1993; 2:341–348.

25

Costs of Evaluating and Treating Patients with Cutaneous T-Cell Lymphoma

Debra L. Breneman, Judi A. VanHorn, and John C. Brenemen *University of Cincinnati, Cincinnati, Ohio*

INTRODUCTION

As we are acutely aware, cost containment has become a key issue in health care systems (1–3). As health care budgets come under increasing scrutiny, we will be called upon to identify which therapeutic approaches can achieve specified objectives at the least cost (4–6). The goal in the 1990s is to provide optimum cost effective care for patients without compromising quality.

In making diagnostic and therapeutic decisions we are first and foremost guided by medical and psychological considerations relating to what we believe is best for the patient. If a treatment is warranted on these grounds, we should do our best to deliver it. However, in the delivery we have an obligation to keep cost to a minimum. This chapter will outline the costs of staging and treating a patient with cutaneous T-cell lymphoma of the mycosis fungoides type. There are a tremendous number of variables relating to the actual cost incurred by an individual patient. Costs vary not only between institutions, cities, and states, but also between individual physicians, laboratories, and pharmacies, and even from week to week. In order to obtain a better understanding of the costs of caring for patients with mycosis fungoides, the costs of evaluating and treating patients in the Cincinnati area in the fall of 1994 were examined. It should be noted that even within the greater Cincinnati area there is a wide variation in the costs of evaluating and treating patients with cutaneous T-cell lymphoma. However, the numbers used in this chapter can provide a general idea of what costs may be in a given area. It should also be noted that the costs listed in this chapter are those actually billed to the patient. This information is utilized because billed costs are easier to use in comparing one modality to another. For instance, the cost of treating a patient with topical mechlorethamine relates primarily to the cost of the medication, whereas treating a patient with PUVA involves the costs of the medication, the treatment administration, and the phototherapy unit. A significant portion of the cost involved in treating a patient with radiation is due to the expense of the necessary equipment and facilities. Systemic chemotherapy costs include those for the medications as well as their administration.

DIAGNOSTIC AND STAGING EVALUATION

There are a number of tests that can be utilized in evaluating a patient with suspected mycosis fungoides. In some patients, only a skin biopsy may be indicated, whereas in others a complete staging evaluation may be appropriate. Tests that may be indicated as part of an evaluation include skin biopsy, screening laboratory studies, blood evaluation, imaging studies, and lymph node and bone marrow evaluation.

Cutaneous histology remains the gold standard in establishing the diagnosis of mycosis fungoides. The skin biopsy is generally performed by a dermatologist. The cost of the surgical procedure itself in 1994 was \$70.00, with additional specimens costing \$46.00. If the skin biopsy was performed as part of an initial evaluation, the cost of the evaluation ranged from \$46.00 to \$163.00. Skin biopsies were evaluated initially by hematoxylin and eosin examination. If this examination was done in a dermatology laboratory, the cost was \$60.00. The cost to have it performed in a surgical pathology laboratory was \$278.00. This included a \$138.00 technical fee and a \$140.00 professional fee. If immunohistochemistry phenotyping was performed, the surgical pathology fee was \$660.00 (\$350.00 technical fee plus \$310.00 professional fee). If T-cell receptor gene rearrangement analysis was indicated, the cost was \$356.00, which included a technical fee of \$256.00 and a \$100.00 professional fee. If B-cell studies were also desired, the technical fee was \$278.00 and the professional fee was \$100.00. Therefore, the total cost of evaluating a skin specimen including the surgical procedure, histology examination (using surgical pathology fees), immunohistochemistry phenotyping, and T-cell receptor gene rearrangement analysis was $1,364.00.

Screening laboratories including a complete blood count with differential and liver and bone profiles are generally obtained as part of the initial evaluation of a patient with mycosis fungoides. Costs were: complete blood count with differential, $29.00; liver profile, $21.00; bone profile, $17.00; and venipuncture, $7.00. The total cost of screening laboratory studies was $74.00.

A variety of tests may be utilized in evaluating the presence or absence of blood involvement in patients with mycosis fungoides. The test most commonly used is a Sézary cell preparation, at a cost of $220.00. This cost consisted of an $80.00 technical and $140.00 professional component. Flow cytometry immunophenotyping may sometimes be helpful at a cost of $1,264.00 ($96.00 technical fee plus $1,168.00 professional fee). The cost of T-cell receptor gene rearrangement analysis performed on the blood was $356.00. Thus, the total cost of fully evaluating a patient for blood involvement utilizing Sézary cell preparation, flow cytometry immunophenotyping, and T-cell receptor gene rearrangement analysis was $728.00.

Imaging studies may be utilized in staging patients with mycosis fungoides. A chest x-ray is the most commonly used imaging study, at a cost of $92.00. This included a $62.00 technical component and a $30.00 professional component. If a chest CT scan was used instead, the cost was higher. CT scans of the abdomen and pelvis are occasionally used in staging patients with mycosis fungoides. The cost of an abdominal/pelvic CT scan utilizing contrast was $632.00. This included a $444.00 technical component and a $188.00 professional component. Therefore, the total cost of imaging studies including chest x-ray and abdominal/pelvic CT scan was $724.00.

In select patients, results of lymph node studies can be very helpful in assessing disease extent and occasionally in making a diagnosis. A large portion of the cost was for the surgical procedure itself, particularly if performed in an operating room. The surgeon's fee of $475.00 included a $125.00 fee for consultation and a $350.00 fee for the procedure. The cost of utilizing the operating room was $1,261.00. Charges for supplies, drugs, and preoperative and postoperative care were $1,103.00. Although the procedure was done under local anesthesia, an anesthesiologist monitored the patient at a cost of $420.00. Cost of histological evaluation of a lymph node was $278.00 ($138.00 technical plus $140.00 professional fee). Immunohistochemistry phenotyping was $660.00 ($350.00 technical plus $310.00 professional fee). Flow cytometry immunophenotyping was $2,432.00 ($192.00 technical plus $2,240.00 professional fee). The cost for T-cell receptor gene rearrangement analysis was $356.00 ($256.00 technical plus $100.00 professional fee). The total cost for complete lymph node evaluation was

Table 1 Costs of Completely Evaluating and Staging a Patient with Mycosis Fungoides[a]

Skin biopsy	**$1,364.00**	
Procedure		$ 70.00
Histology		$ 60.00[b]
		$ 278.00[c]
Immunohistochemistry phenotyping		$ 660.00
T-cell receptor gene rearrangement analysis		$ 356.00
Screening laboratories	**$ 74.00**	
Complete blood count		$ 29.00
Liver profile		$ 21.00
Bone profile		$ 17.00
Venipuncture		$ 7.00
Blood evaluation	**$1,840.00**	
Sézary cell preparation		$ 220.00
Flow cytometry immunophenotyping		$1,264.00
T-cell receptor gene rearrangement analysis		$ 356.00
Imaging studies	**$ 724.00**	
Chest x-ray		$ 92.00
CT scan abdomen/pelvis		$ 632.00
Lymph node studies	**$6,985.00**	
Procedure		$ 475.00
Operating room		$1,261.00
Supplies, drugs, preoperative and postoperative care		$1,103.00
Anesthesiologist		$ 420.00
Histology		$ 278.00
Immunohistochemistry phenotyping		$ 660.00
Flow cytometry immunophenotyping		$2,432.00
T-cell receptor gene rearrangement analysis		$ 356.00
Bone marrow studies	**$3,413.00**	
Procedure		$ 399.00
Histology		$ 278.00
Flow cytometry immunophenotyping		$2,736.00
Total	**$14,400.00**	

[a] Most patients do not require all of these tests/procedures.
[b] If done in dermatopathology laboratory.
[c] If done in surgical pathology laboratory.

$6,985.00. This amounted to approximately one half of the entire cost of completely staging a patient with mycosis fungoides.

Bone marrow evaluation can be useful in establishing whether or not visceral spread was present. The cost of the procedure, performed by an oncologist, was $399.00. This included a $150.00 consultation fee, a $174.00 technical fee, and a $75.00 professional fee. Histological examination cost was $278.00 ($138.00 technical plus $140.00 professional fee), and flow cytometry immunophenotyping cost was $2,736.00 ($216.00 technical plus $2,520.00 professional fee). Therefore, the total cost for bone marrow evaluation was $3,413.00.

The total cost for a complete diagnostic and staging evaluation for a patient with mycosis fungoides, including skin, blood, lymph node and bone marrow evaluation, and screening laboratories and imaging studies was $14,400.00 (Table 1).

THERAPY OF THE PATIENT WITH MYCOSIS FUNGOIDES

There are many therapeutic options in treating patients with mycosis fungoides. These can broadly be divided into three main types: topical, systemic, and miscellaneous therapies. Topical therapies include topical corticosteroids, topical chemotherapeutic agents, phototherapy, and radiotherapy (Table 2). Systemic therapies include single-agent cytotoxic chemotherapy, combination cytotoxic chemotherapy, interferons, and retinoids (Table 3). Miscellaneous therapies include photopheresis and bone marrow transplantation. Of note, the costs of therapies administered by patients at

Table 2 Costs of Topical Therapies Available for Treating Patients with Mycosis Fungoides[a]

Therapy	Dose/Concentration/ Frequency	Cost
Mechlorethamine hydrochloride (aqueous)	10 mg/day	$560/28 days
Mechlorethamine hydrochloride (ointment)	0.02%	$120/28 days
Carmustine (aqueous)	10 mg/day	$364/28 days
Carmustine (ointment)	10 mg%	$93/28 days
UVB	Three times weekly	$264/28 days
PUVA	Three times weekly, 30 mg	$504/28 days
Total skin irradiation	3600 cGy	$12,336
Local radiotherapy	800 cGy	$1,186

[a] Costs (except for local radiotherapy) are based on whole skin treatment.

Table 3 Costs of Systemic Therapies Available for Treating Patients with Mycosis Fungoides

Therapy	Dose/Route	Cost
Methotrexate	50 mg po	\$124/28 days
Methotrexate	50 mg IM	\$164/28 days[a]
Methotrexate	50 mg IV	\$1,060/28 days[a]
Fludaribine monophosphate	42.5 mg IV	\$2,985/28 days[a]
2-Chlorodeoxyadenosine	6.8 mg IV	\$10,906/28 days[a]
Deoxycoformycin	8.5 mg IV	\$12,356/28 days[a]
Combination chemotherapy	Variable	Varies with regimen used
Interferon-alfa	3×10^6 U SQ	\$612/28 days
Interferon-alfa	18×10^6 U SQ	\$3,636/28 days
Isotretinoin	70 mg po	\$308/28 days
Etretinate	70 mg po	\$224/28 days

[a] Includes costs of medication and administration.
po = Per orally; IM = intramuscularly; IV = intravenously; SQ = subcutaneously.

home, including most topical and oral medications as well as self-injected medications, are not covered by some insurance policies. Thus, the patient is responsible for the entire cost of therapy. Conversely, parenteral therapies administered in a hospital or physician's office are more likely to be covered by a patient's insurance.

Topical Therapy

Topical Corticosteroids

Topical therapies are commonly used in treating patients with early stage mycosis fungoides. Although routinely used in clinical practice as sole or adjunctive therapy, particularly in patients with early skin disease, there have been very few published studies on the use of topical corticosteroids in mycosis fungoides (7). The cost of a 60-g tube of a topical corticosteroid ranged from approximately \$5.00 to more than \$30.00, depending on the particular agent used. A 60-g tube will last an average patient approximately 2 days if used to cover most of the skin surface. Specific costs in the fall of 1994 were (1) 1% hydrocortisone ointment, 60 g—\$5.45; (2) 0.1% triamcinolone ointment, 80 g—\$5.85, one pound—\$24.69; and (3) clobetasol propionate ointment, 60 g—\$31.70.

Topical Chemotherapy

Two chemotherapeutic agents are commonly used topically in treating patients with mycosis fungoides: mechlorethamine hydrochloride and carmustine (BCNU). In a study by Vonderheid and coworkers in which 324 patients were treated with topical mechlorethamine hydrochloride, complete responses were obtained as follows: 80% Stage I-A, 68% stage I-B, 61% stage II-A, 49% stage II-B, and 60% stage III (8). A sustained complete response was obtained in 10.5% of patients for at least 8 years, possibly representing a cure in these patients. Some of these patients may have actually had parapsoriasis, and some patients also received concomitant therapies.

Most studies utilizing mechlorethamine hydrochloride topically have used it in an aqueous solution. The solution is prepared daily by the patient at home using 10 or 20 mg of mechlorethamine in 40–60 ml water. An ointment preparation may also be used, commonly utilizing 0.02% mechlorethamine in aquaphor. The cost of aqueous mechlorethamine, 10 mg/day, is $20.00 per day and $560.00 per 28 days. The cost of the 0.02% ointment preparation is $180.00 per pound, leading to a patient cost of approximately $120.00 per 28 days. Thus, ointment preparation is significantly less expensive than the aqueous preparation.

Carmustine is another topical chemotherapeutic agent utilized in the treatment of mycosis fungoides, although it is less frequently used than mechlorethamine. In a study by Zackheim in which 143 patients were treated with topical carmustine, complete response rates were as follows: 86% stage I-A, 47% stage I-B, 55% stage II-A, 17% stage II-B, 21% stage III, and 0% stage IV (8). The median time to complete response was 11.5 weeks, and the freedom from relapse at 5 years was 18%, occurring more commonly in patients with early stage disease. The response to carmustine appears overall to be similar to that obtained with mechlorethamine. In utilizing topical carmustine, a stock solution of 1 mg/cc carmustine in alcohol is prepared by the pharmacist. To administer 10 mg/day, the patient mixes 1 teaspoon of the stock solution in 2 oz of water. This is applied daily generally for 4–12 weeks. Retreatment can be performed after a rest period if necessary. The cost of the stock solution, utilizing 100 mg carmustine in 50 cc alcohol, was $130.00. For the patient to apply 10 mg/day, the cost was $13.00 per day and $364.00 per 28 days. For 20 mg/day application, the cost was $26.00 per day and $728.00 per 28 days. Carmustine may also be administered as an ointment preparation. The cost of carmustine ointment, 20 mg%, was $140.00 per pound. Interestingly, the cost of 30 g was also $140.00. As carmustine is supplied in 100 mg preservative-free vials only, the patient is charged for the entire vial whether or not the whole amount is utilized.

Phototherapy

Phototherapy is commonly utilized in treating the cutaneous manifestations of mycosis fungoides. Both UVB and PUVA phototherapy can be used.

In a study in which 31 patients were treated with home UVB, Resnick and Vonderheid achieved complete responses in 74% of patients treated (9). Complete responses occurred mostly in patients with patch stage skin disease. Median time to complete response was 5 months, and median duration was 51 months. There was a sustained disease-free interval of greater than 58 months in 23% of patients.

The cost of in-office UVB was $22.00 per treatment. If given three times weekly, the cost was $264.00 per 28 days. The cost of a typical home UVB unit was $1,400.00.

In a series of 82 patients treated with PUVA by Roenigk and coworkers, 88% of those with limited plaque disease obtained complete clearing as compared to 51.9% with extensive plaque disease and 0% with tumors (8). Mean time to complete response was 8 weeks for patients with limited plaques and 30 weeks for those with extensive plaques. Mean complete response duration was 13 months for those with limited plaques and 11 months for those with extensive plaques.

The cost of PUVA, administered three times weekly, was $42.00 per treatment and $504.00 per 28 days. This included the cost of methoxsalen 30 mg, which was $11.00 per treatment, and the cost of UVA administration, which was $31.00 per treatment.

Radiation Therapy

The neoplastic cells in cutaneous T-cell lymphoma are radiosensitive, and, therefore, total skin irradiation as well as local irradiation are effective treatment modalities for these patients.

In a study by Hoppe and coworkers, 192 patients were treated with total skin irradiation (8). Of those patients with T1 skin disease, 98% achieved a complete response, representing the highest reported complete response rate with any treatment modality. Of patients with T2 disease, 71% obtained a complete response. Thirty-six percent of patients with T3 disease and 64% with T4 disease obtained a complete response using this modality. Of these same patients, 50% of the patients with T1 disease remained disease-free at 10 years, compared to 20% of the patients with T2 disease.

It has been shown that patients receiving at least 3000 cGy to the total skin surface have a higher long-term response rate than patients treated with lower doses (8). Usual treatment regimens consist of administering 3000–3600 cGy over 8–12 weeks. Two thousand centigray may be administered palliatively. The cost of administering 3600 cGy to the entire skin surface was $12,336.00. The cost of administering 2000 cGy was $5,771.00.

Local radiotherapy is commonly used in treating individual tumors or ulcerating plaques and generally leads to rapid and effective local control.

This is administered to individual lesions in 1–15 fractions. The administered dose varies with the fractionation but generally ranges from 800 to 3000 cGy. The cost also varies with the dose and fractionation used. The cost of 800 cGy administered in one fraction was $1,186.00 and of 2000 cGy administered in five fractions was $2,066.00.

Systemic Therapy

Systemic therapy is commonly used in patients with advanced skin disease or visceral disease, but at times may be used in patients earlier in the course of their disease (8).

Systemic Cytotoxic Chemotherapy

Cytotoxic chemotherapy is commonly used in patients with advanced cutaneous disease or in patients with visceral involvement. Using single-agent cytotoxic chemotherapy, objective response rates of 60–70% have been reported with complete response rates of 15–25% (8). The median response duration is less than 6 months. A number of cytotoxic agents have been used as monotherapy in treating patients with cutaneous T-cell lymphoma. These include mechlorethamine, cyclophosphamide, chlorambucil, methotrexate, cisplatin, prednisone, VP16, vincristine, adriamycin, and bleomycin (7,8). Newer agents include fludaribine monophosphate, deoxycoformycin, and 2-chlorodeoxyadenosine (10–12).

Methotrexate is a chemotherapy agent that has been used by dermatologists and rheumatologists for many years as well as by oncologists. In a study by Zackheim in which 17 patients with Sézary syndrome were treated with methotrexate (doses ranged from 2.5 to 80 mg/week), 76% obtained an objective response, with 41% achieving a complete response (13). The median response duration was relatively long at 38 months. Improvement occurred both in the skin and the blood.

The cost of 50 mg methotrexate administered orally, given as tablets, was $31.00 per dose and $124.00 per 28 days. If given in the liquid form, the cost was $5.00 per dose. If administered intramuscularly, the cost per dose was $5.00 for the drug and $36.00 for administration, with a total cost of $41.00 per dose and $164.00 per 28 days. The cost of intravenous methotrexate, administered by a hospital intravenous therapy nurse, was $265.00/dose. This included $5.00 per dose for the drug, $160.00/dose for administration, and $100.00/dose for the oncologist's professional fee. The cost per 28 days was $1,060.00.

The cost of other medications used as single agents varied with the drug used. Of the newer agents, fludaribine monophosphate is relatively less expensive. For 42.5 mg (25 mg/m^2 utilizing a 1.7 m^2 average-sized person) the cost was \$337.00 per dose for the drug. The cost of intravenous administration was \$160.00 per dose with an additional \$100.00 per dose oncologist professional fee, giving a total cost of \$597.00 per dose. For a cycle of fludaribine monophosphate (5-day infusion every 28 days), the total cost was \$2,985.00 per cycle.

Utilizing 2-chlorodeoxyadenosine at a dose of 6.8 mg (4 mg/m^2, 1.7 m^2 person), the cost was \$965.00 per dose. The cost of administration was \$343.00 per dose. With the \$250.00 professional fee component, the total cost per dose was \$1,558.00. The cost per cycle of 2-chlorodeoxyadenosine was \$10,906.00 (7-day infusion, 28-day cycle).

Deoxycoformycin is an expensive drug used in treating cutaneous T-cell lymphoma at a cost per dose of \$2,864.00 (5 mg/m^2, 1.7 m^2 person). The cost of the drug at lower doses was the same. As the drug is supplied in 10-mg preservative-free vials, any unused drug must be discarded and therefore is charged to the patient. Adding an administration fee of \$160.00 and an oncologist professional fee of \$65.00, the total per-dose cost of deoxycoformycin was a hefty \$3,089.00. The cost of four doses over 28 days was \$12,356.00.

Combination Cytotoxic Chemotherapy

In using combination chemotherapy, multiple drugs are utilized to inhibit different phases of the cell cycle (7,8). Objective responses with this modality in treating patients with mycosis fungoides have been reported in the range of 60–100% (8).

There are numerous combination chemotherapy regimens currently in use which could have potential utility in treating patients with mycosis fungoides. CHOP, a regimen that has been used for many years in treating a variety of lymphoreticular malignancies with relatively low toxicity, consists of a combination of cytoxan, adriamycin, vincristine, and prednisone (14). Assuming a 1.7 m^2 patient, the following dosing regimen would typically be used: cytoxan 750 mg/m^2 IV day 1 (1275 mg), adriamycin 50 mg/m^2 IV day 1 (85 mg), vincristine 1.5 mg/m^2 IV day 1 (2.55 mg), and prednisone 100 mg/m^2 (170 mg) po qd × 5. This regimen is generally cycled every 28 days. The cost of these drugs per cycle was cytoxan \$61.00, adriamycin \$324.00, vincristine \$72.00, and prednisone \$40.00. Administration costs of \$253.00 with an additional professional component of \$175.00 lead to a total cost per cycle of \$925.00.

Interferons

Bunn and colleagues treated 20 patients with cutaneous T-cell lymphoma with high-dose interferon therapy. Maximally tolerated doses of interferon alfa-2a 50 × 10^6 U/m^2 were given intramuscularly three times weekly (8).

Objective responses were obtained in 45% of the patients treated, with complete responses achieved in 15%. The median response duration was 5.5 months. Subsequently, low- and intermediate-dose regimens have been used with similar if not higher response rates. Using intermediate-dose interferon alfa-2a 3–36 × 10^6 U per day, objective response rates have been reported in approximately 60% of patients, with complete response rates in 19% (8). A low-dose interferon regimen may consist of administering 3 × 10^6 U subcutaneously three times weekly.

The cost of interferon alfa-2a 3 × 10^6 U was $51.00 per dose, which if given three times weekly was $612.00 per 28 days. The cost of 18 × 10^6 U was $303.00 per dose, which if given three times weekly was $3,636.00 per 28 days. If interferon was administered subcutaneously at home, the only other cost was that of the syringes and alcohol pledgettes. However, some insurance plans do not cover the cost of the medication if it is administered at home. If the interferon was administered subcutaneously by an intravenous therapy nurse, there was a one-time technical charge of $100.00 for patient instruction and the first injection. Following that, the charge per injection was $36.00. There was also an oncologist professional component fee of $25.00 per injection. Therefore, the cost to have the injections performed in an intravenous therapy unit for the first 28 days, including a $496.00 technical fee and a $300.00 professional fee, was $796.00.

Retinoids

Several of the retinoids have been studied in the treatment of mycosis fungoides, with isotretinoin and etretinate being most commonly utilized.

Kessler treated 25 cutaneous T-cell lymphoma patients with isotretinoin 1 mg/kg/day (8). Forty-four percent achieved an objective response, and 12% a complete response. The median duration was 8 months. Large comparative studies have not been performed, but etretinate and isotretinoin probably have similar efficacy in mycosis fungoides.

The cost of isotretinoin 70 mg is $11.00 per day and $318.00 per month. Etretinate 70 mg is slightly less expensive at $8.00 per day and $240.00 per month.

Miscellaneous Therapies

To undergo photopheresis, also known as extracorporeal photochemotherapy, patients are treated with leukopheresis following ingestion of methoxsalen. The buffy-coat lymphocytes are exposed to UVA light in a photopheresis device. The photoirradiated cells are then reinfused into the patient. This is generally performed on 2 consecutive days at 4-week intervals.

In a study by Edelson and coworkers in which 37 patients were treated with photopheresis, an objective response rate of 64% was achieved, with a complete or near-complete response rate of 27% (8). The responses occurred in 3 of 8 patients with plaques or tumors and in 24 of 29 patients with exfoliative erythroderma.

The cost of a 2-day in-hospital cycle of photopheresis ranged from $4,500.00 to $6,000.00.

Autologous bone marrow transplantation is highly experimental in the treatment of patients with cutaneous T-cell lymphoma. In a study by Bigler and coworkers, six patients were treated with autologous bone marrow transplantation (8). Two of these patients were alive and disease-free one year following transplantation.

The cost of autologous bone marrow transplantation was roughly $120,000.00, with an average hospital stay of 31.5 days.

Miscellaneous Costs

The cost of hospitalization for administration of chemotherapy, if required, for an average length of stay of 3.64 days was $8,000.00. This cost included room, board, ancillary services, and chemotherapy medications and was averaged over a large number of patients.

A number of costs were not included in the figures reported in this chapter. Physicians' fees for following patients while on treatment were not included because of the number of variables involved. For instance, radiotherapy and chemotherapy costs include costs of administering the treatments but do not include the professional fees for following patients while on therapy. In some instances these fees can be substantial. Costs of laboratory monitoring, used particularly with systemic treatment modalities, were not included. The costs of treating adverse reactions resulting from therapy were also not included.

CONCLUSION

There are a number of tests and procedures that may be utilized in diagnosing and staging patients with mycosis fungoides. Many effective treatment modalities are available, particularly in treating patients with early disease. Diagnostic and therapeutic modalities are becoming increasingly more numerous and sophisticated.

Because mycosis fungoides is generally a chronic disease, treatment may be prolonged over years or even decades. As physicians, we have an absolute obligation to do what we feel is best for the patient. In addition, we also have an obligation, as best we can, to keep costs to a minimum.

REFERENCES

1. Ellis MS. Stemming the tide of health care costs. J La State Med Soc 1991; 143:29–36.
2. Tuman KJ, Ivankovich AD. High-cost, high-tech medicine: Are we getting our money's worth? J Clin Anesth 1993; 5:168–177.
3. Buchan J. Cost-effective caring. Int Nurs Rev 1992; 39(4):117–120.
4. Lipton HL, Bird JA. Drug utilization review in ambulatory settings: state of the science and directions for outcomes research. Med Care 1993; 31:1069–1082.
5. Kilbreth E, Cohen AB. Strategic choices for cost containment under a reformed U.S. health care system. Inquiry 1993; 30:372–388.
6. Yarbro JW. Changing cancer care in the 1990s and the cost. Cancer 1991; 67:1718–1727.
7. Wieselthier JS, Koh HK. Sézary syndrome: diagnosis, prognosis, and critical review of treatment options. J Am Acad Dermatol 1990; 22:381–401.
8. Holloway KB, Flowers FP, Ramos-Caro FA. Therapeutic alternatives in cutaneous T-cell lymphoma. J Am Acad Dermatol 1992; 27:367–378.
9. Resnik KS, Vonderheid EC. Home UV phototherapy of early mycosis fungoides: long-term follow-up observations in thirty-one patients. J Am Acad Dermatol 1993; 29:73–77.
10. Kemme DJ, Bunn PA. State of the art therapy of mycosis fungoides and Sézary syndrome. Oncology 1992; 6:31–41.
11. Edelson RL. Treatment of cutaneous T-cell lymphoma. Curr Probl Dermatol 1990; 19:226–237.
12. Foss FM, Ihde DC, Breneman DL, Phelps RM, Fischmann AB, Schechter GP, Linnoila I, Breneman JC, Cotelingam JD, Ghosh BC, Steinberg SM, Lynch JW, Phares JC, Stocker JL, Bastian A, Sausville EA. Phase II study of pentostatin and intermittent high-dose recombinant interferon alfa-2a in advanced mycosis fungoides/Sézary syndrome. J Clin Oncol 1992; 10:1907–1913.
13. Zackheim HS, Epstein EH. Low-dose methotrexate for the Sézary syndrome. J Am Acad Dermatol 1989; 21:757–762.
14. Abel EA, Wood GS, Hoppe RT. Mycosis fungoides: clinical and histologic features, staging, evaluation, and approach to treatment. CA Cancer J Clin 1993; 43:93–115.

26

Strategies for Managed Care Programs to Manage Skin Disease

David J. McLean *United HealthCare Corporation, Golden Valley, Minnesota*

INTRODUCTION

To better understand how managed care programs should manage skin diseases, it is important to review and summarize key aspects of the managed care industry. The industry has grown aggressively over the past 10 years. Larger and more dominant health care systems have evolved on a national and regional basis. New products, services, and technologies have been developed to meet the rising demand of a more sophisticated health care consumer.

Managed care strategies are focusing much more on managing specific conditions. This chapter will review four key areas to summarize how programs in managed care are developing to improve the management of specific conditions such as diseases of the skin. The four sections covered include:

Managed care industry status
Focus on condition management
Patient-centered services
Demonstration of value

MANAGED CARE INDUSTRY STATUS

The managed care industry has evolved significantly over the past 20 years. In the early years (1970s and early 1980s), the first-generation emphasis was on driving down unit cost of provider systems by the steerage of patient volume to providers. Emphasis was on building provider networks and negotiating reimbursement rates. HMO approaches focused on staff models, group practices, and independent practice associations (IPAs). Preferred provider organizations (PPOs) were developed in response to HMOs to provide more access and less patient restriction. The focus was still on negotiating contractual discounted rates in return for an anticipated growth in patient base.

As the industry grew and managed care organizations were playing a larger role of insuring health coverages, a second generation developed (mid-1980s). More efforts were being devoted to the measurement and monitoring of quality and cost. Initiatives were started to develop outcome measures for care at the same time payors were continuing to demand solutions to rising health care inflation.

The early part of the 1990s has initiated a third generation that has begun to focus on the demand for treatment. Previous emphasis has been on the unit cost side of health care and on efforts to better manage the utilization of high-cost services such as hospital admissions and length of stays. As more care is being delivered on an outpatient and ambulatory basis, there are more opportunities to improve the delivery of care by focusing on the utilization of services.

Managed care services have been developed to reduce the demand on the treatment system. Services have been developed that assist patients in understanding how to access the delivery system and how to better educate themselves with regard to their health. Emphasis has been on how to maximize effective use of medical treatment systems and not burden the system with unnecessary usage. The underlying focus still has to be on improving quality and service results and providing for appropriate cost management. Studies are documenting overall quality of care performance among health plan programs (1).

The third generation is still in its early stages. Data and information requirements are much different. Information-management technologies are growing in an effort to analyze patient utilization, provider practice patterns, and the usage of health care services by disease state or medical condition.

Market trends seen on the purchaser side of health care benefits are emphasizing the use of best practice HMOs, seamless integration of certain benefit carve-out programs such as utilization management, mental health, and pharmacy. Purchasers have become much more sophisticated in their knowledge and understanding of the health care system as health benefits are continuing to become a larger portion of their cost of doing business. Demands coming from payors are focusing on (1) quantifiable results, (2) access and flexibility, and (3) demonstration of value. Research is showing how market competition affects cost and quality of care (2, 3). The managed care industry is continuing to develop products and services that will meet these demands of the payor customers.

Managed care services are also being targeted for selected market segments. Each of these market segments has specific requirements that the managed care industry will need to address. These market segments include:

Large self-funded employers, who are pushing for best practice HMOs and demonstration of value added results.

Middle and small insured employers are looking for price relief on health care premiums that have been increasing faster than the overall industry.

Medicare beneficiaries are being offered more HMOs to choose from as the federal government continues to try to control Medicare expenditures.

Medicaid programs are being given more authority at the state level to find solutions to provide coverage under managed care options.

International initiatives are being pursued by a few managed care companies as other countries are finding that the pressures developing in their own health care system are similar to those seen in the United States.

The managed care industry is continuing to evaluate and develop systems, services, and technologies to better meet the needs of the payor customers and the consumers who utilize services. Early approaches focused on unit cost and utilization management of institutional services. There is more emphasis on and investment in the management of specific patient conditions and the appropriate utilization of services. Strategies for these disease- or condition-specific approaches are being developed in order to provide consistency in the assessment, approach, and delivery of service for a wide variety of disease states and conditions. As managed care strategies develop to manage conditions such as skin diseases, these strategies will fit into a common framework that is developing to manage other diseases such as asthma, low back pain, congestive heart failure, and depression.

FOCUS ON CONDITION MANAGEMENT

Managed care initiatives of the 1990s are focusing on "disease management," "condition management," or "demand management." Some of these terms may mean different things to different constituencies. For purposes of discussing strategies to manage skin diseases, the term "condition management" is used to frame the review of how this part of the industry is changing. In this section, the following topics will be addressed: historical focus, industry transition criteria, models, and clinical pathway approaches.

Historically managed care organizations have identified the major components of services as:

Physician services
Hospital services
Pharmacy services
Administration

Contractual arrangements are made to manage each of these components with an emphasis on unit costs of services such as physician fee schedules, capitation rates, hospital per diems or per stay rates, drug cost discounts, and overall discounts based on volume of services provided. Priorities center on unit cost, utilization rates of high cost services, claim reimbursement auditing, and variances in treatment patterns. Managing the total cost of services has focused on:

$$[\text{Unit cost} \times \text{rate of usage}] + \text{administration} = \text{total payor cost}$$

The major emphasis has been on managing unit cost with less emphasis on managing the rate of usage.

Until recently, the emphasis of health care service organizations has been on type of service and place of service, and not on the disease, diagnosis, or episode of condition. Health care service organizations are changing their original focus from being either insurance based or provider based to a combination of these. More provider organizations are taking on more financial risk for services rendered, and financial risk-taking organizations are integrating closer with provider systems.

Information technologies have provided for on-line and point-of-service connections primarily for billing purposes. Data base technologies are providing for more access to larger fields on data related to claims experience. Provider network systems are developing the capabilities to exchange information that is more clinically based. These information linkages will provide an infrastructure to exchange relevant patient-specific clinical information among participants in the health care delivery system.

To effectively manage the care of patient populations by condition type, the emphasis must shift to:

Integrating cost and utilization data
Developing an information data base that is comprised of pertinent patient and claim information
Implementing intervention approaches to optimize patient treatment results by condition

Condition management is generally defined as an integrated information-based process involving the continuing improvement of all aspects of health care for a specific condition—prevention, treatment, and management of care. Conditions that are typically chosen for development meet the following criteria:

High prevalence
High cost
National standard of care
Impactability

The systems that are developing in the industry to manage care by condition are integrating information and patient-intervention approaches. Claim-based data files provide methods to identify high-risk patients. Using national standards of care to develop clinical pathways, assessments can be performed to determine appropriate levels of intervention. Appropriate interventions are necessary to improve care, increase compliance, and prevent acute episodes for chronic conditions. A major tool of condition management programs is education of the patient and the provider.

The development of clinical pathways from agreed-upon national standards of care is critical in the evolution of condition management programs. These pathways establish what should be performed and the frequency for the following service areas:

Physician office visits
Laboratory tests
X-rays
Consultant/Specialist usage
Pharmaceutical usage
Durable medical equipment
Ancillary services

These clinical pathways provide health care professionals with a "road map" to monitor the clinical services being provided to patients with the specific condition.

The early development of condition management programs in managed care have focused on chronic conditions that match the criteria of high prevalence, high cost, national standards, and impactability. Conditions that have been targeted include:

Congestive heart failure
Asthma
Low back pain
Pregnancy/Preterm birth
HIV/AIDS
Diabetes
Burns
Cancer
Depression

There have not, as yet, been widespread efforts to develop comprehensive condition management programs for skin diseases. Various diseases of the skin have a high prevalence, but do not always incur high costs per patient or episode of care when compared to the other conditions listed above. The high-frequency diagnoses seen in managed care populations include:

Rash
Acne
Moles
Skin lesions
Dermatitis
Warts
Psoriasis

Managed care industry initiatives for diseases of the skin have, to date, focused on referral protocols to dermatologists, protocols related to coverage determinations (medical vs. cosmetic), claim review auditing, and patient education materials. Selected studies have been performed that compare Medicare HMO populations diagnosed with skin cancers (4). The industry needs to go beyond these early-generation initiatives. Skin diseases do have high prevalence and lend themselves to impactability that calls for more focus on prevention and education. Certain skin conditions should have more industry and consultant agreements established for national standards of care. Treatment options for precancerous skin lesions (actinic keratosis) and the excision of moles based on squamous cell carcinomas are examples of two areas where more industry standards work needs to be done.

PATIENT-CENTERED SERVICES

A key feature in the development of strategies to manage specific conditions is how services are targeted for and delivered to patients. As the industry is evolving, three areas are important for condition management program development efforts: access to services, use of appropriate medical resources, and participative decision making.

Access to Services

Networks

Managed care organizations have operated in a variety of models ranging from restricted provider networks that rely on primary care referrals to specialists to networks with a completely open panel approach that allow direct access to specialists. Surveys have compared patient satisfaction and access to care between health plans and traditional coverages (5, 6). Managed care product structures are moving towards much more open panel choice or network option-out choices at a higher co-pay or co-insurance. Patient access to providers at a primary care point or to specialists is important, particularly for diseases or conditions that have high prevalence, such as diseases of the skin.

Provider Services

Managed care organizations in designing performance measures for provider networks will focus on availability of services, best practice measures of performance by specialty area, patient satisfaction survey results, and overall clinical performance measures that are profiled by specialty area.

Information and Education Services

A fundamental need in managing specific conditions is providing appropriate and timely information to better educate the patient on specific conditions. Managed care organizations have been developing more services to provide more general health information to populations in advance of requiring services. A key objective in condition management initiatives is to be able to provide targeted education services and to be able to measure the results of improved levels of care based on better educated patients.

Access to services for condition management programs needs to focus on best practice provider networks, measurements of service performance, measurements in education levels, and improved levels of care through the measurement of patient outcomes.

In the development of further strategies to manage the diseases of the skin, industry efforts need to focus on the appropriate level of access to providers at both the primary care level and the specialty level. The industry will over time develop more tools for profiling best practice approaches for both primary care providers and dermatologists treating skin diseases. Information and education services will be more broadly available to patients. Emphasis for skin diseases needs to be placed on many of the preventative programs that can benefit patients and make better use of medical resources.

Use of Appropriate Medical Resources

Patient-centered services must focus not only on the access to care, but also on making sure that access is available to the appropriate medical resources. Managing patients with specific conditions requires not only that the system can identify the patients, but also that once the patient is identified, the patient's needs will be matched with appropriate medical services. It is counterproductive to have primary care providers managing patients that clearly have specialty needs. It is equally inappropriate to have specialty provider resources being consumed by patients who could be managed by primary care providers.

High-Risk Patient Identification

The first step in the process is to identify patients who are at high risk. Technologies and reporting systems are evolving that can search claim data bases to identify patients with significant medical needs. These claims analyses are done by condition based on claims utilization experience and other patient-specific medical history information. After high-risk patients are identified, assessment can be made as to the appropriate intervention and channeling can be provided to the appropriate medical providers.

Appropriate Use of Providers

The evolution of provider systems from pure discounting contracts to provider systems that demonstrate a best practice approach is where the industry is moving. Measurements of what constitutes "best practice" are developed by specialty area. The eventual definition of "preferred providers" will be demonstrated through the actual practice patterns of care rather than discount levels or fee schedules.

Referral systems and parameters must be in place to make sure that primary care providers know when to make appropriate referrals to specialists. Protocols should be in place to know what diagnostic tests should be performed by primary care providers prior to the referral to a specialist. Disease specialists are the more appropriate providers to manage specific conditions when the patient's clinical status dictates that level of care. It is an inappropriate use of specialists' resources when conditions can be managed appropriately under an alternative method.

Integrating Care

There is a growing role for nursing care to assist in matching patient medical needs with appropriate medical resources. Patient needs can be identified and best practice providers can be identified. There is a growing potential in condition management programs for the role of the nurse to serve as the integrator of care.

Services of the nurse role can range on a continuum from episodic general health information to specific information related to a given disease state, to a full medical management information approach that assigns a nurse to a patient to assist both patient and providers in managing the patient's medical care needs.

The integrating role of a nurse in a condition management model will demonstrate value by:

Educating patients regarding care options
Eliminating inappropriate services
Improving the compliance of monitoring programs, diagnostic tests, and treatment regimens
Integrating a fragmented health care system
Creating better health care consumers
Demonstrating quantifiable results

Managed care efforts will use many of these condition management approaches of appropriate medical resources usage to manage diseases of the skin. Being able to screen claims data bases to sort out the patients who may be at higher risk for certain types of skin conditions will be a first step. Providers' systems will require appropriate referral protocols among primary care physicians and dermatologists. The role that nurse information services and medical management systems can play in facilitating appropriate patient education and use of services will demonstrate value in how patient populations with selected skin conditions are managed when measured by cost and quality outcomes.

Participated Decision Making

A major reason for reorienting the health care system by specific condition is to engage the patient much more in the process of managing their care. Information and education play a significant role in improving the health status of patients with the defined condition. Patients who are further educated become more involved in their own care and in appropriate lifestyle changes that may be necessary.

The delivery systems are providing more information to patients. Alternatives need to be presented to patients when choices are available so that patients can take an active role in the decision process regarding treatment options. Patients will take more responsibility for their own care when the information about their condition is understood and they achieve a readiness to make changes in the management of their care and in their lifestyle.

Many diseases of the skin lend themselves to better prevention programs, improved compliance of treatments, and appropriate monitoring and follow-up care by providers. In order to accomplish these steps, patients must be engaged to participate in the decision process of managing their medical care.

DEMONSTRATION OF VALUE

The payors of health care benefits are demanding more accountability of the health care delivery system to demonstrate the value of services rendered. Since managed care organizations hold the contracts with payors, the responsibility rests with the respective managed care organization to develop the systems, the process, and results of measuring value of services delivered to patient populations. Value measurements in the industry are evolving to focus on total costs of services and on quality outcome parameters. Condition management programs require the measurement of outcomes to continually improve program tools and components to assure that impact is made on the specific condition. Value measures typically focus on reduced use of inappropriate services, improved compliance with guidelines, and increases in patient and provider satisfaction levels.

Data bases of information that are developed for condition management programs offer opportunities to demonstrate value in different ways. Three areas that claim data bases can be used: (1) predictive profiling, (2) population-based clinical reviews, and (3) pharmaceutical research.

Predictive Profiling

Claim data bases offer opportunities to construct claim pathways from medical and pharmacy claims to identify patients who are at high risk for defined impactable conditions. Based on claims experience, levels of severity can be established to identify those individuals who can be ranked based on their risk level. Being able to identify patients prospectively allows a condition management program to reach out and involve the patient earlier in their disease state, which can reduce the intensity of care over time.

Claim data bases also offer profiling capabilities for analyzing provider practice patterns. The establishment of appropriate practice patterns also allows providers to be analyzed and compared with peers based on population-based claim experience. This offers the opportunity to compare providers based on agreed upon standards, and identify best practice performance by providers.

Population-Based Clinical Reviews

Using information from a variety of sources such as claims experience, consultant/specialty guidelines, provider practice experience, and patient surveys can establish improved national standards of care by condition. Managed care organizations are expanding the focus by condition to seek agreements on care protocols for condition management programs being developed. These national standards of care become the quantifiable benchmarks for measuring performance by providers and health care outcomes of patients.

Pharmaceutical Research

Managed care data bases offer future opportunities to enhance pharmaceutical research initiatives. Medical and pharmacy claims can provide for population-based analytical techniques to aid in drug design and development. This can lead to the prospective identification of therapeutic agents. In addition, these data base tools and technologies can also be used in the future management of clinical trials and in postmarketing surveillance efforts.

Managed care initiatives will advance the information systems and technologies for condition management programs. These advancements will offer quantifiable methods for measuring and demonstrating value. These approaches will further advance how managed care programs will focus on diseases of skin. The ability to profile patients based on patterns of dermatological care will identify patients who may be in need of more assistance in managing their particular condition.

The expansion of national standards of care for key dermatological conditions will help provide standardization. This will allow delivery systems to reduce the level of variability in how treatment is provided for defined conditions.

Access to managed care data bases will provide for effective methods to enhance how pharmaceutical companies can conduct design initiatives, development programs, clinical trials, and surveillance for dermatological agents.

CONCLUSIONS

The managed care industry is in the early stages of developing and implementing programs to manage care by condition. These programs require information systems that can capture, analyze, and report information related to a patient's medical condition. Establishment of national standards of care, the identification of specialist providers, information, and education programs, along with nurse intervention services, are all important components in building a condition management program.

These condition management program components all have applicability to the management of skin diseases. Managed care organizations can use many of the technologies and approaches being used with other conditions to provide for more comprehensive strategies in managing diseases of the skin.

REFERENCES

1. Miller RH, Luft HS. Managed care plan performance since 1980: A literature analysis. J Am Med Assoc 1994; 271: 1512–1519.
2. Levit KR, et al. Health care spending in 1994: Slowest in decades. Health Affairs 1996; 15: 130–144.
3. The Impact of Managed Care on the U.S. Market. Costa Mesa, CA: KPMG Peat Marwick, 1996.
4. Riley GF, et al. Stage of cancer and diagnosis for Medicare HMO and fee-for-service enrollees. Am J Public Health 1994; 84: 1598–1604.
5. Donelan K, et al. All payer, single payer, Managed Care, no payer: Patients' perspectives in three nations. Health Affairs 1996; 15(2): 254–265.
6. 1995 Consumer Survey: Summary Report of Health Plan Category Comparisons. St. Paul: Minnesota Health Data Institute, 1996.

27

Strategies for Primary Care Physicians to Manage Contact Dermatitis

David M. Pariser *Eastern Virginia Medical School, Norfolk, Virginia*

DEFINITION

Contact dermatitis (CD) may be defined as an inflammation of the skin that results from the interaction of the skin with a chemical substance. CD is only one of many such interactions. Others include urticaria, pigmentation disorders, photosensitization, acneiform eruptions, atrophy, and purpura. CD is characterized clinically in the acute phase by the presence of vesicles and histologically by spongiosis and intracellular edema and in the more chronic phases by erythema, scaling, and other secondary changes.

In general, CD is divided into two major pathways—irritant contact dermatitis (ICD) and allergic contact dermatitis (ACD).

SCOPE OF THE PROBLEM

Contact dermatitis is one of if not the most common skin problem in industrialized societies, and it has been estimated that there is up to 10% prevalence. It is among the top 20 reasons for a visit to a primary care physician/provider (PCP) (1). CD is often seen in the workplace and represents a significant cause of lost days from work. As would be expected, certain occupations where exposure to chemicals occurs represent the highest incidence of CD (2). Most contact dermatitis (about 80%) falls into the category of irritant dermatitis (ICD), whereas a smaller fraction (about 20%) is allergic in origin and, therefore, antigen specific. ICD is caused by direct damage to the skin from the external substance without prior sensitization. There is considerable overlap in the clinical presentation of ICD and ACD. In fact, some substances may act as allergens in some instances and as irritants in other instances, the difference being concentration dependent as well as host specific.

DISEASE MECHANISMS

ACD is a classic delayed hypersensitivity reaction, so-called Type IV immunological reaction, and is mediated by cellular immunity rather than by antibodies. For a patient to develop ACD, there must be a *sensitization phase* where the allergen, usually lipid soluble and of low molecular weight, is taken into the Langerhans cells of the epidermis in the form of a hapten, where it is chemically altered and/or conjugated to a new molecule to form the actual antigen. This antigen on the surface of the Langerhans cells is presented to specific helper T cells, which, along with interleukin-1, activate T cells, which then secrete interleukin-2 and causes proliferation of specific T cell clones that circulate throughout the body.

In the *elicitation phase* of ACD, the same hapten diffuses into the Langerhans cells, is again taken up by the cell, where it is processed, but this time the complex interacts with the cloned T cells in the skin or in lymph nodes or both. Further reactions occur in the skin involving interleukin-1 stimulating the T cells to produce interleukin-2, which leads to further proliferation and expansion of desensitized T-cell populations in the skin. Other mediators of inflammation are involved, which activate mast cells and macrophages as well as histamine and leukocytes, and these lead to vascular dilatation, increased permeability, and the clinical response of inflammation and cellular destruction.

EVALUATION OF THE PATIENT WITH SUSPECTED CONTACT DERMATITIS

The diagnosis of contact dermatitis in any individual patient may be simple and straightforward, or it may be complicated and elusive. Clinicians are often able to make the diagnosis in some cases of contact dermatitis by history and physical examination alone. But a complete evaluation of patients with contact dermatitis requires in many cases a thorough knowledge of (1) the extent and prevalence of the myriad of chemical substances in the environment that can become cutaneous allergens or irritants, (2) clinical presentation of the various cutaneous eruptions that may be caused by contact allergens or irritants, (3) diagnostic techniques needed to diagnose contact dermatitis, which may include skin biopsy, patch, or other skin tests, and (4) therapy, including allergen avoidance, barrier treatments, topical and systemic anti-inflammatory drugs, and other measures.

Often the patient presenting with a dermatitis, particularly in the primary care setting, may not be so straightforward. On a clinical basis, it is often impossible to distinguish contact dermatitis from other eczematous eruptions such as atopic dermatitis, seborrheic dermatitis, nummular dermatitis, inflammatory diseases such as rosacea, systemic allergic reactions, psoriasis, vulvodynia, and infectious dermatoses such as tinea pedis and others (3,4). Some skin diseases, notably atopic and stasis dermatitis, are notorious for the development of superimposed CD (5). When there is a proximate history of allergen contact and development of dermatitis and when the dermatitis is in a distribution that matches the contact, the diagnosis is easy. In the real world of seeing patients in the office, this distinction is not always quite so clear. In most cases, the eruption of ACD is characterized by erythema, papules and/or vesicles, and sometimes bullae, depending on the intensity of the allergic reaction. Certain areas of the skin are more prone to vesicle formation (e.g., the trunk and extremities), whereas other areas (e.g., the genitalia and eyelids) usually produce erythema without vesicles. Chronic ACD shows as clinical findings scaling, papules, and lichenification but not often vesicles. In the acute phase of contact dermatitis, histological examination shows intracellular edema and spongiosis. And while not completely diagnostic, this picture on a clinical presentation usually suffices. In chronic ACD, however, the histological features become much more nonspecific and, in most cases, a skin biopsy is done not to make a diagnosis of ACD but to rule out other causes of a differential diagnosis for any particular patient.

PRIMARY CARE MANAGEMENT

The primary care physician should suspect acute or subacute ACD in a patient who has an eruption of relatively recent onset, i.e., up to a few weeks or months, where the dermatitis is *not* symmetrical from one part of the body to another, when other causes of asymmetrical dermatitis such as dermatophyte infections have been ruled out, when the physical findings just described are seen, and particularly when there is a history of a contact substance or when the distribution of the dermatitis indicates that there could have been so. In a situation of a more chronic dermatitis that has been present for more than a few months, the diagnosis of chronic ACD should be considered, particularly when the dermatitis involves the hands and/or feet or the face, specifically the eyelids (6).

PRIMARY TREATMENTS

In a clinical situation, as noted above, many primary care physicians will be able to make a presumptive diagnosis of acute or chronic ACD and begin an empiric course of treatment. Even if a definite cause of the ACD has not been determined, or if the dermatitis is ICD or some other steroid-responsive dermatosis such as nummular, atopic, dyshidrotic, etc. is in fact the diagnosis, the primary care physician will not go too far wrong by commencing standard treatment. For the purposes of primary care, the vast majority of patients who fit into this category of presumed contact dermatitis will be treated with topical corticosteroids as the primary therapeutic agent (7). Care must be given to use steroids of appropriate strength and of appropriate vehicle, considering the intensity of the dermatitis to be treated and the anatomical location, age of the patient, and amount of corticosteroid to be applied. In acute ACD, when treated topically, relatively potent corticosteroids are needed to achieve a result. The application of steroid in ointment form is often preferable. Care must be taken not to use superpotent steroids on the face, neck, or intertriginous areas or in children, and care should be given such that the safety limits are not exceeded in terms of the amount used at one time (generally less than 45 g per 2 weeks) or the preparation is not applied for too long a period of time. Also, ointment vehicles may not be the best to use in a situation where the dermatitis may have some secondary clinical infection.

Adjunctive treatment for patients with mild to moderate ACD, particularly of the subacute and chronic type, may include soaks to induce drying of vesicles when present, systemic antibiotics if clinically infected, antihistamines to relieve pruritus, and occasionally ultraviolet light treatment. In a patient with acute ACD, particularly with vesicles, administration of oral corticosteroids in the patient with no contraindications is the quickest way to achieve symptomatic improvement. For the averaged-sized adult, prednisone in a dose of 60 mg/day for 7–10 days is usually needed. One of the most common errors of primary care physicians is the undertreatment of acute contact dermatitis with systemic corticosteroids (8); prescription of the usual "dosepak" provides an insufficient amount of steroid for too short a time to provide meaningful improvement in many cases.

WHEN TO REFER

It is the patient who falls into the above description but yet who is not satisfactorily improved with treatment as mentioned who requires further investigation, often by a dermatologist. One reason why this type of patient may not be improving would be that the original diagnosis of contact dermatitis was incorrect and the patient has some other non–steroid-responsive condition such as dermatophyte infection, pityriasis rosea, or pyoderma. Another reason would be that the patient is still contacting the allergen.

The American Academy of Dermatology referral guidelines for inflammatory dermatosis state that (9):

> Inflammatory dermatoses are difficult to distinguish from each other and from certain malignant skin lesions. With appropriate training, a primary care physician may be able to diagnose common inflammatory dermatoses ("rashes") such as contact dermatitis, drug and other allergic eruptions, seborrheic dermatitis, atopic dermatitis and dyshidrotic eczema. Referral is suggested if: 1) the diagnosis is in question or, 2) there is lack of satisfactory response to treatment after a reasonable amount of time (usually 1 to 2 weeks).

REFERRAL STRATEGIES

Once referred to a dermatologist, a more thorough work-up may be conducted if needed. However, the primary care physician with an interest in managing contact or industrial dermatoses and with knowledge of more detailed evaluation techniques could perform much of what has been described in his or her office. However, in clinical practice, most primary care physicians do not have the interest, knowledge, or equipment available to do detailed contact dermatitis evaluation, particularly patch testing.

When a patient is referred to a dermatologist, often a more detailed allergen history may be taken and, hopefully, at least some suggestion as to a cause of the dermatitis may be forthcoming. Also on a clinical basis, the dermatologist may be able to make an alternate diagnosis such as atopic dermatitis, stasis dermatitis, pustular psoriasis of the hands or other hand dermatitis, seborrheic dermatitis, tinea pedis, corporis or manuum or nummular eczema.

The mainstay of the work-up, however, will be patch testing, a procedure by which specific cases of ACD can be diagnosed. In general, a patient will be considered for patch testing if there is a suggestive history or distribution of the dermatitis, if a specific antigen is suspected, if there is an occupationally related dermatitis, or if the patient indicates exposure of chemicals at work. Also, patch testing is used in established cases of atopic, stasis dermatitis and some cases of hand dermatitis not responding to treatment or getting worse despite what seems to be appropriate therapy, since ACD often occurs in the background of one of these other forms of dermatitis. The details of the indications for testing procedures and interpretation of patch testing are discussed in other chapters in this text. However, some comments are in other specifically from a primary care physician's point of view.

The actual performance of a patch test is not technically difficult. Test systems such as the T.R.U.E. Test are simple and easy to apply and have made standardized office patch testing more readily available to the busy office practitioner (10). The reading and interpretation of patch tests is somewhat subjective. Studies have shown that the reading and interpretation of patch tests varies, especially among inexperienced evaluators. Also, reproducibility of patch testing is a problem and in many cases allergen and technique dependent, making as much standardization as possible highly desirable (11,12). The difficulty arises, however, in knowing which patients will benefit by patch testing; difficulty also occurs in interpreting results—both positive and negative. Although it is true that a positive patch test proves that the patient is allergic to the allergen tested, it does not prove that that allergen caused the current dermatitis under investigation. The clinician and the patient must find a historical link between the known allergic substance and the current dermatitis for the test to have any meaning.

When the patient has been tested, when an allergen has been determined, and when the historical correlation between the contacted allergen and the existing dermatitis has been established, the best treatment is to remove exposure to the allergen if at all possible. This is usually done by avoidance of the substance, but some patients may achieve allergen avoidance through the use of barrier creams, particularly in the case of poison ivy and poison oak dermatitis in patients who must work in or around these substances. The use of barrier creams for other common forms of contact dermatitis such as nickel allergy in jewelry and forms of chronic hand dermatitis does not seem to be as effective (13). The real problem in the clinical setting, however, is that identification and/or removal of the allergen is not often possible and, therefore, the dermatitis will need to be treated on a more long-term basis.

The mainstay of treatment of chronic contact dermatitis, whether allergic or irritant, in situations where the allergen cannot be avoided or where diagnosis is suspected based on morphology and distribution of lesions but yet when a specific contact allergy has not been detectable by patch or other testing, continues to be the application of topical corticosteroids. In the case of chronic contact dermatitis as opposed to acute cases, generally topical steroids of less potency are used than are used for acute ACD because of the need for longer-term treatment. Since chronic contact dermatitis exhibits secondary findings such as lichenification, scaling, and fissuring, emollient forms of topical corticosteroids are usually employed. It is best when possible to select a topical steroid in an ointment base that has no preservatives since the use of such preservatives or other additives can produce a complicating factor in some patients who have chronic contact dermatitis. Other symptomatic modes of treatment such as systemic antipruritics, usually antihistamines, and other topical antipruritics are often used in cases of chronic contact dermatitis. Ultraviolet light therapy may be beneficial to many patients as well. The use of other nonsteroidal anti-inflammatory agents, however, seems not to help very much in chronic contact dermatitis.

SUMMARY

The investigation of a patient with contact dermatitis may be rewarding or frustrating. When the diagnosis of contact dermatitis is suspected by history, when an allergen is found by patch testing, and when the patient's dermatitis is relieved by avoidance of the allergen, a rewarding result is obtained for both the physician and the patient. However, when the original diagnosis is elusive, when contactants are suspected but not found, when elimination of suspected allergen does not produce amelioration of the dermatitis, or when treatments fail, both patients and physicians may be frustrated. A good working relationship between a primary care physician and a consultant dermatologist may expedite work-up and treatment for these patients.

REFERENCES

1. del Savio B, Sheretz EF. Is allergic contact dermatitis being overlooked? Arch Fam Med 1994; (6): 537–543.
2. Meding B, Barregard L, Marcus K. Hand eczema in car mechanics. Contact Dermatitis 1994; 30(3): 129–134.
3. Zug KA, Palay DA, Rock B. Dermatologic diagnosis and treatment of itchy red eyelids. Surv Opthalmol 1996; 40(4): 293–306.
4. Perniciaro C, Bustamante AS Jr, Gutierrez MM. Two cases of vulvodynia with unusual causes. Acta Derm Venereol 1993; 73(3): 227–228.
5. Klas PA, Corey G, Stors FJ, Chan SC, Hanifin JM. Allergic and irritant patch test reactions and stopic disease. Contact Dermatitis 1996; 34(2): 121–124.
6. Pariser DM, Caserio RJ, Eaglstein WH. Techniques for Diagnosing Skin and Hair Disease. New York: Thieme, 1986.
7. Ramsing DW, Agner T. Efficacy of topical corticosteroids on irritant skin reactions. Contact Dermatitis 1995; 32(5): 293–297.
8. Pariser RJ, Pariser DM. Primary care physicians' errors in handling cutaneous disorders. J Am Acad Dermatol 1987; 17(2): 239–245.
9. Guidelines for Dermatology Referrals in a Managed Care Setting. Schaumburg IL: American Academy of Dermatology, 1995.

10. Scheman A. Contact allergy testing alternatives: 1996. Cutis 1996; 57(4):235–240.
11. Brasch J, Henseler T, Aberer W, Bauerle G, Frosch PJ, Fuchs T, Funfstuck V, Kaiser G, Lischka GG, Pilz B, et al. Reproducibility of patch tests. A multicenter study of synchronous left- vs. right-sided patch tests by the German Contact Dermatitis Research Group. J Am Acad Dermatol 1994; 31(4):584–591.
12. Bruze M, Isaksson M, Edman B, Bjorkner B, Fregert S, Moller H. A study on expert reading of pathch test reactions: inter-individual accordance. Contact Dermatitis 1995; 32(6):331–337.
13. Gawkrodger DJ, Healy J, Howe AM. The prevention of nickel contact dermatitis. A review of the use of binding agents and barrier creams. Contact Dermatitis 1995; 32(5):257–265.

28

Understanding Managed Care Contracts

Lisa J. Kaplan *American Academy of Dermatology, Schaumburg, Illinois*

INTRODUCTION

The recent growth of managed care organizations has provided many opportunities to physicians and physician groups interested in participating in managed care contracts. Today, dermatologists are faced with a dual challenge of practicing quality medicine and staying in business. In many areas of the country, managed care organizations are merging with each other, and many are promoting strict gatekeeper systems where access to specialty care is limited. As specialists, dermatologists are forced to learn the business of managed care and try to negotiate favorable arrangements in order to stay afloat. Some dermatologists practice in areas where managed care has not yet entered the marketplace. Others are being forced to sign contracts for less money in order to stay competitive. No matter where dermatologists practice today, it is important to learn about managed care in order to maintain the viability of the specialty in this rapidly transforming market.

Deciding to participate in a managed care plan is a personal decision. Such factors as practice goals, income requirements, personal autonomy, and age should be taken into consideration. The most difficult hurdle for a dermatologist is accepting that he or she will lose a certain amount of freedom in a managed care setting. Dermatologists will still retain control, but after signing any managed care agreement, the dermatologist is forced to make decisions that follow the health plan's protocol.

The manner in which dermatologists receive patients dramatically changes in the managed care environment. Because of the rapid changes, dermatologists are forced to deal with such issues as contract analysis, review, and negotiation. In the past, it was common for physicians to sign contracts that were reimbursed at a discounted fee-for-service. Contracts were and still are very long, difficult to understand, and full of ambiguous language that may confuse even physician's personal attorneys. Today, the rules of the game have changed with the addition of capitation and risk-sharing contracts. Dermatologists must carefully review every definition and every paragraph of any proposed managed care contract before signing and becoming legally bound. Because of the difficulty in understanding some of the ambiguous language, contracts should also be reviewed by an experienced managed care attorney who is familiar with the nuances of managed care. Signing a contract without expert legal advice can be an invitation to disaster since these contracts can represent a significant portion of a dermatologist's livelihood. This chapter is designed to help dermatologists navigate the often bumpy waters of a managed care contract.

Unfortunately, there is no generic contract language, but there are many standard issues to guard against and have the managed care organization explain. Before signing any type of managed care contract, keep in mind the following negotiation principles: the more information you have about the organization, the more leverage you might have during the negotiation process; always ask questions and ask for clarification of key terms and definitions: compromise when possible; know what points are deal breakers; and never sign a contract without obtaining professional advice from an attorney, consultant, or actuary. Finally, be prepared to negotiate aggressively if possible by having pertinent information from your practice ready, including your overhead, utilization, and costs per procedure and per patient.

Thoroughly investigate any managed care plan you are thinking about joining. Start by obtaining financial reports, calling the state insurance department for information about the plan, and obtaining plan directories. Ask the managed care organization for a copy of its provider manual. Find out what the plan's reputation in the community is, who the key employer groups are, and the size of the plan. What type of referral guidelines if any are in place and what type of financial incentives are offered to participating physicians. Talk to other participating physicians to find out what the plan's reputation is for working with physicians, the plan's reliability, and the payment philosophy.

When applying for participation with a health plan, be prepared to do lots of paperwork. The plan will want a complete application, which is often quite lengthy, in addition to other documentation. Examples of other required documentation include copies of your board certificate, DEA license, state license, and proof of malpractice insurance. The managed care organization may require that you have a certain amount of liability insurance as well as other criteria. Find out what these criteria are prior to signing a contract.

Once you have completed the preliminary analysis, you are ready to evaluate the contract. First, make sure the contract is written clearly so that you understand your obligations. If the contract is unclear, find out if it can be changed. Know how the contract will affect your costs.

FEE SCHEDULES

When negotiating a fee-for-service contract, ask to see the fee schedule prior to signing the contract. If the plan will not show you the fee schedule, ask for the reimbursement, by CPT code, of the most commonly billed codes. Make sure the fee schedule is attached to the contract. Contracts frequently refer to documents such as the fee schedule as "incorporated by reference," meaning that these documents, although not attached, are considered to be part of the contract. Do not sign a contract prior to reviewing anything "incorporated by reference." You will still be legally bound even if the documents are not attached to the contract and even if you have not read them. Find out how the fee schedule is determined by the health plan, for example, what type of actuarial formula they might use to determine physician reimbursement. Sometimes fee schedules are modified. Make sure you know whether the plan has the unilateral power to modify the fee schedule or if you get to review the changes first. Also, make sure you know how often the fee schedule is going to be updated, how you will be informed, and in what time period.

DEFINITIONS

All contracts should have a definitions section in order to clarify the meaning of each and every contractural term discussed in the body of the contract. This helps avoid potential disputes regarding the meaning of those terms in the future. Sample definitions include capitation, copayment, emergency, service area, and out-of-area. All major terms in the body of the contract should be clearly defined in the definitions section of the contract.

COVERED SERVICES

All basic covered services should be succinctly and clearly defined in the contract, preferably by CPT code. Make sure the services set forth in the contract are services you perform. Unless specifically stated, assume all services are covered. You will be legally obligated to perform all services or pay someone else to perform them unless the contract specifically states otherwise. It is also important to differentiate between covered services and noncovered services. Physicians should try to retain the right to bill for noncovered services since anything patients elect to have done that is not specifically covered by the health plan is the patient's responsibility.

CARVE OUTS

When negotiating a capitation contract, it is advisable to carve out of the capitation as many of the time-consuming, expensive procedures as possible. In addition, any services a physician does not perform should be carved out as well. Any carve-outs may still be performed, but the contract should include specific language on how the carved-out procedures will be reimbursed. Common carve-outs for dermatology include Mohs, laser therapy, large excisions, and complex closures.

MEDICALLY NECESSARY

Distinguishing between medically necessary and medically unnecessary is crucial in a managed care contract. Medically necessary are the services performed by the provider that the plan determines to be needed. Medically unnecessary are those services the plan determines not to be needed and that the plan will not reimburse for. Find out in advance what the plan's expectations are. This is crucial when addressing issues such as dermatopathology, which a plan may or may not acknowledge as being medically necessary. Make sure dermatopathology is discussed during the negotiation period in order to find out prior to signing a contract whether it is a reimbursable service.

TERM AND TERMINATION

One of the most important and legally binding areas of a managed care contract is the term and termination section. If anything goes wrong, for example, if a practice is losing money or if you are unhappy with the plan's protocol or reimbursement, this section may or may not allow you to terminate a contract quickly, easily, and without penalty. Make sure the entire duration of the contract is clear.

AUTOMATIC RENEWAL

Some contracts have an automatic renewal and others have an annual CPI (consumer price index) increase attached. An automatic renewal contract rolls over on the anniversary date of the contract without mandating an additional contract to be negotiated or signed. This can be a double-edged sword. If you are happy with the reimbursement from a particular plan, an automatic renewal is beneficial because it locks in the reimbursement. If things are not going well and there is an automatic renewal clause in the contract, the participating dermatologist is locked in to the unfavorable rate for the duration of the contract, which could last for several years. Sometimes a clause can be included in the contract, allowing for a renegotiation prior to the automatic renewal date.

Standard termination language includes a definite time period in which either party must give a written notice in order to terminate the contract. This time period can range anywhere from at least a 30-day written notice to more, depending on the health plan. Make sure the time period is reasonable and that the contract reflects the exact requirements for termination. Many health plans include language that might say either party can terminate with written notice "without cause." Without cause means that either party can terminate the contract without stating a reason for the termination.

Legislation is currently being introduced in several states to prevent the use of without-cause language. This clause allows managed care organizations to terminate physicians without giving them any reason for the termination. After many years of participation or many long-term relationships with patients, receiving a termination letter without explanation can be very upsetting for physicians. The legislation, if approved, will mandate that health plans in that particular state give a reason whenever they terminate a physician from their health plan. Consequently, a physician who chooses to withdraw from a health plan would also have to state a reason when giving the appropriate notice.

Make sure that the time period requirement in the termination section of any managed care contract is reasonable. Often contracts address continuity of care during the roll-out period from the time notice of termination has been given to the actual termination date. Routine language often states that the physician must continue to treat existing patients until alternative arrangements are made by the health plan. The contract should state that the same reimbursement provisions will continue during the roll-out period. Also, check to see if the contract provides an opportunity to cure a default prior to being terminated or if the plan retains the right to terminate without hearing any physician input.

CLAIMS

Claims are a key area of managed care contracts because this section affects your payment. All contracts should specify a time period within which a physician can submit a claim. The failure to submit a timely claim may result in a denial or financial penalty. Many contracts refer to a "clean claim," which is the type of claim a plan requires to be submitted. Contracts should always include a detailed definition of a "clean claim" including the type of form and the information required by the plan. The plan's requirements should be compatible with your billing system and should be reasonable. The time period to submit a claim as well as the time period in which the plan has to pay the physician should be reasonable. More than 45 days to wait for payment is usually considered unreasonable.

Language that states the plan will use its "best efforts" to pay a physician is an example of the often vague and ambiguous language that may be included in managed care contracts. This language allows a plan to use any number of excuses for not making timely payments since they are using "best efforts." Some plans offer financial incentives to practices that can alleviate paperwork and submit their claims electronically. Any financial incentives should always be clearly set forth in a contract so there is no future potential dispute.

ELIGIBILITY

Eligibility can be a sore spot in the contracting process because managed care organizations often make it the physician's responsibility to check and verify eligibility each time a patient walks through the door for service. Prior to signing a contract, make sure the plan explains the eligibility requirements so that the appropriate office staff may correctly verify eligibility for all patients requesting services. The plan should clarify whether an ID card, patient listings, 24-hour phone line, or referral forms are the preferred method of verifying eligibility. If the health plan expects you to verify eligibility from patient listings, the plan should set forth a protocol for how often the listings will be updated and distributed to your office.

Managed care organizations also should explain what protocol is used to deal with noneligible patients. Sometimes a plan later determines that a patient is no longer eligible for services and will want to take back money from a practice that rendered services to the patient, even though the office did nothing wrong. The health plan my conclude the patient knows that he or she was not eligible at the time services were rendered and therefore were obtained fraudulently. The physician then, according to the plan's protocol, becomes responsible for billing the patient directly for the services rendered in good faith. Often this leads to a lot of time-consuming work in which it is difficult to obtain reimbursement. A helpful provision to alleviate this guarantees that the plan pays the physician for all services rendered in good faith to the noneligible patient after following the correct protocol for that plan and based on incorrect information supplied to the physician from the plan. For example, a patient listing that was not updated or accurate could cause a practice to conclude that a patient was eligible when in fact that patient terminated several weeks earlier. Occasionally this can be negotiated and included in contracts as long as the physician makes a good faith effort to bill and collect payment directly from the patient. Many contracts that include this type of language consider two attempts to recover money from patients to be adequate, but this is not always negotiable.

UTILIZATION MANAGEMENT AND QUALITY ASSURANCE

Utilization management and quality assurance are areas that should be of concern to everyone during the contracting process. There will most likely be a prospective, concurrent and retrospective review of the care rendered, so it is vital for you to know who will conduct such a review and how it will be accomplished. Include in the contract a reasonable mechanism for appeal. When signing a managed care contract, you become contractually obligated to abide by the protocols of the health plan, so it is crucial that you have a complete understanding of what the protocols are. At the very least, the contract should have a summary of what the utilization review process is as well as the specific details about the process, such as whether there is physician involvement in the review and an opportunity for appeal.

Contracts should ideally address the ownership of all the medical, financial, and other proprietary information of the physician. Preferably, the contract should specifically state that the physician owns the physical records documenting services rendered to patients. All contracts should set forth a procedure for the managed care organization to access patient and quality assurance information in a manner consistent with the principles of patient confidentiality, e.g., requiring patient consent and demanding special sensitivity to the disclosure of records in areas such as HIV. Contracts should treat as confidential and treat as proprietary any financial, strategic, utilization review, and quality assurance data and protocols including the pricing and other terms of the contract. The terms should remain between the dermatologist and the health plan. Also, the scope of access to each party's materials should be defined in the contact such as advance notice not to interrupt normal business activities and identifying who will pay for copying charges.

GRIEVANCE PROCEDURES

Grievance procedures regarding patients are often set forth in policies separate from the contract. These policies should be reviewed prior to signing the contract. Usually contracts include arbitration as an option and should always clearly define the terms and conditions including the ultimate financial responsibility of each party. There should always be an acceptable method of resolving disputes including an appeal process. If there is a disagreement with the plan, a denial of a claim, or an administrative decision regarding the physician's participation, the contract should clearly state the recourse open to the physician.

HOLD HARMLESS

There may be two hold harmless clauses in a contract: one is negotiable and often one is not. A paragraph could prevent a physician from charging a patient anything for covered services except for a deductible or copayment. The physician agrees to hold harmless and indemnifies the patient for any and all charges if the health plan fails to pay the bill. Usually this is not a negotiable clause and physicians will never be allowed to bill patients directly. The second and most important hold harmless clause to be aware of and to negotiate out of a contract is any language in which the physician holds harmless or indemnifies the health plan. This means that a physician is accepting the plan's liability as well as the physician's own liability even if the plan's protocol is followed or if liability occurs due to a procedure or practice of the plan. A physician could be subjected to litigation for circumstances and acts beyond his or her control. Malpractice insurance may not cover a physician if this type of clause exists in a contract.

WITHHOLDS

Withholds are common but irritating components of managed care contracts. The payor holds back a portion of reimbursement as a reserve to cover unexpected expenses. Contracts should specify how much is being withheld, when, and under what conditions the withhold is refunded. Also the specific terms of when the withhold refund is due and what financial formula the plan uses in circulating the withhold should be clearly defined as well as a list of services that are applicable to the withhold.

MARKETING

Health plans are responsible for marketing their participating physicians to employer groups and their employees. Prior to signing a contract, the plan's representatives should explain how the physician will be marketed to employer groups as well as referring physicians. Noncompete clauses, also known as restrictive covenants, are appearing more and more frequently in managed care contracts. The laws are decided on a case-by-case basis regarding these clauses. The rule of thumb is that they should not be too limiting in geographic region or too long in duration. Most important, the restriction should not prevent a physician from earning a living.

GAG CLAUSES

Gag clauses prohibit certain communications and conversations with patients. These are most often designed to prevent physicians from discussing the plan in a negative way with patients. A gag clause may be particularly burdensome since a plan may terminate a physician immediately for a violation. These type of restrictions are problematic because they put restraints on what type of conversations can occur between physicians and their patients. Examples include restricting a physician from telling patients about alternative methods of treatment, that the physician is capitated, or that the physician has terminated from the plan. Review the contract carefully for these clauses since they can be very limiting.

CONCLUSION

No matter what your personal preferences are, your options may be limited depending on the penetration of managed care in your city. Other factors such as a strong corporate presence, number of other dermatologists, and even the number of hospitals will play a role in determining whether to sign up with a particular managed care company. It is inevitable that changes in the health care delivery system will demand that dermatologists work more closely with primary care physicians. Finding opportunities to participate in managed care organizations may vary depending on the different factors occurring in any particular region. Dermatologists must stay informed in order to stay competitive. Educating primary care physicians and health plan executives on dermatology will lead to a control of overutilization and management problems and help dermatologists interact successfully with the managed care system. It is important for dermatologists to remember, in this ever-changing world of managed care, that they are the best trained specialists to appropriately diagnose and treat diseases of the skin. Continue talking to patients and to health plans directly. Get involved with your state societies and legislators. Most important, negotiate with as much advice and information as possible.

29

Pharmacy Benefits Managers

Tools Used to Control Selection and Utilization of Dermatological Products

Kent H. Summers *Eli Lilly and Company, Indianapolis, Indiana*

OVERVIEW

Managed care organizations (MCOs) have grown and evolved into entities that attempt to balance patients' simultaneous and conflicting desires to both preserve their freedom of provider selection and reduce costs. MCOs often use pharmacy benefits managers (PBMs) to administer the pharmacy component of the benefit. These PBMs use a variety of mechanisms to control the cost and utilization of drug products by MCO patients. Most notably, this includes the selection of products for inclusion in restrictive formularies. Health outcomes research can be used to assist product selection decisions by documenting the comprehensive value of pharmaceutical products. However, many MCO decision makers are unable to incorporate this information into their decisions related to the selection pharmaceutical products for formulary inclusion. This is particularly true in the case of dermatological products. These limitations in the use of health outcomes research and some potential suggestions will be explored.

MANAGED HEALTH CARE

The roots of today's managed health care organizations can be traced back to the 1930s. Sidney Garfield, a physician, contracted to deliver combined industrial accident and personal medical care for 5000 workers building a fresh-water aqueduct across the California desert to Los Angeles (1). In 1938, the industrialist Henry Kaiser invited Dr. Garfield to deliver health care services to employees and dependents working on the Grand Coulee Dam. Based on this successful experience, Kaiser transplanted the Garfield program to his shipyards in California, Oregon, and Washington during World War II. In the 1950s and 1960s, a number of prepaid group medical practices developed in California. However, the growth of these practices and the Kaiser Health Plan was limited by physicians' reluctance to join group practices and their aversion to management by nonphysicians. The opportunities provided by independent, private practice provided many physicians the financial security that enabled them to avoid joining these early MCOs.

The term, MCO is used to broadly identify those entities providing medical (with or without pharmacy) benefits to an enrolled patient population, using some mechanisms to control the cost, utilization, and quality of care. Thus, MCOs may have patients enrolled in managed indemnity, preferred provider organization (PPO), or health maintenance organization (HMO) plans.

The term "health maintenance organization" was coined by the physician Paul Ellwood in the early 1970s (2). He used the term as part of a strategy to win Nixon administration support and congressional approval to finance the development of prepaid care as an alternative to the predominant fee-for-service (FFS) reimbursement mechanism. This effort culminated with Richard Nixon signing the Federal HMO Act of 1973. The Act authorized $325 million for grants and loans to encourage the start of HMOs (3). The set of federal regulations pursuant to the Act prescribed a broad range of benefits which HMOs *must* offer in order to qualify for federal funds. These restrictions hindered the initial growth of HMOs, and 1976 amendments to the Act considerably loosened the requirements for federal qualification.

Thus, the HMO Act of 1973 heralded the beginning of rapid growth of MCOs. Traditional health care in a FFS environment is actually *medical* care, not *health* care. Traditional care is problem-oriented and focuses on treating patients after they become ill. Prepaid health care, on the other hand, possesses a financial motive for keeping patients healthy and avoiding their unnecessary utilization of medical resources.

Organizational Structure of Managed Care

Managed care is provided by providers and administrators operating in a variety of organizational structures. These structures range from managed indemnity programs to tightly controlled staff-model HMOs. A brief description of selected organizational structures follows.

Preferred Provider Organizations

PPOs use a select panel of professionals and institutions to deliver care. The services provided by the individuals and institutions in this panel are monitored for quality and cost efficiency. Providers and institutions who cannot achieve required levels of quality and/or efficiency may not be retained on the panel. Enrolled patients are channeled toward these providers through benefit structures that include a financial penalty for the use of physicians and pharmacies not in the panel. Use of panel providers may involve patients spending a minimal co-pay for visits, while the use of non-panel physicians and pharmacies (i.e., "out-of-network" providers) may require the patient to pay all charges. In exchange for this increased volume of patients (or protection from patient and revenue loss), providers accept FFS reimbursement that is discounted from their usual fees.

Health Maintenance Organizations

The hallmark of HMOs is the use of prepaid, capitated contracts for the payment of health care services. Capitation rates are negotiated for the defined population and are paid to the HMO regardless of patients' utilization of services. This form of financing has become very attractive to employers since it reduces their exposure to financial risk (i.e., variations in health care expenditures). As this risk shifts to HMOs, they have a financial motive for keeping patients healthy and out of the medical treatment system.

Health maintenance organizations are categorized according to their mode of operations. There are four general models of HMOs: independent practice associations (IPAs), network, group, and staff models. Figure 1 provides a depiction of these four basic models. However, a growing number of plans are multimodal or hybrid operations, combining aspects of more than one model.

Independent Practice Associations:

These organizations consist of a loose federation of autonomous physicians practicing alone or in small, single-speciality groups. They contractually agree to treat patients enrolled in the HMO on a FFS in their private

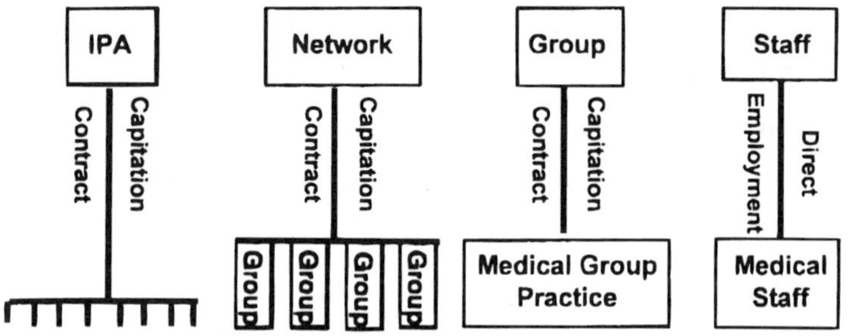

	IPA	Network	Group	Staff
Physician Contracts:	Individual contracts with IPA	Multi-specialty groups contract with HMO	Physicians' group contract with HMO	Direct HMO Employees
Physician Compen-sation:	Usually Fee-For-Service (FFS)	Each group's pooled income	Salary + group incentives	Salary
Practice Setting:	Private office, some pre-paid patients	Group offices, mixture of pre-paid and FFS patients	Group's office, mostly pre-paid patients	Clinic, all pre-paid patients

Figure 1 Forms (models) of health maintenance organizations.

offices. The IPA organization assumes the financial risk via capitated contracts to finance health care, while paying providers on a FFS basis. Thus, the IPA is vulnerable to excessive cost escalation, with limited ability to control it.

Network Models:

These HMOs use capitation contracts with multiple, independent medical groups. The physicians working for these medical groups usually have some of their income tied to their groups' ability to efficiently provide services.

Group Models:

These HMOs negotiate contracts with large, multispeciality medical groups. The groups, which are typically physician partnerships, may be legally and fiscally separate from the HMO but operate as captive service suppliers. Physicians typically are reimbursed on a salary or salary plus profit-sharing basis.

Staff Models:

These HMOs directly employ physicians and can most readily control physician behavior in their use of costly products and services. Physicians' salaries may vary, based on activity (average patient load) or on contribution to the HMO's profitability (profit sharing).

The Need for Managed Care

The means used to finance health care has contributed to the growth in costs. Historically, health care was financed largely by indemnity insurance organizations that reimbursed providers for care given to members enrolled in the plan. These organizations provided security to patients by shielding them from the catastrophic financial impact of hospitalizations. They functioned by pooling patients' financial risks and paying the claims for health care services rendered. These purchasers of health care were not greatly interested in efforts to control the utilization or cost of health care since costs were not rising rapidly. The job of indemnity insurers was to pay, without question, providers' claims for the services provided. Consequently, indemnity insurance programs minimized patients' and physicians' concerns about the use of increasingly expensive health care services and products.

Costs grew as indemnity insurance financing provided the illusion that unlimited resources were available to satisfy patients' unlimited demand for services. In addition, patients came to expect comprehensive hospitalization and out-patient care as a basic right. Many employers in the 1960s and 1970s found that offering concessions in tax-advantageous health insurance benefits was often preferable to giving wage increases. In addition, the Medicare program (financed and administered via insurance mechanisms) increased the public's perception of their *right* to readily available health care with minimal personal cost. Consequently, our reliance on financing health care costs by indemnity insurance has contributed to the rise in health care costs.

Cost and Utilization Controls for Managed Care

MCOs exist in a continuum ranging from managed indemnity programs to group or staff model HMOs. Figure 2 provides a comparison of these organizations, contrasting patients' freedom to choose their providers vs. the organizations' abilities to control costs. Managed indemnity occurs in insurance programs with some mechanisms to control costs and/or utilization. PPOs combine some utilization controls with discounted providers' reimbursement paid on a FFS basis. Staff model HMOs, on the other

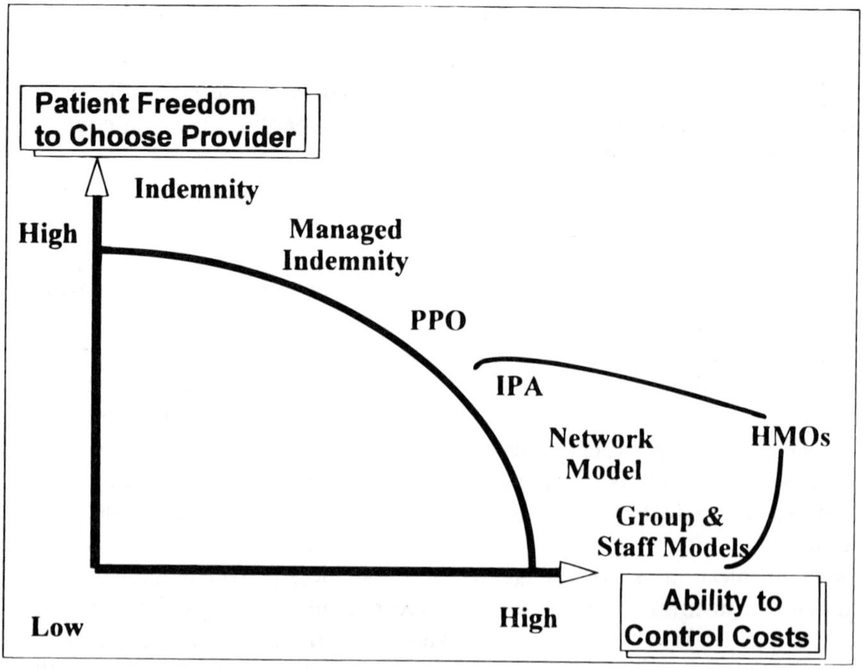

Figure 2 MCOs: patient choice vs. savings ability.

hand, can offer significant cost control through the actions of salaried physicians. However, these organizations provide patients little choice in selecting their physicians. We may expect future growth to occur in these organizations based on the importance of patient choice vs. the need to control costs.

Table 1 depicts specific cost and utilization control methods used by MCOs. Managed indemnity programs control utilization primarily through the use of mandatory second opinions and preauthorizations. These cost-control mechanisms help to avoid unnecessary hospitalizations and other costly service utilization through a priori review of the proposed services' appropriateness. In addition to preauthorization, retrospective utilization review is used to identify excessive and unwarranted use of services. Payment denial for these services occurs where it is deemed appropriate. Criteria for denying payment often include tests for medical necessity. Denials may also occur when there is no government approval for the use of medical services and products (e.g., the denial of payment for experimen-

Table 1 Cost and Utilization Controls Used by Managed Care Organizations

Type of MCO			Cost and utilization control methods
	↓	Managed indemnity	Mandatory second opinions, preauthorizations Retrospective utilization reviews (and claims denials)
	↓	Preferred Provider Organizations (PPOs)	Channeling to panels of selected health care providers Prospectively determined, discounted remuneration paid to providers on a FFS basis Quality monitoring; provider evaluation and credentialing
Health Maintenance Organizations	↓	Independent Practice Associations (IPAs)	Bundled services; capitation
		Network models	Reports documenting physician groups' utilization
		Group, staff models	Salaried physicians

tal uses or in situations for which there is no FDA-approved indication). The lack of medical community acceptance of the treatment as a standard of practice may also provide a basis for payment denial.

Future Growth

MCOs face many challenges in their quest to become or remain successful. Remaining unresolved is the dilemma regarding patient choice vs. ability to control costs. MCOs seem to have appealed mostly to a market niche that places primary focus on cost containment. Consequently, competition among MCOs has centered on their "per member per month" (PMPM) charges. MCOs employ a wide variety of cost-control mechanisms to compete in this market. In some cases, this frugality has resulted in member dissatisfaction related to access (the lack of convenient availability of network providers) and frustration with coverage limitations for expensive new technologies (e.g., the use of formularies to limit access to the more expensive new drug products). Nonetheless, benefits managers who represent employers' interests in purchasing health care services seem likely to continue in their quest to satisfy employees demand for less costly coverage. The benefit designs most likely to grow in the future will be decided by the public's trade-off preferences concerning cost control vs. freedom in provider selection (Fig. 2).

Quality may become a more important factor in future competition among MCOs. With the changes that have occurred in the provider market, one could reasonably argue that most price concessions for provider services have reached a limit. The next area of focus for MCOs may be utilization. Therefore, future activities may focus on demand management in the form of disease prevention and management programs, as well as implementation of programs designed to gain physician adherence to treatment guidelines.

It may be that our ability to reduce costs will eventually reach a plateau beyond which additional efforts produce diminishing returns. We have already experienced this phenomenon in hospitals in their response to the Medicare Prospective Payment System. In this system, Diagnosis-Related Groups (DRGs) are used to pay hospitals' services for Medicare beneficiaries. This arrangement represents a form of managed health care in that it uses prospectively determined prices for bundled services to determine provider reimbursement. Initially, many hospitals experienced a dramatic drop in their patients' average length of stay (ALOS). However, this indicator of improved efficiency seems to have reached a plateau in recent years. We may find an analogous situation in the ambulatory patient environment. The question remains, how will MCOs compete when we reach the limits of our ability to squeeze more efficiency out of the health care system? Given similar costs among competing suppliers of health care, purchasers may make their choices based on quality indicators, including patient satisfaction with the care given by the various providers and minimization of aggravation by administrative cost-containment tactics.

Recent growth has occurred primarily in the PPO and IPA plans. This is due in large part to the freedom of patients to choose their providers. However, this comes at a reduced ability to control costs. Many MCOs are struggling to control costs in these types of plans. An interesting arrangement has become established in the California market. Physician groups known as "managed medical provider organizations" (MMPOs) have established themselves as self-contained entities with reasonable ability to control costs. They contract with MCOs in a network model arrangement. Some of these MMPOs have challenged MCOs through direct contracts with employer groups, thereby avoiding the costs of MCOs as "middlemen." MCOs counter that under such arrangements, MMPOs should adhere to state regulations and file required documents with the state insurance commission. Regardless of the outcome of this dispute, MMPOs and network model HMOs seem to represent a growing segment of managed care.

THE PHARMACY BENEFIT IN MANAGED CARE ORGANIZATIONS

Availability of the pharmacy benefit has played an important role in the growth of managed care. Patients have grown to appreciate the convenience of using a card and minimal co-pays to obtain prescriptions. Acceptance of this benefit has resulted in its becoming an integral part of the health care package. Benefits managers working for large employers often find that employees will not permit the exclusion of this component from their health care package.

Much growth has occurred in the area of "carve-out" pharmacy benefits provided through a network composed of existing retail pharmacies. Pharmacy carve-outs are sold as riders to existing medical plans. They represent stand-alone programs that may be added to the basic medical benefits package. Pharmacy benefits managers (PBMs) offering carve-out programs often focus their competition on the price of the pharmacy component. This requires negotiations for lower pharmacy dispensing fees, increased use of generic products, and the avoidance of reimbursement for expensive medications. Use of generic alternatives is encouraged through the use of variable patient co-pays (e.g., the patient pays a higher co-pay for the brand-name product, when a generic equivalent is available) and pharmacy incentives, such as increased dispensing fees for generic products. Formularies, or preferred product lists, are used to encourage the dispensing of lower-cost alternatives to expensive prescription products. Thus, competition in this "carve-out" environment is based on the PBMs' ability to reduce costs in the pharmacy component alone.

Pharmacy services also can be provided through "in-house" pharmacies. These are captive pharmacies, operating on the premises of the HMO. Such arrangements typically occur in group or staff model HMOs where pharmacists service the needs of patients seeing physicians in a clinic-type setting. The ability to maintain continuity in the provision of care (i.e., controlling the spectrum of services utilization) and to capture data creates an environment most capable of appreciating the comprehensive value of pharmaceutical products.

MCOs, either directly (in-house pharmacies) or through a PBM (community pharmacies organized into a network), control drug costs through the use of a variety benefit design variations and administrative tactics. These include (4):

Co-payments—fixed or variable payments for prescriptions designed to control utilization, or in the case of variable co-payments, shift utilization to preferred products (e.g., $10 co-payment for formulary drugs, $25 for nonformulary items)

Deductibles—designed to minimize administrative costs (claims payments) for MCO plan members who use prescription products sparingly

Prior-approval protocols (e.g., preauthorization or "pre-auth")—designed to avoid excessive utilization of products that might be used for conditions not generally accepted as cost-efficient or medically necessary (e.g., requiring documentation of growth hormone deficiency due to idiopathic causes, cranial insult, renal insufficiency. Turner's syndrome, or Silver-Russell syndrome prior to approval of payment for somatrem or somatropin—this provides a means to deny payment for normal variant short stature or athletic performance enhancement)

Generic enforcement—designed to maximize potential savings from the use of less expensive multisource products in the place of more expensive brand-name products

Formulary enforcement—designed to maximize utilization of products deemed by the MCOs' Pharmacy & Therapeutic Committees to be most cost-effective

Thus, MCOs and PBMs employ a variety of benefit designs and administrative tactics to maximize savings while minimizing plan member dissatisfaction.

The pharmacy benefit requires the availability of computerized systems to handle the massive quantities of claims for prescriptions dispensed. These systems have evolved in many cases to eclipse the sophistication of medical claims reimbursement systems. The first step in the development of pharmacy benefits involved an evolution of the systems to rapidly and efficiently pay claims for prescriptions dispensed. The universal claim form used to manually submit bills for third-party payment of prescriptions has been largely replaced by on-line, computerized claims adjudication systems that immediately recognize patient eligibility. These systems have gone a long way in reducing the rejection of claims for ineligible patients. The continuum of tools available to PBMs to control drug utilization can be seen in Figure 3. This figure demonstrates the reliance on sophisticated computer systems as PBMs use increasingly restrictive tools.

Pharmacy Benefits Managers' Control of Product Selection and Utilization

Survival of MCOs is dependent on their ability to use limited resources to satisfy the unlimited demand of enrolled patient populations for high-quality care. This represents a classical resource allocation dilemma, one

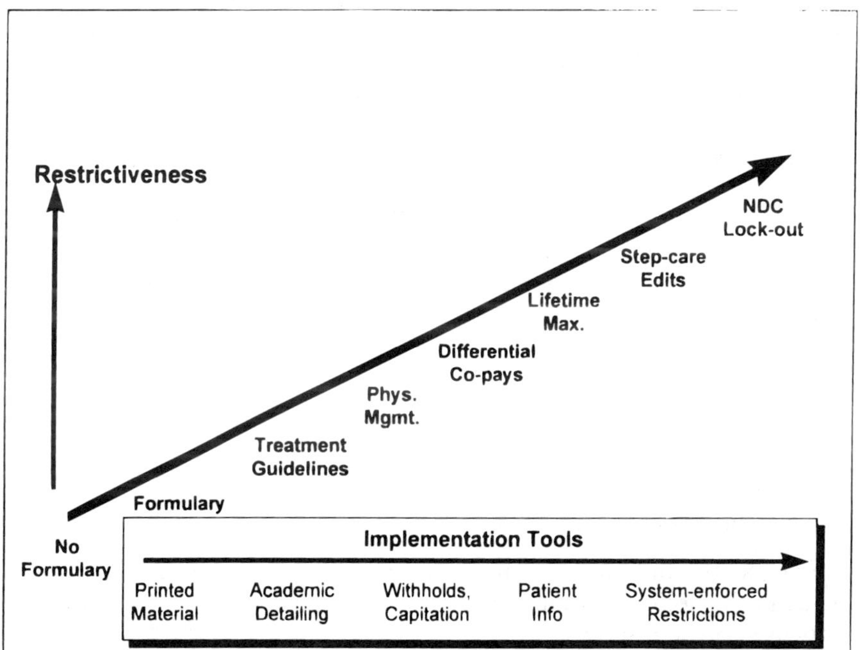

Figure 3 Continuum of drug utilization control tools.

that would seem to benefit from information provided by economics research. Pharmacoeconomics has developed as a means to document the value of pharmaceutical products through the identification, measurement, and analysis of the costs and consequences of drug therapy. Health outcomes research includes this as well as other components of health services research. Consequently, outcomes research (OR) represents a general category that includes pharmacoeconomics. Such studies can be used in making decisions that have a more scientific basis.

Health care providers traditionally have selected products and services based on what they believe is best for the individual patient. The growth of MCOs has led to an increased centralization in this decision-making process. Further, the selection of products and services is based on what appears to be best for the beneficiary population, not necessarily individuals. Making decisions that are population-based rather than individual patient–based represents a fundamental change in outlook health professionals need to select products and services. Approaching decisions from this different perspective can produce conflicting conclusions since priorities and preferences of individuals may differ from that of an organization (5). Since the impact of these decisions is much greater than those made for individual patients, much more information is needed to make good product selections. This increases the difficulty MCO administrators face when making product selection decisions.

OR can be used to demonstrate the comprehensive value of drug therapy. It identifies and measures the costs and consequences of drug therapy alternatives. Costs (and savings) include both direct and indirect resources consumed in providing therapy (6). Consequences, or outcomes, may fall into three categories: economic, clinical, and humanistic (7). OR studies have demonstrated that the substantial direct costs of expensive drug therapy can be offset by equal or greater reductions in other direct institutional and patient costs associated with therapy. The analyses used in OR research include:

cost-identification analysis
cost-minimization analysis
cost-effectiveness analysis
cost-utility analysis
cost-benefit analysis

Consequently, the information provided by OR research can be used to assist in the decision-making process to select drug products to be used by patient populations.

OR information has become increasingly available and will play a major role in drug product selection decisions around the world. In Australia, pharmaceutical manufacturers must include an economic analysis in each new submission for inclusion on the government's list of subsidized drugs (8). In Canada, provinces use formulary lists to indicate their acceptance of products reimbursable under the subsidized drug benefit program. The province Ontario has put forth guidelines to guide pharmaceutical manufacturers in preparing economic analyses for inclusion in their submission to the provincial review committees. In France, Spain, Sweden, the Netherlands, and the United Kingdom, economic analysis is encouraged to assist in reimbursement and co-payment decisions by the national health insurance systems. The United States however, has no such national health insurance system making formalized, singular decisions regarding drug product coverage.

Formularies

In the United States, individual MCOs use formulary lists to communicate the specific drug products considered acceptable for coverage. Formularies are a tool used by Pharmacy & Therapeutic (P&T) Committees to manage the quality and cost of drug therapy provided by MCOs (9). Increased economic pressures on MCOs have caused them to increasingly use formularies and practice guidelines as cost-containment tools (10). MCO P&T Committees should take into account the following when selecting drug products (11).

1. Efficacy
2. Safety
3. Costs
4. Patient acceptance
5. Ease of use
6. Dosage forms
7. Preparation requirements
8. Stability and storage requirements
9. Reputation of manufacturer and services it provides

Hence, the optimal selection of pharmaceutical products by P&T Committees is a complex, multifaceted proposition.

The incorporation of these considerations into product-selection decisions requires the application of a rational, systematic process. Decision analysis has been proposed as a systematic approach to permit an explicit, orderly, and careful consideration of a variety of issues when making decisions under conditions of uncertainty (12). Multiple Attribute Utility Theory (MAUT) has been proposed as a decision analysis method in which numerous variables that may affect a decision are identified, characterized, and compared (13,14). The use of such efforts to make good formulary decisions occurs in the larger, more sophisticated MCOs where technology assessment subcommittees provide the P&T Committee relevant information in this area (15). Good examples of organizations that use systematic decision making include Thomas Jefferson University Hospital, United Health Care, the Pharmacoeconomic Center in Fort Sam Houston, and King County Medical Blue Shield in Washington. In many MCOs, however, the full use of decision analysis-techniques does not routinely occur because they require specialized skills and the processes must be consistently applied. The salary structures in many MCOs do not permit the development and retention of individuals possessing such skills. Further, inappropriate and irrational decisions often arise from P&T Committee members' falling prey to decision fallacies such as tradeoff contrast, extremeness aversion, and risky shift (5). Consequently, multiple factors are often not included in product selection decisions. This results in irrational and "partial" decisions employing a suboptimal consideration of relevant factors.

The incorporation of cost considerations, in addition to clinical attributes, into the decision-making process represents a challenge for many P&T Committee members. P&T Committees have traditionally evaluated products based on clinical attributes. Information for formulary decisions comes from clinical studies documenting the safety and efficacy of drug products under ideal circumstances. Concerns about bias in industry-sponsored studies is allayed by adhering to a policy of limiting studies considered to include only randomized, controlled trials (RCTs) published in peer-reviewed journals. With this approach, physicians and pharmacists serving on P&T Committees can compare products using a minimal level of competence in the areas of statistics and research design. However, such studies do not provide optimal information for making decisions regarding the performance of products in actual use (i.e., effectiveness). OR provides the information regarding product effectiveness needed for good administrative decisions. However, the techniques used in OR research have not been standardized and universally accepted, as has the RCT in clinical research. Therefore, P&T Committee members cannot easily discern good studies: those free of bias and providing the best information possible, given the inherent limitations of "naturalistic" research. Therefore, many P&T Committee members tend to reject information provided from OR research and revert to the security of using clinical studies in product selection decisions.

Many OR studies provide information that is not relevant to MCO decision makers. Some OR studies document premium-priced products' ability to provide economic advantages some years in the future. However,

P&T Committee members in MCOs are most concerned with reducing direct medical costs in the current year. The premium a MCO would have to pay for such products would represent an investment in the success of a competing MCO, as patients often switch among these organizations. For the same reason, P&T Committee members find it difficult to justify acceptance of expensive products based solely upon improvements in quality-adjusted life years (QALYs) using patients' willingness-to-pay measurement approaches. The willingness-to-pay measurement technique is not relevant for patients unaccustomed to directly paying for health care. Rather, P&T Committee members would be most attracted to relative benefits in the form of reduced direct medical costs in the short-term.

OUTCOMES RESEARCH AND DERMATOLOGICAL PRODUCT SELECTION

Time limitations force many P&T Committees to focus their attention on those products with the potential to have the biggest impact on program savings. The first consideration is to determine which products are frequently prescribed and/or represent large expenditures of the pharmacy budget. Many MCO and PBM managers believe that savings can result from the imposition of formulary restrictions limiting coverage to a select number of products within therapeutic classes where several alternatives exist. Products in therapeutic categories with many product alternatives often receive attention from P&T Committees. Therefore, ACE inhibitors, calcium channel blockers, histamine H_2-receptor antagonists, and HMG-CoA reductase inhibitors are common objects of committee reviews. Products in these classes are commonly prescribed and represent significant expenditures for pharmacy budgets. OR is important to the market success of these products to document the value of these products relative to competitors within the therapeutic class.

Dermatological products have not been the focus of many formulary restrictions because they usually represent a limited number of prescriptions and a relatively small portion of the pharmacy budget. However, many P&T Committee members may not appreciate the importance of subtle differences in dermatological products. OR can be used to document the financial and humanistic impact of these differences, thereby avoiding the placement of restrictions on premium-priced products. Alternatively, the introduction of innovative (and expensive) new products can benefit from more rapid formulary acceptance with the availability of good OR.

OR needs to be properly designed and applied to realize optimal impact on formulary decisions. Effective OR demonstrates the impact of products on direct medical costs in a short time period. Such information can be used to leverage the concerns of those responsible for the medical budget where the use of less expensive pharmaceutical products may lead to increased expenditures on the medical side. In other words, OR may be used by medical directors to force PBM administrators to refrain from decisions that might benefit the pharmacy budget at the cost of raising the medical budget (i.e., formulary inclusion of lower priced, less effective products and exclusion of higher priced, more effective products). Further, the OR results would need to be published in reputable journals to facilitate credibility and acceptance. Studies also need widespread dissemination in an understandable form that permit incorporation into P&T Committee decisions.

SUMMARY

The growth of MCOs will depend on their ability to balance patients' simultaneous and conflicting desire to preserve their freedom of provider selection and interest in reduced costs. MCOs often use PBMs to administer the pharmacy component of the benefit. These PBMs frequently use restrictive formularies to limit reimbursement to those products deemed to represent the best value. OR can be used to make better product-selection decisions by documenting the comprehensive value of pharmaceutical products. However, many MCO decision makers have difficulty incorporating this information into their decisions. This is particularly true in the case of dermatological products. However, good OR can be used to avoid decisions that might disadvantage an existing product or to enhance formulary acceptance of new products.

REFERENCES

1. Williams G. Kaiser-Permanent Health Plan: Why It Works. Oakland, CA: Henry J. Kaiser Foundation, 1971: 3.
2. Luft HS. Health Maintenance Organizations: Dimensions of Performance. New York: John Wiley & Sons, 1981:1–5.
3. Thorpe K. In: Jonas S, ed. Health Care Delivery in the United States. New York: Springer Publishing, 1986: 166–182.
4. Hieber KA. Pharmacy benefit administration options. J Managed Care Pharm 1996; 2(3): 272–278.
5. Larson LN, Bjornson DC. Interface between pharmacoepidemiology and pharmacoeconomics in managed care pharmacy. J Managed Care Pharm 1996; 2(3): 282–289.
6. Weinstein MC. Principles of cost-effective resource allocation in health care organizations. Int J Technol Assess Health Care 1990; 6: 93–103.
7. Kozma C, Mauch D, Reeder CE, Lawrence J. The ECHO model. Clin Therapeut 1994; 16: 1037–1051.

8. Johnson JA, Bootman JL. Pharmacoeconomic analysis in formulary decisions: an international perspective. Am J Hosp Pharm 1994; 51:2593–2598.
9. Summers KH, Szeinbach SL. Formularies: the role of pharmacy and therapeutics (P&T) committees. Pharm Therapeut 1995; 20(8):534–546.
10. Hatoum HT, Freeman RA. The use of pharmacoeconomic data in formulary selection. Top Hosp Pharm Manage 1994; 13(4):47–53.
11. Sheperd M, Salzman G. The formulary decision-making process in a health maintenance organization setting. PharmacoEconomics 1994; 5:29–38.
12. Calvo S, Fruns D, Dominguez-Gil M. Decision analysis applied to selection of histamine H_2-receptor antagonists for the formulary. Am J Hosp Pharm 1990; 47:2002–2006.
13. Thompson D, Oster G. Cost-effectiveness of drug therapy: application of the concept part 1. Hosp Ther 1990; 5:663–679.
14. Schumacher G. Multiattribute evaluation in formulary decision making as applied to calcium-channel blockers. Am J Hosp Pharm 1991; 48:301–308.
15. Schrogie JJ, Nash DB. Relationship between practice guidelines, formulary management, and pharmacoeconomic studies. Topics Hosp Pharm Manage 1994; 13(4):38–46.

30

Future Directions

Elizabeth F. Sherertz *Bowman Gray School of Medicine of Wake Forest University, Winston-Salem, North Carolina*

What are our goals of treatment for skin disease?
What is important to patients?
What are the costs of disease and treatment?

The questions must continue to be asked as we enter the next millennium in dermatological care. Dermatologists have been teased that their field is perfect because their patients neither die nor get better, so there is a fairly constant population to serve. Of course, patients with skin diseases *do* get better, and symptoms and signs not evident on the surface are often the major therapeutic concerns for both patient and doctor. Despite our supreme medical advancements, health quality remains at the center of each visit, and economic questions often become a consideration.

It is tempting to suggest that quality of life and economics could be combined with laboratory measures to yield an evidence-based approach that could reduce dermatology to a series of algorithms. This is not a good idea—life-quality symptoms pertaining to emotional and social issues cannot be reduced to yes–no decision making. The essence of human communication must remain in health care. Attention to life quality and economic detail will facilitate the network of communication.

The future direction of care management of skin diseases must include:

1. *Education*: Building on this contemporary foundation of quality of life and economic information, there must be a broadened awareness of the importance of these concerns.
2. *Expansion*: The communications network, starting with the patient, needs to identify quality and morbidity measures that have not yet been studied adequately but that reflect very real disease impact.
3. *Refinement*: The current techniques are somewhat crude. As we gain experience in sociological, psychological, and bioeconomic research, there needs to be a customized adaptation of research techniques and instruments to evaluate particular issues. Standardization is difficult, and there needs to be an understanding of the limitations of intangible measures without underestimating their value.

It may not be an understatement to conclude that quality of life and skin health are essential elements for the future of dermatology.

Appendix

Key References of Life Quality Instruments Developed for Skin Diseases

The list below contains many of the instruments that have been validated to detect quality of life impacts from skin diseases, and that are described in this volume. The reader is encouraged to contact the developers to obtain formal psychometric data and use parameters. The type of skin disease each measure was developed to assess and/or has been validated for use is indicated by the following abbreviations:

AV = acne vulgaris
CD = contact dermatitis
PS = psoriasis
AD = atopic dermatitis
O = other dermatoses

MULTIDIMENSIONAL QUALITY OF LIFE INSTRUMENTS

Children's DLQI—Lewis-Jones, Finlay AY. The Children's Life Quality Index (CDLQI): initial validation and subsequent use. Br J Dermatol 1995; 132:942–949. [**AV**, **CD**, **PS**, **O**]

Skindex—Chren MM, Lasek RJ, Quinn LM, et al. Skindex, a quality of life measure for patients with skin disease: reliability, validity and responsiveness. J Invest Dermatol 1996; 107–713. [**AV**, **CD**, **PS**, **O**]

The Psoriasis Life Stress Inventory—Gupta MA, Gupta AK. The Psoriasis Life Stress Inventory: a preliminary index of psoriasis-related stress. Acta Derm Venereol (Stockholm) 1995; 75: 240–243. [**PS**].

Acne Disability Index—Motley RJ, Finlay AY. How much disability is caused by acne? Clin Exper Dermatol 1989; 14: 194–198. [**AV**]

Dermatology Specific Quality of Life Questionnaire—Anderson R, Rajagopalan R. Development and validation of a quality of life instrument for cutaneous diseases (DSQL). J Am Acad Dermatol, July 1997. [**AV**, **CD**, **AD**, **PS**, **O**]

Psoriasis Disability Index—Finlay AY, Kelly SE. Psoriasis: an index of disability. Clin Exp Dermatol 1985; 12: 8–11. [**PS**]

The Dermatology Life Quality Index—Finlay AY, Khan GK. The Dermatology Life Quality Index: a simple practical measure for routine clinical use. Clin Exp Dermatol 1994; 19: 210–216. [**AV**, **CD**, **AD**, **PS**, **O**]

EXAMPLES OF DISEASE GRADING MEASURES

PASI—Fredriksson T, Pettersson U. Severe psoriasis: oral therapy with a new retinoid. Dermatologica 1978; 157: 238–244.

Self-Assessed PASI—Feldman SR, Fleischer AB, Reboussin DM, Rapp SR, et al. The self-administered psoriasis area and severity index is valid and reliable. The Society for Investigative Dermatology, 1996: 183–186.

Acne Severity Index—Allen BB, Smith JG. Various parameters for grading acne vulgaris. Arch Dermatol 1982; 118: 23–35.

The Cook Scale—Cook CH, Centner RL, Michaels SE. An acne grading method using photographic standards. Arch Dermatol 1979; 115: 571–575.

Index